Readings in

SPEECH
AND
HEARING

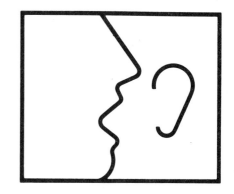

Special Learning Corporation

42 Boston Post Rd. Guilford, Connecticut 06437

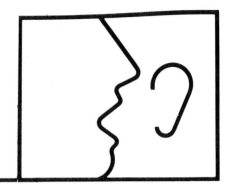

Special Learning Corporation

Publisher's Message:

The Special Education Series is the first comprehensive series designed for special education courses of study. It is also the first series to offer such a wide variety of high quality books. In addition, the series will be expanded and up-dated each year. No other publications in the area of special education can equal this. We stress high quality content, a superb advisory and consulting group, and special features that help in understanding the course of study. In addition we believe we must also publish in very small enrollment areas in order to establish the credibility and strength of our series. We realize the enrollments in courses of study such as Autism, Visually Handicapped Education, or Diagnosis and Placement are not large. Nevertheless, we believe there is a need for course books in these areas and books that are kept up-to-date on an annual basis! Special Learning Corporation's goal is to publish the highest quality materials for the college and university courses of study. With your comments and support we will continue to do this.

John P. Quirk

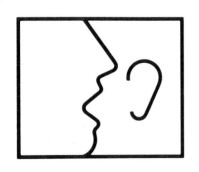

First Edition

2   3   4   5

ISBN No.   0-89568-005-X

SPECIAL EDUCATION SERIES

- Autism
* ● Behavior Modification
  Biological Bases of Learning Disabilities
  Brain Impairments
- Career and Vocational Education
  Child Abuse
  Child Development
  Child Psychology
  Cognitive and Communication Skills
* ● Counseling Parents of Exceptional
  Children
  Creative Arts
  Curriculum and Materials
* ● Deaf Education
  Developmental Disabilities
* ● Diagnosis and Placement
  Down's Syndrome
- Dyslexia
  Early Learning
  Educational Technology
* ● Emotional and Behavioral Disorders
  Exceptional Parents
* ● Gifted and Talented Education
* ● Human Growth and Development of
  the Exceptional Individual
  Hyperactivity
* ● Individualized Educational Programs

- Language & Writing Disorders
* ● Learning Disabilities
  Learning Theory
* ● Mainstreaming
* ● Mental Retardation
- Motor Disorders
  Multiple Handicapped Education
  Occupational Therapy
- Perception and Memory Disorders
* ● Physically Handicapped Education
* ● Pre-School Education for the
  Handicapped
* ● Psychology of Exceptional Children
- Reading Disorders
  Reading Skill Development
  Research and Development
* ● Severely and Profoundly Handicapped
  Education
  Slow Learner Education
  Social Learning
* ● Special Education
* ● Speech and Hearing
  Testing and Diagnosis
- Three Models of Learning Disabilities
* ● Visually Handicapped Education
* ● Vocational Training for the Mentally
  Retarded

● Published Titles   * Major Course Areas

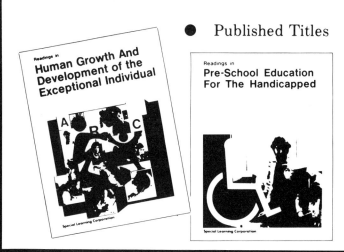

Readings in
Human Growth And
Development of the
Exceptional Individual

Readings in
Pre-School Education
For The Handicapped

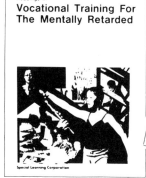

Readings in
Vocational Training For
The Mentally Retarded

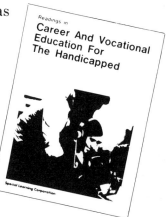

Readings in
Career And Vocational
Education For
The Handicapped

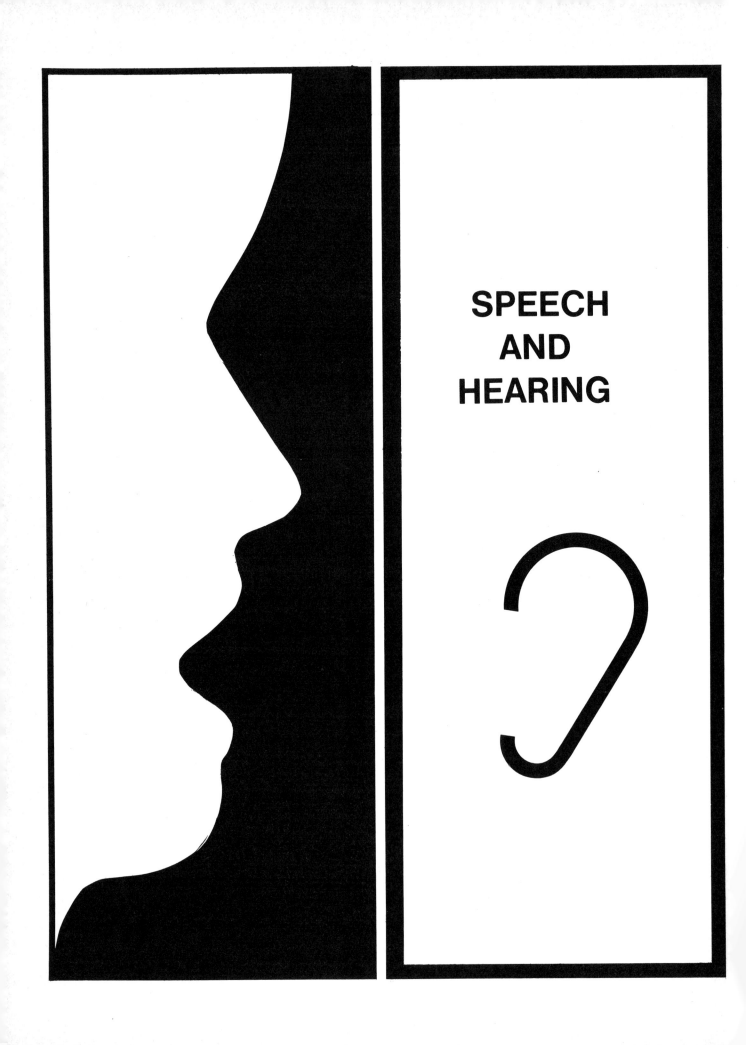

SPEECH
AND
HEARING

CONTENTS

1. Auditory Impairment: Diagnosis and Assessment

Glossary of terms   viii
Topic Matrix   ix

Overview   2

1.   **"A Look at the Future for a Hearing** 4
Impaired Child of Today," John C. Croft,
Ph.D., The Alexander Graham Bell Association for the Deaf, Inc., 1974.
Training programs for deaf children can become more numerous only if parents exercise their aggressiveness concerning the type and amount of social, educational, and audiological opportunities and services available in their own community.

2.   **"The Auditory Approach,"** *The Volta Review*, Vol. 75 No. 6, 1973. 10
Discussions of the different types of professional experience available in auditory procedures are covered through a broad spectrum of residual hearing and language techniques.

3.   **"Auditory Behavioral Responses of** 21
some hearing infants," The Alexander Graham Bell Association for the Deaf, Inc., 1969.
Behavioral response data which attempts to predict responses of hearing infants as a function of age and sex are discussed in this article.

4.   **" 'I Heard That!' Auditory Training At** 25
Home," Joan C. Rollins, *The Volta Review*, 1972.
Techniques are described to help parents develop an awareness of sound within the home combining a trained sense of hearing with a sense of sight for the hearing impaired child.

5.   **"Loop Auditory Training Systems for** 29
Preschool Hearing Impaired Children,"
Mark Ross, Ph.D., The Alexander Graham Bell Association for the Deaf, Inc., 1969.
Some previously undiscussed problems of using loop systems with preschool children are discussed in a pro and con format through creative clinical research views.

6.   **"Auditory Dysfunction Accompanying** 32
Noise-Induced Hearing Loss," Robert C. Findlay, *Journal of Speech and Hearing Research*, Vol. 41 No. 3, August 1976.
Two groups of 16 young male subjects with normal low- and midfrequency hearing are compared on a series of tests with two forms of competing noise.

7.   **"The Fine Art of Auditory Training, or Is** 38
Anyone Listening?" Frank B. Withrow, Ph.D., *The Volta Review*, Vol. 76, No. 7, 1974.
The importance of the development of a child's residual hearing is discussed as the foremost component of any educational program for the hearing impaired.

2. Speech Disorders: Pathology and Classification

Overview   42

8.   **"Tongue Thrust: A Point of View,"** Marvin L. Hanson, *Journal of Speech and Hearing Research*, Vol. 41 No. 2, May 1976. 44
The author presents evidence supporting the validity of therapy for tongue thrust through myofunctional treatment methods.

9.   **"Effect of Vicarious Punishment on Stut-** 54
tering Frequency," Richard Martin, Samuel Haroldson, *Journal of Speech and Hearing Research*, Vol. 20 No. 1, March 1977.
This investigation explores the effects of response-contingent stimulation of twenty adult stutterers through use of videotape techniques.

10. **"Listeners' Impressions of Speakers** 59
With Lateral Lisps," Ellen-Marie Silverman, *Journal of Speech and Hearing Research*, Vol. 41 No. 4, November 1976.
Research was conducted to determine whether the lateral lisp calls adverse attention to the speaker and thus constitutes a speech defect.

11. **"Word Frequency and Stuttering: The** 63
Relationship to Sentence Structure,"
Irwin Ronson, *Journal of Speech and Hearing Research*, Vol. 19 No. 4, December 1976.
This experiment was designed to determine the relationship between word frequency and stuttering within simple-active-affirmative-declarative, negative, and passive selected sentence types.

12. **"Stuttering: Discoordination of Phona-** 68
tion With Articulation and Respiration,"
William Perkins, Joanna Rudas, Linda Johnson, Jody Bell, *Journal of Speech and Hearing Research*, Vol. 19 No.3, September 1976.
Complexity of phonatory coordination with articulatory and respiratory processes yield consistent effects on stuttering in this observation by the authors on the subject of stuttering.

13. "Verbal versus Tangible Reward for 78
Children Who Stutter," Walter H. Manning, Phyllis A. Trutna, Candyce K. Shaw,
Journal of Speech and Hearing Research, Vol.
41 No. 1, February 1976.
Behavior modification programs for children
who stutter are discussed with the question
of whether rewards should be verbal or of a
tangible nature.

14. "Acquisition of Esophageal Speech Sub- 86
sequent to Learning Pharyngeal Speech:
An Unusual Case Study," John T. Togerson, Daniel E. Martin, *Journal of Speech and
Hearing Research*, Vol. 41 No. 2, May 1976.
A presentation of a difficult clinical technique that successfully changes pharyngeal
voice production to esophageal voice production through the inhalation method of air
intake.

FOCUS 90

3. Linguistic Development

Overview 92

15. "Speech Is More Than Mere Words," 94
June Mather, The Alexander Graham Bell
Association for the Deaf, Inc., 1970.
The author suggests that a child's abilities
might be expanded, enlarged, and encouraged through gestures, sounds, words, or
phrases in order that the goal of speech might
be reached.

16. "Vocabulary Development of Educable 100
Retarded Children," Arthur M. Taylor,
Martha Thurlow, James E. Turnure, *Exceptional Children*, Vol. 43, No. 7, April 1977.
This study represents an important link between laboratory research on learning strategies and the development of instruction.

17. "Aphasia in Children, Diagnosis and Ed- 103
ucaton," Edna K. Monsees, The Volta
Bureau, 1957.
Normal, hearing handicapped, and aphasic
children are grouped together in an educational program where their educational
needs and abilities provide the stimulus for
suitable diagnosis.

18. "Murdering Our Mother Tongue," Edwin 108
Newman, *Reader's Digest*, Vol. 105 No. 632,
December 1974.
This well known news correspondent and
commentator offers us a look at the decline of
language in our society through speech and
writing.

19. "Home Language Training Program for 110
Dysacusic and Aphasic Children," Ed-
ward G. Scagliotta, The Alexander Gaham
Bell Association for the Deaf, Inc., 1966.,

A home training program for dyacusic and
aphasic children and their parents is covered
through auditory training, voice, speech, and
language development.

20. "A Tangibly Reinforced Speech Recep- 114
tion Threshold Procedure for Use With
Small Children," Frederick N. Martin,
Sherry Coombes, *Journal of Speech and
Hearing Research*, Vol. 41 No. 3, August
1976.
Methodology of evaluating the hearing
thresholds of very young children is discussed from the view point of the audiologist.

21. "Helping Your Child Speak Correctly," 118
John E. Bryant, Public Affairs Pamphlet,
1974.
The author outlines in detail what a parent
can do to insure correct speech devlopment
in their children.

22. "Word Retrieval of Aphasic Adults," Ro- 124
bert C. Marshall, *Journal of Speech and
Hearing Research*, Vol. 41 No. 4, November
1976.
A study highlighting the careful analysis of an
aphasic patient's verbal habits by the clinician is discussed and evaluated.

23. "Folk Linguistics: Wishwashy Mommy 129
Talk," Cheris Kramer, *Psychology Today*,
Vol. 8, No. 1, June 1974.
This article offers us a linguistic look at
female forms of language through stereotype
roles of speech and language research.

24. "Linguistic Performance in Vulnerable 133
and Autistic Children and Their Mothers," Sheldon M. Frank, M.A., M.D., Doris
A. Allen, E.D.D., Lorrayne Stein, and Beverly Myers, *American Journal of Psychiatry*,
August 1976.
The authors studied the language patterns of
schizophrenic mothers and their four year old
children, as compared with speech patterns
of normal mothers and children and normal
mothers with autistic children.

4. Educational Services: Resources and Therapies

Overview 140

25. "Learning to Listen in an Integrated 142
Preschool," Doreen Pollack and Marian
Ernst, *The Volta Review*, 1973.
Integration of hearing impaired children into
preschool classes is discussed along with
parental and teacher guidelines as to effective implementation of the program.

26. "Teaching Aural Language," *The Volta* 149
Review, 1968.
Teaching concepts of aural language for the
hearing impaired child are presented in this
article.

27. **"Characteristics of an Adequate Auditory/Oral Program–A Guide for Parents and Educators,"** *The Volta Review*, Vol. 77, No. 7, 1975.   152
35 priority recommendations for an adequate auditory/oral program for parents and educators are outlined.

28. **"Innovation in Speech Therapy: A Cost Effective Program,"** David J. Alvord, *Exceptional Children*, Vol. 43, No. 8, May 1977.   156
Results of a program for the treatment of mild to moderately speech disordered children through the use of trained paraprofessional aides are discussed in this speech therapy program.

29. **"Acquisition of American Sign Language by a Noncommunicating Autistic Child,"** Robert L. Fulwiler, Roger S. Fouts, *Journal of Autism and Childhood Schizophrenia*, Vol. 7 No. 2, 1977.   161
Through perceptual and language oriented experiments, it was found that autistic children benefitted both auditorially and visually.

30. **"Information Processing of Visually Presented Pictures and Word Stimuli By Young Hearing Impaired and Normal Hearing Children,"** Ronald B. Kelly, Tomlinson-Keasley, *Journal of Speech and Hearing Research*, Vol. 19 No. 4, December 1976.   167
This study compares the hearing impaired and normal hearing subjects in order that normal developmental courses of information processing might be followed up.

31. **"Teaching the Nonverbal Child,"** Ruth E. Bender, *The Volta Review*, 1968.   176
The nonverbal child with a variety of handicaps is helped through teacher guidelines for effective language development.

5. Medical, Technological and Psychological Rehabilitation

Overview   182

32. **Hearing Aids Children Wear: A Longitudinal Study of Performance,"** G. David Zink, M.A. ©1972 The Alexander Graham Bell Association for the Deaf, Inc.   184
This two-year study evaluates and monitors electroacoustic performance characteristics of hearing aids worn by children.

33. **"Don't Be Afraid To Wear a Hearing Aid,"** Charlotte Himber, *Retirement Living*, Vol. 15 No. 5, May 1975. ©1975 Retirement Living.   192
A whole new world can become available to the hearing impaired by the use of a hearing aid.

34. **"Recognition of Verbal Labels of Pictured Objects and Events by 17 to 30 Month-Old Infants,"** Leila Beckwith, Spencer K. Thompson, *Journal of Speech and Hearing Research*, Vol. 19 No. 4, December 1976. ©1976 Journal of Speech and Hearing   195
Research.
Effects of child rearing practices on the acquisition of receptive vocabulary comprehension and production are examined at length by the authors.

35. **"How to Protect Your Hearing,"** Ken Anderson, *Retirement Living*, Vol. 15 No. 5, May 1975. ©1975 Retirement Living.   202
Early and frequent exams of hearing will detect hearing loss, thus making correction and treatment easier and perhaps less costly.

36. **"Research Implications for Communication Deficiencies,"** John H. Hollis, Joseph K. Carrier, Jr., *Exceptional Children*, Vol. 41 No. 6, March 1975. ©1975 The Council for Exceptional Children.   204
Four decades of chimpanzee research relevant to the prosthesis of communication deficiencies are discussed, along with results of research and its implications of communication deficiencies in the retarded and deaf.

37. **"Applying Technology to Special Education,"** *American Education*, February 1972. ©1972 United States Department of Health, Education and Welfare.   211
Through the use of electronic technology, the perceptual skills and mobility of handicapped children are being improved.

38. **"Noise,"** Lawrence S. Burns, *Horizon*, September 1977. ©1977 American Heritage Publishing Company.   214
1 in 20 persons suffer a hearing loss through noise in today's living from cars, trucks, sirens, planes, subways, buses and jackhammers.

39. **"Language Training for the Severely Retarded: Five Years of Behavior Analysis Research,"** Lee K. Snyder, Thomas C. Lovitt, James O. Smith, *Exceptional Children*, Vol. 42 No. 1, September 1975. ©1975 The Council for Exceptional Children.   217
A timely series of 23 studies which raises hope for two-way communication avenues to be opened to those who have been shut out for too long.

40. **"Subtitles for TV and Films,"** *American Education*, Vol. 13 No. 2, March 1977. ©1977 American Education Association.   221
The latest technical advances along with the changing attitudes of the 70's have combined to allow the hearing impaired to enjoy films and television which had previously been denied them.

41. **"Time-Intensity Trade for Speech: A Temporal Speech – Stenger Effect,"** Michael J.M. Raffin, David J. Lilly, Aaron R. Thornton, *Journal of Speech and Hearing Research*, Vol. 19 No. 4, December 1976. ©1976 Journal of Speech and Hearing Research.   226
A clinical view of experimentation with time-intensity trade for speech acquisition through psychophysical procedures.

Index   238

Appendix   241
Comments Please   245

GLOSSARY OF TERMS

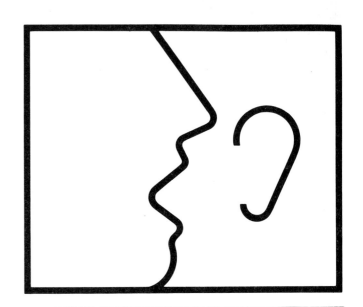

aphasia Loss or impairment of the ability to use oral language.

articulation The movements of speech organs employed in producing a particular speech sound or consonant.

audiometer Instrument for testing acuity of hearing.

auditory association Ability to relate concepts presented orally.

auditory closure The ability to recognize the whole from the presentation of a partial stimulus.

auditory reception The ability to derive meaning from orally presented material.

auditory sequential memory The ability to reproduce a sequence of auditory stimuli.

aural training Of or pertaining to stimulus training perceived by the ear.

autism A childhood disorder rendering the child noncommunicative and withdrawn.

cleft palate Congenital fissure of the roof of the mouth, often associated with cleft lip (harelip).

conductive hearing loss A condition which reduces the intensity of the sound vibrations reaching the auditory nerve in the inner ear.

decibel A relative measure of the intensity of sounds, zero decibel represents normal hearing.

dysarthria Difficulty in the articulation of words due to invovlement of the central nervous system.

grammatic closure Ability to make use of the redundancies of oral language in acquiring automatic habits for handling syntax and grammatic inflections.

intonation Rise and fall in pitch of the voice in speech.

larynx The modified upper part of the windpipe; the organ of the voice.

linguistic development Of or relating to language acquisition or linguistics.

lipreading A technique used by the deaf to understand inaudible speech by interpretation of lip and facial movement.

mastoidectomy Surgical removal of the mastoid cells of the temporal bone in the ear.

otosclerosis The formation of spongy bone in the capsule bone in the ear.

pitch The fundamental frequency of voiced speech.

pharynx That part of the throat that leads from mouth and nose to the larynx.

phonation The production of speech sounds.

phoneme A speech sound or closely related variants commonly regarded as being the same sound.

sensory-neural hearing loss A defect of the inner ear or the auditory nerve transmitting impulses to the brain.

sound blending Ability to synthesize the separate parts of a word and produce an integrated whole.

stuttering A speech impediment in which the even flow of words is interrupted by hesitations, rapid repetition of speech elements, and-or spasms of breathing.

syntax That part of a grammar system which deals with the arrangement of word forms to show their mutual relations in the sentence.

verbal expression Ability to express one's own concepts verbally in a discrete, relevant, and approximately factual manner.

TOPIC MATRIX

Readings in *Speech and Hearing* provides the college student in special education a comprehensive overview of the subject. The book is designed to follow a basic course of study.

COURSE OUTLINE:

Speech for the Hearing Impaired

I. Principles and Techniques in Teaching the Hearing Impaired

II. Developing Oral Communication Skills

III. Development of Voice Quality, Pitch, Rhythm

Readings in Speech and Hearing

I. Auditory Impairment: Diagnosis and Assessment

II. Speech Disorders: Pathology and Classification

III. Linguistic Development

IV. Educational Services: Resources and Therapies

V. Medical, Technological and Psychological Rehabilitation

Related Special Learning Corporation Readers

I. Readings in Special Education

II. Readings in Autism

III. Readings in Mental Retardation

IV. Readings in Diagnosis and Placement

V. Deaf Education

VI. Readings in Mainstreaming

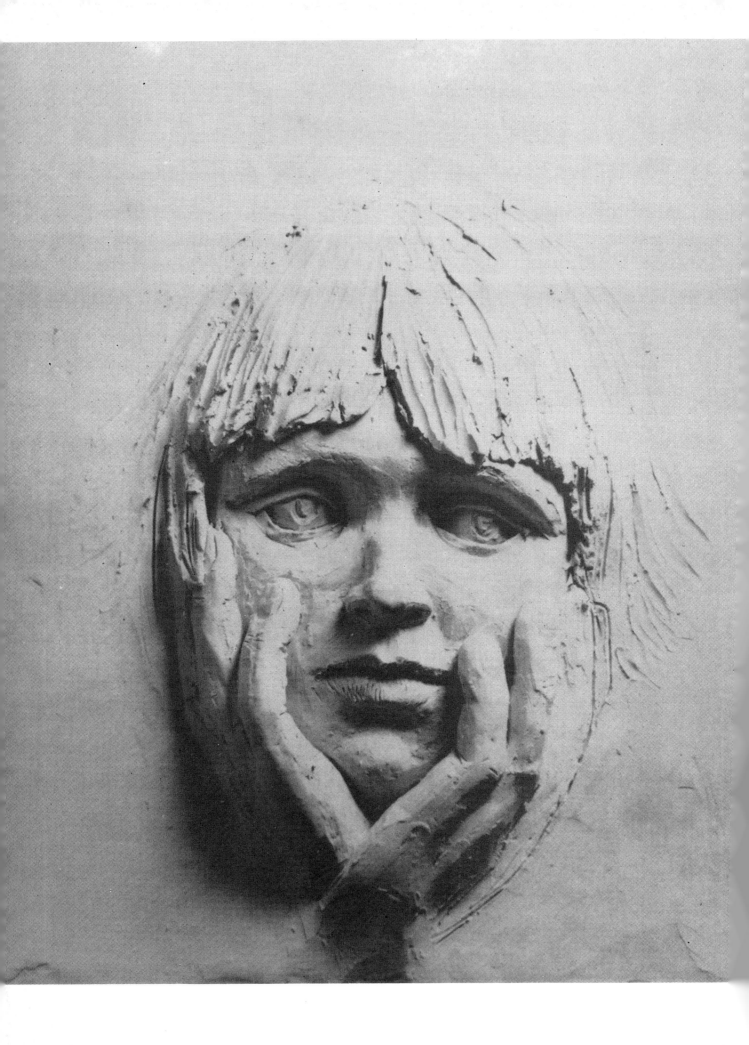

PREFACE

Today, linguistic and auditory skills cannot be taken for granted. It is becoming more widely recognized that training of these skills, including speech pathology is as fully essential to present day education as training in the traditional educational mode. The number of children who are affected by speech and hearing disorders in the United States constitute the largest group of exceptional children. Today, linguistic and auditory skills cannot be taken for granted. It is becoming more widely recognized that training of these skills, including speech pathology is as fully essential to sound present-day education as training in the traditional educational modalities. Current awareness points out the fact that for the children who are affected by auditory or linguistic handicaps, our schools have little to offer that is more important than appropriate speech correction.

This situation is now being faced frankly and constructively in most states, with speech correction courses now being included as a requirement for certification. This need is further felt by those whose responsibility lies in the training of classroom teachers and those who must prepare students to effectively function as speech pathologists.

The articles contained within this anthology offer an informative statement of the educational needs and basic philosophy for those who are acquainted with the problems of speech and hearing handicapped children.

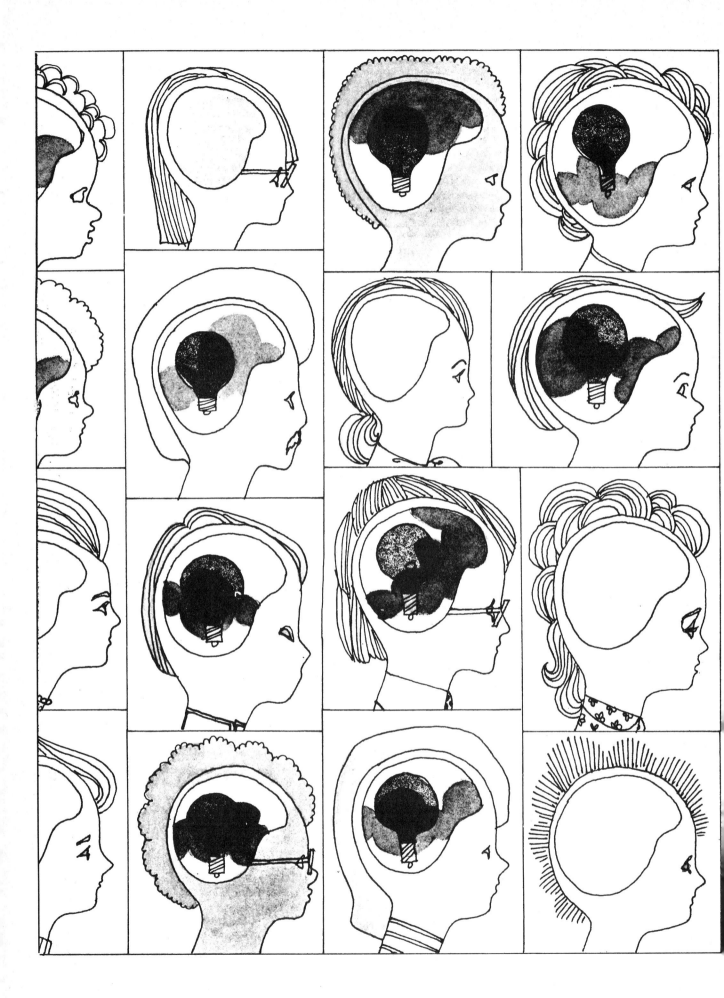

Auditory Impairment: Diagnosis and Assessment

The auditorially impaired have only recently emerged as a clearly defined group. Prior to the turn of the century, those children with the milder hearing impairments were enrolled in regular public school classes, and achieved whatever success they could with the teaching methods that were being employed for the normal child. The more seriously hearing impaired children were placed in schools and classes for the deaf. This lack of distinction between the two disabilites has persisted over into current programming. A landmark decision was made in Detroit in 1912 that began the move to more carefully assess the hearing impaired child, and employ proper placement procedures. It was at that time that the administration of the Detroit Day School for the Deaf became aware that there were some students in the school who were in fact, hearing impaired, not deaf, and that some speech and meaningful interpretations were possible for them. A special study was begun, and the beginning of separate classes for the hearing impaired was begun. This movement spread to other cities which were having similar experiences.

In recent years, C.D. O'Connor and A. Streng have suggested four classifications for children with hearing impairments. Group A includes children with a slight hearing loss up to 20 decibels, and therefore able to make a fair adjustment in regular classes. Group B consists of those children with 25 to 50 or 55 decibel loss, and show need for help in speech reading, a possible placement in a hearing impaired classroom. Group C includes children with 55 or 60 to 65 or 75 decibel loss, who will be placed in hard-of-hearing classes with the aid of hearing amplification, so as to take advantage of speech reading. At the most extreme end of the scale is Group D with a 70 to 75 decibel loss. These children are unable to have a practical hearing of speech and language so that they must be taught by methods applicable to deaf children.

The classroom teacher today must be aware of the nature of a child with an auditory impairment. These children will demonstrate physical symptoms, such as tilting their head at unusual angles to receive better sound, earaches, mouth breathing, or running ears. They may demonstrate defects in speech, peculiar pitch in the voice, or the lack of an adequate flow of language. Their school performance may be poor, and their social interaction lacking.

The future of the auditorially impaired child lives in the hands of those professionals performing diagnostic testing and assessment procedures. This child can no longer be grouped together as a homogeneous sector of exceptional children.

A Look at the Future for a Hearing Impaired Child of Today

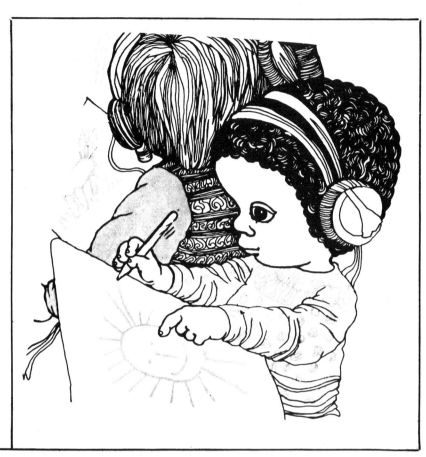

— John C. Croft, Ph.D. —

As parents and educators of hearing impaired children, let us look at the future awaiting our deaf children of today. We *do* know that they will be adults in the future; also we know that there will be a strong need for rapid communication from man to man and from man to machine. The future exists *now* in scattered bits and pieces, and we must remember this when educating our deaf children. We have very little reason to believe that hearing impaired children today must be trained and educated like a deaf adult *was* when he was a child.

I do not know whether what I am about to describe concerning a child's future will be typical. It certainly *could* be, but that will depend on the choices parents make in raising and training their deaf children. According to the U.N. Committee on Human Rights, all parents have the right to choose the education for their children — a right which should be exercised by parents whether the child is deaf or not. As parents have this right to choose, it would be highly desirable to make that an active choice, not an unwitting one. There is training now available which if followed carefully should enable the hearing impaired child to remain fully in a hearing/speaking world.

the auditory approach

What about opportunities for deaf children which do exist now yet still seem to be out of the mainstream of educational thought and practice? Recently (February 1973) a conference was held in Pasadena, California,

"A Look at the Future for a Hearing Impaired Child of Today," John C. Croft, Ph.D., The Alexander Graham Bell Association for the Deaf, Inc. ©1974 The Alexander Graham Bell Association for the Deaf, Inc.

(International Conference on Auditory Techniques), to bring together research and practice, the world over, related to an auditory approach. The science of the auditory approach has enabled us to break away from the viewpoint that the deaf must remain deaf and are educable only in an entirely deaf environment. Rather, the emphasis is on teaching the hearing impaired child to communicate through the means of an auditory input. This involves: 1) early intervention, 2) full-time use of carefully selected, wide-range amplification, 3) constant exposure to normal speech and language, and 4) special techniques to develop auditory processing. When hearing aids are used as a tool to reach the child's brain with clear sound, intelligible and normal speech will result.

The Acoupedic program in Denver, Colorado, which has existed for over 25 years, is designed to reach acoustically handicapped children who have been detected in infancy and involves the basic ingredients of an auditory approach*:

1. Early detection of the hearing impairment
2. Early fitting of hearing aids
3. A unisensory approach
4. A normal learning environment
5. The use of an auditory feedback mechanism
6. Development of language following normal patterns
7. The parent as the first model of communication
8. Individualized teaching.

With these opportunities, "Deaf Children *Are* Learning to Hear." This is such a profound and important statement that the Alexander Graham Bell Association has chosen it as one of the slogans for their *Hearing Alert!* program, and lapel buttons and bumper stickers are now conveying the message throughout the United States and Canada.

These are a few of the things existing now which will become even more typical as parents actively seek and choose them. Let me turn now to our own deaf child, Jane, to illustrate some of the choices we made and some of the results of those choices. Although our experience is totally a Toronto experience, it is not necessarily the *common* Toronto experience. There is situated in Toronto the Metropolitan Toronto School for the Deaf — a free, tax-supported, *oral,* day facility, well-equipped and staffed only by highly certified personnel. Here, or at a satellite school in the suburbs, or in a number of classes for the hard of hearing scattered throughout the metropolitan area, most of Toronto's deaf children beyond the age of 3 receive their education.

our family's experience — making the choice of "normality"

However, it is a *normal* childhood, as well as a normal adulthood, that has been our primary goal for Jane. We learned early, from many sources, that it takes an enormous amount of motivation, intelligence, and physical stamina for a child with a severe, congenital hearing loss to integrate from a special, small class (where she is spoken to in carefully phrased, basic sentences by a specially-trained teacher over special auditory equipment) into a normal classroom of 30 active children who are spoken to in complex sentences by a teacher who may or may not be in a position to be easily lipread. We felt quite certain from the outset that Jane would never really become good "integration material." Therefore, it seemed that our only alternative, given the goal we had, was never to segregate her in the first place. And so she has never attended a class for the deaf.

Jane was born deaf as part of the syndrome associated with maternal

---

*For further information about the Acoupedic program, see *Educational Audiology for the Limited Hearing Infant,* Doreen Pollack. Springfield, Ill.: Charles C Thomas, 1970.

1. AUDITORY IMPAIRMENT

rubella, which my wife contracted during her first five weeks of pregnancy. Exactly how deaf Jane is will never be known, for the method in which she has been trained since the age of 22 months considers degree of "deafness" to be a manipulatable quantity, and an audiogram only the measure of how much hearing a child is using at a particular moment — giving no indication of how much she may be able to develop over the years in a program of intensive listening and intellectual training.

I can state, however, that Jane's first complete audiogram made at 26 months of age after 4 months of intensive, unisensory auditory training shows an aided response in one frequency only, and no response without the aid. So one would probably consider her — deaf.

Yet Jane, at age 7½ (May 1973), seems to be quite minimally handicapped by this hearing loss — which the hospital currently records as averaging 102 dB in the better ear (see Table 1). Her listening habit is well established, and after 5½ years of training her aided audiogram has risen slowly to a level between 15 and 30 dB with the latest SAT* at 0dB. *Yet, she is still wearing her original hearing aid.* With this ability to hear she is, as one would expect, using the telephone and conversing meaningfully with us from another floor in our home.* Needing no loop system nor any other special apparatus to cope in her public school classroom, Jane can readily function there without focus or fanfare, and she operates "quite comfortably" (her vice-principal's term) without extra help from either her teacher or her peers. We have not asked a public school to cope with Jane; instead, we have tried to prepare her with the skills needed for coping in the normal educational system.

developing the characteristics of normal children

We have felt that our child could be helped by being given training in "normality" skills. We began with the gross skills in infancy, refining them according to the ability and progress of the child. For instance, we worked on developing the following characteristics of children whose performance

Table 1.   Audiograms for Jane Croft Over a Five-Year Period

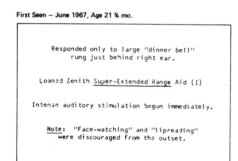

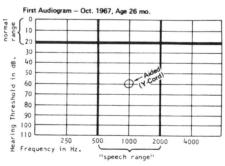

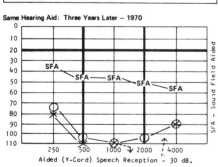

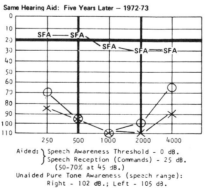

*Speech Awareness Threshold.

*As of August 1973 Jane was binaurally fitted with the Omniton 111F (150 to 5000 Hz with electret mikes) and is now training into her new aids.

6

falls within the "normal" range (after a relatively short exposure to the normal educational process).

1. They use more verbal communication and less gesturing as they grow.
2. They can learn *some* things through their ears alone and don't feel insecure when they can't see the speaker's face clearly.
3. They have learned to separate meaningful sounds from background noise.
4. They have fewer meaningless body movements as they grow older.
5. They neither touch a person to get his attention nor wait until they have that attention before beginning to speak.
6. They have a reasonable attention span for verbal activities and the self-discipline to remain quiet while others are speaking; and they can remain in a group mentally, even though disinterested.
7. They can function as one of a group of 30 without constant adult attention, can take responsibility without constant adult supervision, and can complete school tasks by themselves without constant adult monitoring.
8. People speak to them without waiting for face-to-face contact first.
9. They can follow verbal directions, use common jargon in their speech, and can express themselves both in conversation and in argument.
10. They are treated by peers completely as equals — there exist no "maternal" or "helpful" motives — and are included or excluded in neighborhood activities solely on the basis of peer- or self-selection, not upon any neighborhood mother's suggestion.
11. Daily concern over their performance level doesn't dominate the supper table conversation.
12. They attend school with the neighborhood children, know the local games and ways, and are conversant with the current neighborhood news.
13. They receive only their fair share of family focus, and similar behavior standards are expected of them.
14. All areas in which parents feel the child's performance is below "standard" are not attributed to and excused by a physical problem; the children are not perceived as living in some "magical" world of their own, different, somehow, from the real world.

What we wanted was a normally coping, self-sufficient, nondependent, confident, listening adult; and so we have headed for anonymous normality as quickly as we could get there!

a typical daily routine

Like every other 7-year-old in our neighborhood, at about a quarter to 9 every weekday morning, Jane heads for our local neighborhood school, usually equipped with a skipping rope. Like the other 7-year-olds, she is in the second grade; she is assessed as performing comfortably at about the middle of a class of 35 children, and she's not straining herself to get there. She has a boyfriend and a gang of girlfriends who seem to spend endless recesses skipping rope, reciting:

> Ice cream, candy, peanut' butter, fudge,
> How many boys like (name) so much?
> 1, 2, 3, 4, etc.

Jane, not a very talented skipper, rarely gets beyond six; but she says, philosophically, "That's too many boyfriends, anyway!"

At noon on Mondays she often comes rushing in saying that she has heard over the loudspeaker system that Team B is playing Team A, or C, or D, in the House League at 1:00 — or at 1:10 — and that she must eat immediately and get back early to participate. She is also a Brownie, having recently earned her Golden Bar, and she studies serious ballet at the

1. AUDITORY IMPAIRMENT

studio of a former soloist of the National Ballet of Canada, where she is considered to be doing quite well.

aural training — its numerous benefits for Jane

On Friday afternoons she leaves school 15 minutes early for her weekly "listening lesson" with her buddy, Miss Crawford, at the Hospital for Sick Children in downtown Toronto. For about 10 years now the Hospital for Sick Children has offered a program of aural — AURAL — training taught by Louise Crawford. We are greatly indebted to this training for the following four reasons:

First, it attacked the root of Jane's problem — her inability to hear. Parents who instill in their small children the *habit* of trying to listen first and look second produce children who tend to make almost unbelievable use of that little residual hearing they possess. We accomplished this by constantly directing the child's attention to the sound while not being in a position where she could read our lips. An infant habit is hard to break, and our goal was to establish the infant habit of listening *without looking* at our faces. In other words, one behaves toward the child as a hearing child, not as a deaf child.

Second, this therapy consisted of intense intellectual stimulation given by individual instruction, which we felt was the best use of our small child's time — especially since, like many syndrome children, she had other problems to which we were addressing ourselves at the same time. Under this program, by the age of 6, Jane became intellectually capable of taking her place in the regular school with her own age group.

Third, the training was always given only on her own hearing aid so that a given word always sounded the same way to her. Also, in later years, she would be able to hear the detailed academic instructions in a classroom with no need of additional amplification or a loop system.

Fourth, although carefully guided by weekly visits with the child to the hospital teacher, the day-to-day training was the sole responsibility of the parents and was accomplished in the home. When quite young, our child could have her lesson at *her* best time of day, and Mom, Dad, and often even the older neighbor children knew the current content matter and reinforced the learning in the child's environment all day long. It also helped to ease the fatigue potential for a child who weighed only 24 pounds at age 3.

Beyond age 3, this flexibility of time for lessons became a real blessing to us. It enabled Jane to enter a normal nursery school like any ordinary 3-year-old and to learn to cope amid her normal peers without sacrificing any intellectual training. She learned to imitate normal speech sounds and normal behavioral habits, and it was in this environment that Jane soon learned the normal child's habit of using speech to manipulate playmates and the world. As speech was practiced, it improved all by itself. She also began, along with her peers, to learn to concentrate amid a classroom of 33 other moving bodies (there were four teachers), to follow routines well, and to begin to discriminate with her ears what was speech to be heard and what was merely background noise to be ignored. These invaluable skills, practiced as early as age 3, directly contributed to her ability to succeed anonymously in a regular classroom by age 6.

So, since the age of 3, Jane has led the schedule of a normal child from 9 a.m. to 4 p.m., and we settle down with our lesson usually in the early evening. At the outset, we worked six days a week for half-hour stretches; now we only work about four nights a week, in sessions of no longer than an hour.

the advantages of "anonymity"

The most important result of all this comfortable anonymity in the classroom, we feel, is that as an equal among peers one can readily develop a strong, positive self-image and can experience normal emotional and social growth. We have deprived Jane of any special focus which her degree of loss could easily command, primarily because we feel that it is hard to wean a child from such special attention and also because it can both retard maturity and later lead to a lonely existence. It's lonely to feel too different. Jane knows she has a hearing loss and understands well the problems this brings, but she doesn't feel that this fact about her makes her either inferior or "super-special." There is absolutely no value judgment made in her mind.

So our program for her has really been one of prevention as well as of intense aural and intellectual stimulation. We work hard at the "normality" skills I listed earlier. We feel three points are terribly important to the progress Jane has made.

First, Jane has always heard through both ears: we used a Y-cord until last fall, when we began to utilize the "back up" aid in a binaural system. Second, we have always tried to keep to a minimum the amount of paraphernalia she must carry on her body to lessen the "nuisance factor" of the hearing aids. Fortunately, her aids are small and light; *she* only weighs 43 pounds right now. She wears them in well-fitting, totally enclosed pockets which are an integral part of each piece of clothing she owns, and there is a "window" in the front of each, the size of the microphone. The pockets are placed *high* on her body at the audiologically best spot for her to hear herself and others. The cords go to the back, are pinned there, and then to up the back of the ear to the receivers but, of course, are *not* crossed over. She has never been encumbered by harnesses or dangling wires. Third, we have her aids checked regularly for distortion and make vigilant use of a battery tester. Since Jane was 5 years old, we have owned a nearly identical "back up" aid in case of malfunction.

a place in the hearing/speaking world

The public school experience has helped Jane develop realistic self-knowledge and an accurate self-assessment of her strengths and weaknesses since she is always seen as compared with the norm for her age group. There is no "two-world" or cloistered situation here; there is really only one hearing/speaking world, and Jane is right in the middle of it.

The obvious drawbacks of the route we have taken are: 1) it *initially* requires such a large output of energy on the part of the family — particularly the mother — and 2) audiological attention of the sophistication these children require is *very* hard to come by.

We are now making active choices, literally from day to day, so that as an adult Jane can make them rather than have them made for her because of a linguistic deficit, a psychological impairment, a communication inadequacy, or the arrogance of some professionals. A growing number of families are making the effort these days, feeling that the end result is worth *any* effort.

Training programs such as those described here will be more common only if parents of deaf children actively choose and become more aggressive about the type and amount of social, educational, and audiological opportunities and services which are established in their own locale. The choice is yours, as parents, and you are making a choice whether or not you are aware of it.

The Auditory Approach

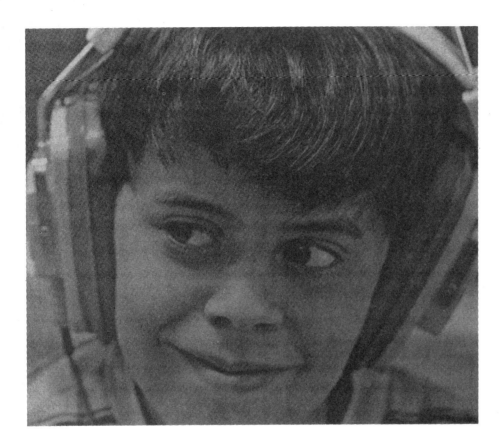

These were some of the comments on the Regional Conference on the Auditory Approach, sponsored by the Alexander Graham Bell Association last May in Alexandria, Virginia. The auditory approach to the education of the hearing impaired emphasizes early detection, use of residual hearing, early and consistent amplification, and, ultimately, integration into the normal-hearing world. It places primary emphasis on *audition* rather than vision in the development of oral communication skills. Unlike traditional oral methods of education, the auditory approach stresses how well the child can use his residual hearing, not how well he can function without it. Many people feel it is one of the most positive and exciting trends in the field of education of the hearing impaired today.

The speakers — Dr. Ciwa Griffiths, Andrew Gantenbein, (Mrs.) Kathryn Horton, Dr. Daniel Ling, Dr. Winifred Northcott, and Dr. Joseph Stewart — represent many different types of professional experience in auditory procedures. Their discussions covered a broad spectrum of what can be accomplished through the use of auditory techniques in a variety of settings. (See following pages.) Several of the speakers

illustrated their presentations with tape recordings, video tapes, and slide presentations. The use of media helped to integrate theory and practice, giving the audience a firmer understanding of both the rationale for the auditory approach and its results — children who make use of every bit of residual hearing in learning language and in living in society.

The following remarks are excerpts from taped interviews with the six speakers at the Conference on the Auditory Approach, Alexandria, Virginia,

"The Auditory Approach, *The Volta Review,* Vol. 75, No. 6, 1973. ©1973 The Alexander Graham Bell Association for the Deaf, Inc.

*Ciwa Griffiths, Ed.D., is Director of HEAR Foundation
in Pasadena, California.*

Q: In your book, *Conquering Childhood Deafness,* you present evidence that if a child's hearing loss is discovered before the age of 8 months and is not caused by rubella or inheritance, the hearing loss may possibly be reversed through the use of hearing aids and auditory training. Have there been any new developments in this area since your book was published?

A. In the history of HEAR Foundation, a total of 106 infants (62%) who were fitted with hearing aids before the age of 8 months eventually discarded their hearing aids. Most of these children wore their aids about 2½ to 8 months with a mean of 5 months for the 106 infants. This does not mean that we put hearing aids on the child and 24 hours later he can hear normally; it is usually a number of weeks or months of wearing aids before the child can discard them. As indicated in the book, this reversal is never possible with rubella babies or those who have inherited deafness.

Our work with infants has been the most exciting for me and is still the part of our program that has been least accepted. People have been loath to put hearing aids on infants until they can precisely assess their hearing levels. They wait for another test and another test, until the child is 9, 12, 15 months old. I feel that you must start immediately — that every 24 hours' delay can be damaging. The oldest child we had who was able to discard his aids was 8 months, 3 days old when he received them. We've had other children 8 months, 6 days old; 8 months, 14 days old; 9 months old; and many older children, and not one of them has discarded his aids. I think that the maturation of the auditory function may complete itself by the eighth month; after that point you can't change anything.

We have not yet learned *why* some children are able to discard their hearing aids if they receive them early enough. Several theories have been proposed, but nobody will really know the answer until a parallel study is done. Dr. Djordje Kostic from Yugoslavia theorizes that at the time when the embryo's brain is beginning to divide into precise cells, there is a possibility that something happens that prevents development of the auditory section. Early amplification then creates a climate in which this development can occur, and the auditory section becomes complete.

I feel that we need new terminology to describe reversible hearing loss in infants. Presently, when a hearing disorder cannot be attributed to a middle ear problem, it is labeled a sensorineural loss. Doctors are perfectly right when they say you cannot change a sensorineural loss. I think, however, that we are looking at something totally different with these infants, and in time we will have vocabulary to take care of this.

Q: **Why do you feel that wide-range amplification is necessary for hearing impaired children?**

A: Hearing aids usually respond only to frequencies from 300 to 3,000 cycles, a narrow frequency band. A normal hearing range is from 0 to 20,000 cycles. So when you put a hearing aid on a deaf child, you are giving him only one-fifth of the spectrum that the normal-hearing child uses to collect data, develop the auditory process, and learn to talk. Normal hearing is a very good mechanism; barring other disabilities, everybody who hears normally learns to talk. I believe that if you are trying to duplicate normal hearing or attain anything close to it, you must use binaural aids and wide-range, compensatory amplification.

When I began the HEAR Foundation in 1954, I started with the same information as anyone else: you put a hearing aid on the child, get him to listen to everything he can, and hope that he will talk. As the children learned to talk, it became obvious to me that all of them were saying *some* sounds, and *none* of them were saying others. As a teacher, I assumed that with individual differences some children should say some sounds, and other children should say other sounds. But when I looked at the response curve of the hearing aids, I realized what the difficulty was: the consonant sounds were not reaching the brain. So I reasoned that if the child could repeat only the sounds that reached the brain, we should try to get *all* sounds to reach the brain.

In Yugoslavia I saw Dr. Guberina's work with wide-range amplification, 20 to

1. AUDITORY IMPAIRMENT

20,000 cycles. The children at his center for the deaf were talking English as well as Croatian, and that impressed me. This led to the development of our wide-range amplification unit, the HEAR Training Unit 1-A. We make a card for each child, put it in the equipment, change the levers, and have a compensatory setting (inverse to the audiogram). We also have formant cards, which, when inserted into the equipment, let the child hear *s* or *ch* or any particular sound louder than any other. We can isolate sounds auditorily and teach the child to repeat them auditorily with the rhythm and inflection of normal speech.

We now have a smaller unit, the HEAR II. It uses the same cards, but is lighter and more attractive and has a module system that can be sent out for repair. We also have a small portable unit with a range of 40 to 17,000 cycles. It weighs about two pounds and is fitted at the factory to each child's loss so that he has his own prescriptive battery-operated amplifier. This unit does not replace hearing aids, but supplements them. Some of the children whose parents have bought this unit are now using it up to eight hours per day, and it makes a great difference in the children's understanding. I have been trying to adapt this kind of amplification from a desk-size unit to one that the child can wear all of the time. I still say that if you supply a child with normal or near-normal hearing all of the time, you will hear a great difference in his ability to accrue normal speech.

Q: **What percentage of children do you feel can benefit from auditory training?**
A: We have not found a totally deaf child — one without any residual hearing — at the HEAR Foundation. I think that every child can benefit from the auditory approach. If a child does not have other learning difficulties, he will hear sound to benefit his voice quality, rate of speech, and factors that contribute toward intelligible communication. But an additional learning disability, parents who don't care or who don't keep the hearing aids in good working order, or other environmental problems will slow down the child's progress, and he may never become an auditory, verbal person. Even very damaged children, however, get a great deal of comfort from hearing. I think, then, that every child benefits from sound, but there are varying degrees of benefit depending on the child.

The auditory approach isn't easy; it isn't magic — it's hard work. But then, having a deaf child is hard work anyway. We feel that our goal is well worth working for.

Kathryn B. Horton, M.A., is Chief of Language Development Programs at the Bill Wilkerson Hearing and Speech Center and Associate Professor at Vanderbilt University, Nashville, Tennessee.

Q: **What is the rationale for early amplification and application of auditory techniques?**
A: A child's acquisition of language and speech occurs so naturally, in most instances, that we take this marvelous process for granted, failing to recognize the critical nature of the first three years of life. Yet during these years, the auditory organization and intersensory patterning which undergird oral language are developed and the process of learning to listen occurs. By the age of 6 the child with normal hearing has passed the critical periods for auditory processing and language learning.

The human infant is a moving, exploring organism. His auditory input is not subject to spatial limitations. He is capable of continually processing his auditory environment irrespective of his spatial orientation to the source of sound. If vision is given primary emphasis for linguistic input, however, we significantly reduce the amount of aural language input to which the child has access. In the early stages of language organization, para-linguistic features — intonation and stress — bear the burden of transmitting meaning. Because a system of signs or manual symbols cannot transmit these features, the hearing impaired infant, preschooler, or older child misses a significant part of communication.

The baby's capacity to stimulate himself by prelinguistic and linguistic sounds helps him to become aware of the regularities of linguistic organization and to monitor his own output of speech sounds. A significant problem for the prelingual hearing impaired child is his lack of auditory feedback from his vocalizations. The auditory-vocal feedback loop, available to the hearing baby, is disrupted at the level of sensation and secondarily reduced at the level of production. The hearing impaired child is additionally impeded by being deprived of the auditory input from his environment, essential to his receptive organization and learning. Failure to compensate for these deficiencies through amplification and auditory training significantly retards, if not prevents, the normal development of language and speech.

Q: **What must be done, then, to provide the child with optimal language learning opportunities?**
A: Identification, assessment, and treatment must be implemented as early as possible, preferably under 12 months of age; assessment and treatment must continue concurrently and intensively. Professionals have begun to recognize the need for early detection and relevant follow-up services. Consequently, a growing number of neonatal and pediatric hearing screening programs and parent-infant programs have been designed to initiate language teaching and learning activities very early in the child's life. The most effective and efficient programs emphasize the home rather than the school and the parents rather than the teacher, with the goal of utilizing every available resource to maximize the early language learning opportunities of the very young deaf child.

The principal teaching targets for children in the 0-3 range should be the parents. This is critical. Parents should be taught to increase their linguistic and auditory input to the child during this time. Programs for children in the 0-6 age span should also give primary emphasis to aural-oral language learning and should be based on normal developmental processes and sequences. All efforts — parental, educational, audiological — must be directed toward the goal of establishing language, the function which lies at the heart of intellectual development.

Q: **What is the audiologist's role in the education of the hearing impaired child?**
A: Continuing and intensive services of the audiologist are critical if the child is to develop fully the use of his residual hearing. The audiologist's provision and monitoring of amplification makes possible the systematic process of associating sound and meaning through which the child learns to make optimum use of his hearing residuum. Too frequently, the roles of educator and audiologist are widely separated, and the audiologist is not available to meet the needs of the very young hearing impaired child, his parents, or his educators. Consequently, the educator often feels that he or she knows, or needs to know, little or nothing about the child's individual amplification system. Therefore, audiological and educational management must be coordinated to make possible an orderly and on-going audiologic schedule which will ensure that the child receives optimum benefit from wearable amplification.

Q: **Do you feel that all children can benefit from the auditory approach?**
A: The majority of severely hearing impaired children previously considered "deaf" have significant degrees of residual hearing, which, if captured early and utilized fully, will facilitate learning of aural and oral language. Amplification through binaural hearing aids should therefore be provided as soon as possible. We feel that *every* child with reduced hearing should be given a chance to benefit from acoustic input; *no* child should be denied the opportunity to use a hearing aid on at least a trial basis.

I do not mean to imply that I think all children have the capacity to learn primarily through an auditory modality because, obviously, there are children who simply do not have sufficient sensory capacity. My contention is, rather, that we have insufficient evidence to warrant making a decision that will deny acoustic-linguistic information to the child under 5 years of age. A decision to follow another educational route must be made, in my opinion, only after the critical auditory and aural period has passed.

1. AUDITORY IMPAIRMENT

Joseph Stewart, Ph.D., is a Communication Disorders Specialist with the Medical Services Branch of the Indian Health Service, Rockville, Maryland.

Q: What do you see as some of the major trends in research in education of the deaf?

A: The majority of the people working in any of the approaches to education of the deaf are not researchers; they are clinicians. There has not been nearly enough publication of anecdotal materials with audiograms, test results, etc. Certainly there has not been enough work in the area of controlled research. One major problem here is one I ran into when I was doing research in this area 10 years ago. To do good, precise research, you have to be able to match children on age, amount of loss, intelligence, socio-economic status, parental motivation, etc. This means that to run even a small study, you have to have a sufficiently large pool of children to draw from. For example, we wanted to do a comparison study of an experimental program in the auditory approach and a traditional oral program. The reaction I received from the administrators of the oral program we approached was that their children had been researched too much already and they didn't see any value in researching them again. We did find a traditional oral program that was very cooperative, but we had to go from Denver to Cleveland to find it.

There is another problem with doing research in this area. Let's say that you have your own clinical facility and you can arbitrarily assign every other child to one approach or another. If everything you have done clinically up to this point tells you that one approach is more beneficial, you have to be more hardhearted than most of us are to put a child in a program which you think will give him inferior results. When we can train laboratory animals to speak, we'll have the problem solved, but right now we are dealing with children. One of the possible ways out of this dilemma is to set up a collaborative type of research activity — perhaps in a different country where they do not have the same resources and where you cannot interfere with the management of the program — and make hearing aids and auditory equipment available to them. This is not an ideal situation, but you are at least letting them make the decision of which child gets into which program. This is also too hardhearted for me, but I think that it may be necessary in order to get the research we need.

Q. In your own experience, have you seen any opposition to early amplification?

A. There have been two main arguments against early fitting of amplification. You cannot put a hearing aid on a baby, it is argued, because 1) it will ruin his hearing, or 2) he can't take care of it. Neither statement has any basis in fact, and there is some very good research that indicates that the hearing aid does not accelerate hearing loss. (Once in a while you will find a child who has a progressive hearing loss. It is very easy to say that the child's hearing worsened because of the hearing aid.) The business of whether or not a child can take care of the aid is totally ridiculous. I don't care whether the child can take care of the aid or not; the important thing is that he has the benefit of amplification. I have seen aids that have been brought back for repair because the child wouldn't take them off, and the mother put the child in the bath with them on. We have had to scrape oatmeal out of hearing aid microphones. This isn't maltreatment. If the child insists on wearing the hearing aids in his bath or when he's eating breakfast, I say fine. The investment in dollars can in no way compare with the investment you have in this child's future lifetime potential. Oddly enough, my experience has been that the child who gets the aid early is often more careful than the child who is older and theoretically more responsible. The former has learned to depend on his aids; he knows what they do for him and what happens when he is not wearing them. While he may be careless, he is not malicious.

Q: Your work primarily concerns hearing loss among American Indians. Is there a particular type of hearing problem prevalent among these groups?

A: Middle ear disease is the most prevalent health problem among American Indians. There are probably a number of reasons for this: standard of living; nutrition; geographic isolation of many groups, particularly in Alaska; lack of medical care; and anatomical and cultural differences. All these factors impede good service delivery. Middle ear disease also interferes with educability; so besides being a health problem, it is an educational problem. About three years ago, the Indian Health Services started a major program for otitis media, which is my primary responsibility.

Q: What sort of approach do you use?
A: We are working from a three-pronged approach: 1) prevention; 2) active treatment of the disease in the acute stage and medical and surgical treatment for the chronic stage; and 3) follow-through rehabilitation. We are working more and more on the development of ancillary paramedical personnel (local Indian or Eskimo people) to work in the communities. We train them in audiometry, tympanometry, speech screening, language screening, hearing aid repair, and earmold fitting. These persons then go back to their communities and become the focal point for the local program. They are rather quickly identified with the community as the persons to whom a parent should take a child with a suspected hearing problem. They do the testing, make the medical referral if indicated, and provide the parents with instructions for the hearing aids and procedures to follow if the aids don't work.

There are several advantages to this approach. First, we don't have enough professional personnel to send to these isolated areas; and even if they were available, we probably wouldn't be making the best use of them. Second, native people are more likely to accept services from another person from the community than from an outsider. Third, the program gives a person who is interested in this kind of work the opportunity to enter a para-professional or even professional career without leaving the community. For example, one of our most outstanding workers in this program will probably be starting her college career in this area very soon. A high school graduate with two children, this young woman showed an amazing talent for doing this type of work and has developed a great interest in it. We hope to train her all the way to being an accredited audiologist, and she in turn can help us train other young Indian people.

Andrew Gantenbein, M.Ed., is Head Teacher at the Berrien County Day Program for Hearing Impaired Children, Berrien Springs, Michigan.

Q: What kinds of audiological services are provided for hearing impaired children at Berrien Springs?
A: All of our children go to an independent speech and hearing association for audiological evaluation. The audiologist selects the aids (most of the children use two) which will give the child the best hearing according to his hearing loss. The school pays for an annual audiological evaluation and, beginning with the 1973-74 school year, will send every child's aids in to be tested on B & K equipment four or five times per year.

We are presently planning to have an audiologist from the Constance Brown Hearing and Speech Center spend a couple of days per week with us to do some field testing and inservice training. There are many times when we would like to have our electronics technicians and our teachers meet with audiologists. We would like to get some of the audiological evaluation out of the soundproof room and into the classroom so that we can concentrate on the functional aspects of hearing. For example, we may know the acoustical characteristics of a room but want to test a child at various distances or with more than one person talking. I do not need to see a phonetically balanced speech reception test score; I want to know what the child does when another child comes into the room and says, "Hi! What are you doing?" We are not fighting with the audiologist, but we have very little use or time for studies of hearing impaired children that make categories of deafness or that study things in isolation. These have not helped our program.

Our children are accustomed to hearing sound through one kind of amplification and in the best conditions we can contrive during the heavy speech and language

1. AUDITORY IMPAIRMENT

learning years. The school buys all the batteries, cords, and receivers. We make our own earmolds and have 20 or 30 loaners so that if something goes wrong with the child's individual aid, the teacher can immediately provide another. If something is wrong with the aid internally, we go to great ends to get the paperwork and the cost cut down so that the child has his own aid back as soon as possible. We feel that the hearing aid for a hearing impaired child is no less important than a pencil for a normal-hearing child; the child has a right to it for educational purposes.

With the advent of the auditory approach we started thinking about something besides the amplification devices — about the environment itself. Signal to noise ratio is as important as the hearing aid, and you must consider this when working with children. Another "law" is that the distance between the speaker and the listener affects the loudness and the frequencies that reach the child. If you stand 30 feet away instead of 3, much less sound will reach the child. Therefore, you must talk louder, and when you talk louder, your vowels come across, and your consonants drop in the aisle. We have had to retrain ourselves to go by the "laws" of signal to noise ratio and distance from speaker.

Our children who have integrated are successful. I think we could enormously improve the acoustics of the regular classroom, but that would be frosting on the cake. The child who uses the auditory function uses it in conjunction with speechreading, and the two together are greater than either one alone.

Q: **Is there much parental involvement in the Berrien Springs program?**
A: There are several kinds of parent involvement. I don't think you should confuse national, state, or local politics with the responsibility the parent has for his child. Outside the home, the first line of parent effort is between the teacher and the parent, the only persons who can effect change. Parents must first handle their responsibility to their child; then, if they want, they can become involved in local or state parent group efforts. No parent in our program is penalized in any way for not coming to meetings. There are only two things the parent is asked to do: keep the hearing aids on the child and work with the teacher on the tape recorder.

At Berrien Springs, the child begins a series of programmed, taped texts on a 52-week per year basis at the age of 4 or 5. The texts use conversational and expressive-needs language and cover 12 basic linguistic patterns. The teacher presents the lesson to the child on Monday morning. The cassette with the directions to the parent then goes home with the child. The teacher simply talks to the parents on the cassette and does not need to bother with written instructions or complicated theory. He can ask the parent to present the lesson as the teacher has said it on the tape. Thus, the parent repeats the exercise with the child and, since the child is already familiar with the exercise from his session at school, the parent can easily see the child's progress.

Success begets success. We get 100% cooperation from our parents with the hearing aids and well over 90% with the cassette tapes. When a parent sees his child functioning with hearing and language, then he will continue. It's as simple as that.

Daniel Ling, Ph.D., is Professor and Director of the School of Human Communication Disorders, McGill University, Montreal, Quebec, Canada.

Q: **Do you foresee any developments in auditory devices in the future?**
A: We greatly need better quality hearing aids that are child-proof, that give better frequency response, that have less distortion, etc. Certain advances — such as the electret microphone — are being made, but we still need better high frequency response in aids, particularly for the great number of children with potential high frequency hearing. Many children are unable to hear the sound *s*, for example, mainly because their hearing aids don't reproduce it adequately.

Q: **What about low frequency response in aids? Have there been any new developments in this area since your 1964 Volta Review article?**
A: The use of low frequency amplification has increased and there are many available aids of this type. But, unfortunately, many people think that if *some* low frequency amplification is good, then *more* must be better. This is by no means the case. The objective is to allow low frequency sounds to be audible — not to amplify them to any great extent. If they're strongly amplified, then the combination of 1) speech sounds in that frequency range and 2) ambient noise can overload the auditory system and mask or cover up sounds in the higher frequencies. This is called "upward spread of masking." It shouldn't occur with the judicious use of extended low frequency response aids, which might pass sound with 5-10 dB gain at 150 Hz. However, it can occur with low boost aids, which may provide 45 or 50 dB of amplification at this frequency. Barbara Franklin of San Francisco State College has found that upward spread of masking may be avoided if you use two hearing aids — one with extended low frequency response and one with normal response — on separate ears. The child with an intact central nervous system can integrate the two signals and benefits more than if he were wearing only one aid.

Q: **What could be done to increase the effectiveness of the auditory approach?**
A: We must find ways to define the child's auditory possibilities and limitations at a much earlier age. This will involve a great deal of audiological research and development of more hearing tests that are applicable to young children. We could also use those aids already at our disposal to much better effect, i.e., design better auditory training programs, ensure that teachers and parents know how to utilize hearing aids, find ways to teach language through the use of residual hearing, and so on. Hearing aids are more than a means to an end; they are an integral part of the hearing impaired child's auditory system, beginning at the microphones of the hearing aids and ending at the cortex. The auditory system of many hearing impaired children will not function normally even with the most appropriate aids. Our training procedures must be geared toward filling the gap between audiometric zero and the hearing levels depicted on audiograms showing aided thresholds.

Unfortunately, audiograms, aided or unaided, show what *cannot* be heard rather than what can. Also, while frequency and intensity are plotted, the third dimension of sound — time — is omitted. Much of our speech recognition is time-based; to hear the difference between "pat" and "bat," for example, we must pick up cues on voicing that may be as short as one-fiftieth of a second. The speed at which particular sounds are released, their rate of utterance, and their duration are extremely important in auditory perception. These factors must be considered in assessing hearing loss, for people with similar audiograms may have very different speech discrimination abilities.

Nor does the audiogram show what differences in intensity, frequency, or time the defective ear can detect at levels of intensity *above* threshold — the levels at which we normally listen. As several experiments show, the ability to detect such differences can improve with training, but I personally doubt whether speech perception would necessarily improve if we trained children to hear just intensity, frequency, or time differences. Speech is a complex combination of these factors, a dynamic ever-changing stream of events; therefore, perception and memory of speech require discrimination of sounds in rapid sequence.

Q: **So, if hearing for speech is the goal, then auditory training programs should concentrate on speech recognition?**
A: Largely, yes. Speech sounds are processed in a different hemisphere of the brain and are much shorter than non-speech sounds such as bells, drums, and whistles. This is not to say non-speech sounds aren't worth hearing. To the contrary, it can be very important for a child to learn to recognize a car horn and fun for a child to hear music; but there's no evidence of direct carry-over into speech perception. Of course, there may be indirect carry-over, such as a better level of general auditory awareness and gross rhythmic concepts, which are at a much more primitive level than fluent speech.

When we learn speech and language, we don't just learn the sounds and the words; we learn the rules for putting them all together based on our experience of speech and

1. AUDITORY IMPAIRMENT

language within a context of *meaning*. Normal-hearing babies learn to talk largely because what their mothers say to them is positively, actively, and interestingly linked to what is going on around them. Teaching speech and language through exercises based on rules is usually dull and largely unsuccessful. In essence, there is no better way for a hearing impaired child to acquire natural language and speech than through its meaningful use under conditions allowing him to hear and use as much of it as possible, as often as possible. Speech and language skills are used primarily for communication, and it is through meaningful communication that they must be acquired and perfected.

Q: **Can the majority of hearing impaired children achieve natural speech and language?**

A: While a relatively small proportion of severely or profoundly hearing impaired children do, in fact, end up with good speech and language, there is much evidence that the hearing impaired children with a normal central nervous system (the majority) have a natural human ability to learn these communication skills. When hearing impaired children are given a fair chance to exploit this ability, a high percentage end up talking well and using normal language.

The "fair chance" implies many conditions, some of which are essentially hard to meet. Certainly the most important are early detection, early diagnosis (which must accompany early training), active and positive involvement of parents at every stage of the child's development, optimum use of residual hearing from early infancy, an environment in which speech is the expected mode of communication, social and educational experience with normal-hearing children, and help from educators who are committed to meeting the total needs of the child. Given these conditions and an intact central nervous system, most hearing impaired children can break through the communication barrier and grow up able to speak, compete, and conform in a world where 999 people in every thousand do not have a hearing problem.

> *Winifred H. Northcott, Ph.D., is Consultant, Early Childhood Education Program for the Hearing Impaired, 0-6 Years, Minnesota State Department of Education, St. Paul, Minnesota.*

Q. **Is there a good possibility that a child given early auditory training will integrate into regular classes?**

A. Although integration is not appropriate for all children, the expectation is that increased numbers of children will be successfully assimilated in regular classrooms in later years. Given the single disability of deafness and an intact sensory nervous system, almost all children hopefully will be integrated by the time they have finished the elementary grades. The question is *when* the child will be integrated. In Minneapolis, very few students remain in self-contained classrooms at the secondary level. One group of children integrates at the preschool level (kindergarten); another group is considered at around third grade level when they are beginning to read inferentially for meaning and to develop systematic word attack skills; others are ready by sixth grade.

Q. **What do you feel a parent could do to ensure his child's success in an integrated classroom?**

A. First, parents must realize the disastrous results of inappropriate placement. The goal should not be that the child automatically will be integrated without looking at him as an individual. It is, in part, a question of whether he is curious and competitive and "turned on" by school. If the parent has false expectations and is pressing for placement that is inappropriate, the professionals must explain to him why the child is not a realistic candidate for integration at that time.

Assuming that there is a general consensus of the staff through testing and observational judgments that the child is ready for integration and that he has been suitably placed in a regular classroom, the parent's first responsibility is to send the child off to school with a good breakfast and without emotional troubles. If possible, a parent should also meet the child at the door when he gets home and ask him, "How did it go today?" – not "What grade did you get on the test?" A parent might say, "I remember you were going to show your book on sports. What did the class say about that?" Or, "Were the kids interested in your rock collection? Which one did they like best?" Talk to him about what happened, not about how well he did.

Second, the parent can relate the academic content of what the child is learning in school to his daily life. For instance, the parent can get the spelling list or vocabulary for the week, not to sit down and study with the child, but to use the new words casually in natural situations.

Third, parents can help by trying to have realistic expectations for the child. They should frequently get together to check out what's "par for the course" for children of similar ages. Deaf children at the proper age should be encouraged to have their own paper route or go downtown alone on the bus. Teen-agers know that their primary status symbol is driving a car; deaf teen-agers drive cars, too (in fact, with a lower incidence of accidents than children with normal hearing). The parent should move the child along toward an independence level appropriate for his age, not his deafness.

Q: **What should a parent expect from the regular school and regular classroom teacher?**
A: The parent should expect to see the teacher, the supporting clinician, and the academic tutor often enough to develop a comfortable, open relationship that permits clarity and understanding. The parent should be able to assess what the teacher has observed about the child and to contribute his own observations about how the child operates at home. The parent should also request information on how the teacher evaluates the child, e.g., whether she grades on a class curve or whether the child is being measured against his own performance.

A parent can also encourage a teacher to have reasonably high expectations for the child. I am troubled as a consultant when I see how many children are allowed to practice aberrant behavior because they are "deaf" and therefore different. As a result, some children with potentially good academic skills and speech intelligibility are reinforced by the teacher to maintain a low frustration level. They develop poor work habits because when they come up for constant reassurance, the teacher will give it, rather than saying, "Sit down and figure it out on your own; then come to me!" The parent should expect that the teacher will treat the child in proportion to his intelligence and with the expectation that he will be assimilated into the class.

Q: **Along with positive relationships among parents, teachers, and children, what other components are necessary for an effective auditory program?**
A: I believe that a state-wide systems approach is essential to mandate comprehensive auditory programs in public schools. The Gentile study* on the characteristics of hearing impaired children in 1970-71 found that audiometric data was not available for children in special education programs for 57% of those under age 3, 47% of the 3-year-olds, 39% of the 4-year-olds, and 35% of the 5-year-olds. When such data is not available, one cannot design an appropriate, sequential set of auditory activities for each child; there is nothing to go on except guesswork. This lack of information argues for a state plan requiring, for instance, that copies of all audiological assessments or diagnostic information be routinely sent to the state consultant and to the local school district.

In only 12 state departments of education are there specifically designated hearing consultants to direct expanded services and programs for the hearing impaired. Such individuals can organize regional and statewide workshops on auditory procedures and formulate state plans describing available educational services and the nature of

---

*Characteristics of Hearing-Impaired Students by Hearing Status, United States, 1970-1971, A. Gentile. Washington, D.C.: Office of Demographic Studies, Gallaudet College, 1973. P. 15.

1. AUDITORY IMPAIRMENT

support that must be given to children in integrated settings.

Workshops are critical to train and retrain those who work with the hearing impaired. For example, orientation of regular classroom teachers really needs to be approached systematically. Workshops can also help train participants in observational techniques on how a child uses his hearing and how a teacher can model and expand the child's expressive language. They can introduce administrators and teachers of regular and special classes in isolated settings to ideas about good acoustic environments, amplification systems, and auditory techniques. Speech clinicians, too, need retraining which emphasizes that speech must be taught in a language setting, that the primary focus must be on what the child hears, and that the material presented must relate to that being taught in the regular classroom. Thus, workshops and retraining programs should include professionals from general education as well as teachers of the deaf. The state consultant, with his or her broad overview of pressing needs and available services, is best equipped to design such a program with the assistance of a broadly based advisory committee.

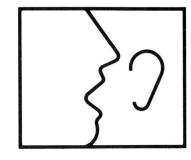

AUDITORY BEHAVIORAL RESPONSES
of some hearing infants

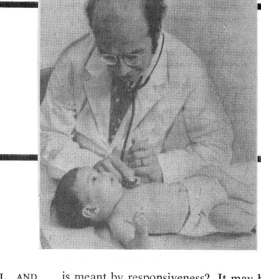

Sanford E. Gerber, Ph.D.

After conducting monthly infant hearing screening clinics for about two years, it seemed advisable to review what we had learned. For no reason other than ease of analysis, we selected the first 100 babies seen in the clinic. All children were tested with one or more of the following stimuli: pure tones, warble tones, narrow band noise, and wide band noise.

Most of the children were lying down during the testing and could be observed through the transparent basket in which they lay. A stimulus was presented to one side of the child and responses were noted by two or three trained observers. When we analyzed the responses of these 100 infants, we were somewhat surprised to learn that there was a marked uniformity of responses. Nine of the 100 infants did not respond at all to any stimuli at any level and upon further examination these all turned out to be profoundly hard of hearing children. The vast majority of the remaining 91 children made one or both of two responses: immobilization or localization. The reliability of these responses was very, very high in the sense that they could be re-elicited with certain stimuli. Statistical analysis of the ages of these infants revealed that those who immobilized were significantly younger than those who localized. Data of this kind on much larger numbers of children will permit us to predict responses of hearing infants as a function of age and sex.

WHILE THE AUDIOLOGICAL AND pediatric literature on the subject of aural behavior of infants and neonates has been growing at great speed the past several years, we continue to be unsure of what to expect aurally from a hearing or from a deaf infant. Physicians, audiologists, speech pathologists, and teachers of the deaf and hard of hearing have repeatedly urged the auditory screening of infants and of neonates. Nevertheless, such screening programs occur only in rare communities (such as Denver).

The clinical importance of early identification of the hearing impaired child should be obvious. Many, but certainly not all (e.g., Goodhill, 1967), authorities on education of the deaf and hard of hearing agree that auditory education should begin in infancy. Robinson (1965), for example, recommended hearing aid fitting and auditory training before the age of two years; and Griffiths (1967) has suggested eight months as the critical age before which auditory training should begin for maximum effectiveness. Silverman (1957), on the other hand, considered that too early amplification would be risky if the infant turned out to be suffering an impairment other than an auditory one.

The truly deaf infant is (or will become) obvious to his parents and other adults in his milieu due to his unresponsiveness. Even so, it is often amazing how old deaf children are before their parents seek assistance. The more important question, ultimately, is: what

is meant by responsiveness? It may be easy to recognize the infant who does not respond, but what about the one who does? What does a hearing baby do to indicate that fact? Or, to phrase it differently, what does the responsive infant do that the unresponsive infant does not?

DEVELOPMENTAL CRITERIA

Hardy (1965) has discussed the developmental process in terms of prelanguage (up to 10 months) and prespeech (up to 24 months) states and the preschool period. Frisina (1963) chose the pediatric definition of neonate up to two months and infant up to 24 months, so that his criteria overlap Hardy's with respect to age. Hardy described the "readiness to listen" in the prelanguage state and the "readiness to talk" in the prespeech state. An infant's readiness to listen is evidenced by his reactions to noise and his responses to acoustic stimuli. His readiness to talk, of course, is made apparent by the fact that he does so.

Frisina (1963) called attention particularly to the physiological responses. While Hardy mentioned that psychogalvanic skin responses may be elicited at the prelanguage state, Goldstein (1963) pointed out that "Very young children are less responsive and conditionable than older children." Kendall (1965), like Frisina, called attention to the reflexive and physiological nature of responses of hearing infants as well as behavioral responses. All three of these writers pointed out that the Moro

1. AUDITORY IMPAIRMENT

and the auropalpebral (APR) reflexes can be educed at birth, and Kendall showed that the electroencephalic response may be observed at one month of age.

Wedenberg (1956) was among the first to observe elicited auditory behavior in human neonates. He observed auropalpebral reflexes in 150 infants all within the first week of life. He thereby demonstrated that the APR is present at or very soon after birth, and that it may be elicited by stimuli of specifiable spectra. In 1960, Fröding confirmed Wedenberg's results on a much larger scale and also demonstrated the clinical utility of the evoked APR. He tested 2,000 infants all within the first half-hour of life, and 96.1 per cent of them had positive APR. Of the remaining 78 children, 73 became positive within a week, four died, and one was later shown to be severely hearing impaired.

It has been the exhaustive work of Eisenberg and her associates (summarized in 1966) which has clearly fixed the developmental criteria as well as delineated the methodological problems. A most outstanding conclusion which she has stated in reference to the newborn is that ". . . he processes intensity pretty much as you and I do."

Limiting our attention to later developmental behavior, Kendall's (1965) table is illuminating. It indicates that at three months a hearing infant will search for sound with his eyes and at five month he will turn his head toward the source. At six months he will respond to quiet sounds and by nine months he can locate them. Frisina (1963) was in general agreement with these data.

SELECTION OF STIMULI

It is one thing to indicate that a hearing infant should behave aurally in a certain way at a certain age, but it is quite another matter to elicit the desired behavior for clinical purposes. What stimuli will cause an infant to behave in a way that would permit observers to determine if he responds to sound?*

* The reader is urged to heed Hardy's (1965) warning: "If a baby does not respond, one cannot conclude that he does not *hear*; only that he does not *respond*."

Hardy (1965) has used a simple wooden clacker to elicit APR and Moro responses in neonates, but insists upon the use of sounds from the environment for testing older infants. As early as eight weeks of age an infant will respond to the sound of familiar toys, his mother's voice, or a spoon rattling in a cup. DiCarlo and Bradley (1961) found that to elicit localization, "White noise proved to be a very effective signal." Kendall (1965) opined, "The ultimate goal is the use of the pure tone audiometer . . ." Griffiths (1967), in fact, has used a specially designed pure tone audiometer. Downs and Sterritt (1964) found that neonates responded to white noise and to a narrow band noise peaking at 3000 Hz. Later, Downs and Sterritt (1967) found similarly reliable responses using a warble tone of 3000 ± 150 Hz. Other investigators have used various whistles, bells, buzzers, and pure tones.

Screening tests, as opposed to diagnostic tests, are intended to serve only a gross purpose. In the present context, one may say that the screening is intended to separate those who are deaf from those who are not deaf. While this is a desirable goal, it would be desirable also to discriminate those who are deaf from those who are hard of hearing and the hard of hearing from the normal. This cannot be done by screening at our present level of sophistication. Nor can we decide what sort of screening test and what test level could lead us to such discrimination. We really don't know what stimuli elicit what responses at what ages. We only have some observations.

RESPONSE RECORDING

The response recording method of choice is one that might be called "consensus audiometry." If two or more observers agree that the infant's behavior was in response to the acoustic stimulus, then that response is recorded. Downs and Sterritt (1964) reported perfect agreement in 62 per cent of observer pairings, and that 96 per cent of the pairings were within one (of five) points on a scale. That was substantial inter-observer reliability, and indicated that trained observers do agree upon behavioral responses to

acoustic stimuli. Eisenberg (1965), on the other hand, has cautioned that ". . . statistical agreement among observers, which measures the uniformity of independent assertions, is not necessarily an index of validity."

The point is that an infant cannot raise his hand when he hears the sound, or point at an earphone, or push a button. But he does make overt responses to sound, and these may be reliably observed. When such responses are not observed, we have an unresponsive child who requires intensive and extensive diagnostic study. Hypacusis is not the only cause of unresponsiveness in infants. On the other hand, it has been our experience that hearing infants agree very well with each other as to how to indicate that fact to observers.

THE INFANT HEARING SCREENING CLINIC

Under the auspices of the HEAR Foundation of the Tri-Counties in Santa Barbara, California, we have held monthly infant hearing screening clinics. These are free and open to the public. We have so far tested about 180 babies. We selected the first 100 babies for statistical observation. These 100 babies constituted the population of this study. It is to be emphasized that we are not reporting research data. What follows is simply a set of observations made on a group of infants under various conditions over a period of time. The reader is cautioned against drawing conclusions of a sort which may be inferred from careful, clinical research.

Subjects

There were 52 boys and 48 girls observed. The boys had a mean age of 228 days while the girls had a mean age of 204 days. The youngest child in the population was a girl aged 32 days and the oldest was a girl aged 524 days. There were no significant differences between the age distributions of the sexes.

Stimuli

Three different stimuli have been used since the clinics began. Since this study is after the fact, that is to say, it is an analysis of what we did, the choice of stimuli was not a parameter. Nevertheless, one observation is in order. We used narrow band noise, wide band noise, pure tones, and warble tones. It has been our experience that the warble tone (3000 ± 150 Hz) is the stimulus of choice in terms of test-retest reliability. We have found that the same baby will give the same response repeatedly to a warble tone, although he will not necessarily repeat a response to the other stimuli. For reasons we cannot now explain, babies seem to like warble tones.

Method

The infant was taken into a small and quiet room with the testers. He was placed in a transparent basket so that he could be comfortable but not obscured from observation. The output of a pure tone source was through a loudspeaker flexibly mounted on the stand which held the basket. The other signal sources were hand held instruments (Vicon Apriton, Tracor Warblet), and the basket permitted positioning these devices according to manufacturers' instructions. In most instances the babies were supine, but occasionally an older baby was obviously happier sitting. Parents were permitted in the room only when subjects were too upset to be tested otherwise.

The signal was presented first to one side of the baby, then to the other. The level used was typically 90 dB SPL. Infants who did not respond to this level were tested at higher levels, but such infants typically did not respond at all.

Impaired Children

Because the clinic is free and open to the public, our overall sample tended to be biased; that is, parents who believe their children may not hear well are more likely to come to such a clinic than are parents who are satisfied with their babies' auditory behavior. For this reason, we found a higher proportion of hearing impaired children than would be found in the population at large. Of the 100 babies, there were nine who made no response to any of the stimuli at any level. Of these nine, eight were products of maternal rubella and one of Waardenburg's syndrome.

Table 1. Mean Ages of Infants in Days

	All	Immobilize	Localize
Male	228	198	289
Female	204	182	255
Both	211	190	272

Responses

Of the remaining 91 children, 78 gave one of two responses; and these two responses, therefore, became the subject of this analysis. Forty-five babies gave the response which we call "immobilization." This response consisted of a cessation of motor activity and an apparent increased auditory awareness. It may be said that the baby literally stopped to listen. This response was very apparent, even in the youngest children and has been observed in an infant at the age of 42 days. The other common apparent response was localization—the baby turns toward the source of sound. This response also was a very obvious one. All responses were noted by at least two observers, and inter-observer reliability has been very high.

It occurred to us to inquire if there were differences between those babies who immobilized and those who localized. Indeed, there was. One would hypothesize that localization is a more mature response than immobilization. This certainly appeared to be the case since the children who localized were significantly ($P > 0.01$ level) older than the children who immobilized (by 34 days). One would also tend to hypothesize that the girls would localize at an age younger than that of the boys. This, however, did not seem to be the case. There were no significant differences between the ages of males and females who immobilized nor between the ages of males and females who localized. On the other hand, if we separate responses by sex, we find that males who turned were significantly older than males who immobilized (91 days) and females who turned were significantly older (73 days) than females who immobilized; and both of these differences were beyond the 0.05 level. These differences may be observed in Table 1, which shows the mean ages by sex and type of response.

CONCLUSION

For clinical purposes, one would want to predict what the response should be as a function of age and sex of the infant. From these data, it has been shown that girls localized at an age younger than that of boys, although there was greater variation. In either sex, the age of localization was older than that of the age of immobilization. Moreover, 78 per cent of the children in an unselected sample gave one or the other of these responses.

It must be emphasized again that these are not research data, but are only observations. The kinds of controls repeatedly urged in the literature have not been strictly observed; nor has this been our goal. Furthermore, one must be continually aware of the values and the limitations of screening. The techniques employed in such a clinic serve only to separate those who respond to rather loud noises from those who do not. We are not able to make finer discriminations. It is to be hoped that research will lead us to wiser selection of stimuli and of test level as a function of the infant's age. Certainly, our observations point to such a desideratum.

ACKNOWLEDGEMENT

The author is most pleased to thank Mrs. Eric Anderson of the HEAR Foundation of the Tri-Counties who has been the second observer, and those students who served as additional observers. Moreover, we are all indebted to our consulting otolaryngologist, Walter H. Martin, M.D., for permitting us to usurp his office in which to hold the clinic.

REFERENCES

1. DiCarlo, L. M. and Bradley, W. H., "A Simplified Auditory Test for Infants and Young Children," *Laryngoscope*, v. 71, 628–646.

1. AUDITORY IMPAIRMENT

2. Downs, M. P. and Sterritt, G. M., "Identification Audiometry for Neonates: A Preliminary Report," *J. Aud. Res.*, 1964, v. 4, 69–80.

3. Downs, M. P. and Sterritt, G. M., "A guide to Newborn and Infant Hearing Screening Programs," *A.M.A. Arch. Otolaryng.*, 1967, v. 85, 15–22.

4. Eisenberg, R. B., "Auditory Behavior in the Human Neonate: I. Methodologic Problems and the Logical Design of Research Procedures," *J. Aud. Res.*, 1965, v. 5, 159–177.

5. Eisenberg, R. B., "Auditory Behavior in the Human Neonate: Functional Properties of Sound and Their Ontogenetic Implications." Paper presented at the annual convention of the American Speech and Hearing Association, Washington, D.C., November 19, 1966.

6. Frisina, D. R., "Measurement of Hearing in Children," in Jerger, J., *Modern Developments in Audiology.* New York: Academic Press, 1963.

7. Fröding, C. A., "Acoustic Investigation of Newborn Infants." *Acta Otolaryngologica*, 1966, v. 52, 31–40.

8. Goldstein, R., "Electrophysiologic Audiometry," in Jerger, J., *Modern Developments in Audiology.* New York: Academic Press, 1963.

9. Goodhill, V., "Detection of Hearing Loss in Neonates." *A.M.A. Arch. Otolaryng.*, 1967, v. 85, 1.

10. Griffiths, C., *Conquering Childhood Deafness.* New York: Exposition-University Press, 1967.

11. Hardy, W. G., "Evaluation of Hearing in Infants and Young Children," in Glorig, A., *Audiometry: Principles and Practices.* Baltimore: The Williams and Wilkins Co., 1965.

12. Kendall, D. C., "The Audiological Assessment of Young Children," *Pediatrics and Disorders of Communication*, reprint number 835 of the Alexander Graham Bell Association for the Deaf, 1965.

13. Robinson, G. C., "Hearing Loss in Infants and Young Pre-school Children," *Pediatrics and Disorders of Communication*, reprint number 835 of the Alexander Graham Bell Association for the Deaf, 1965.

14. Silverman, S. R., "Clinical and Educational Procedures for the Deaf," in Travis, L. E., *Handbook of Speech Pathology.* New York: Appleton-Century-Crofts, Inc. 1957.

15. Wedenberg, E., "Auditory Tests on Newborn Infants," *Acta Otolaryngolgica*, 46, 446–461, 1956.

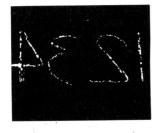

"I Heard That!" Auditory Training at Home

Joan C. Rollins

To persons unfamiliar with deafness, auditory training of deaf children may not make much sense. They might ask, "How can you teach a child to use his hearing when he hasn't any? That's what deafness means."

But a parent of a deaf child knows that most deaf children are not completely deaf, that they have some hearing with which we can work. Some children have more residual hearing than others, but the usefulness of that hearing depends not only upon how much remains, but also upon how effectively the child learns to use it.

A psychologist with whom I am acquainted describes an optimist as a person who would say, "My cup is half full," when a pessimist would say, "My cup is half empty." It is the same cup with the same contents—the difference is in the point of view. This can apply to the utilization of residual hearing. Seeing an audiogram of a moderately deaf child, a parent who is a pessimist might say: "Look at this hearing loss. My child can't hear any sounds softer than 60-75 decibels." But the optimist will look down at the lower portion of the audiogram and see that the cup is part full. He will say: "My child has some hearing for us to work with. Let's do the best we can with that." This residual hearing, even if there is only very little, is extremely precious. It can provide the child with a vital link to the world around him because he can be taught to hear and to understand some of the sounds in that world. It is especially helpful in his language development—both in his understanding of the language of others and in his ability to express himself.

To the hard of hearing child, the sense of hearing, although somewhat impaired, is the main channel through which he will gain understanding. He will also learn to use his vision as an aid to his impaired hearing. But the profoundly deaf child must learn to rely upon his vision as his most useful sense, and he must be taught to utilize his residual hearing as an aid to his understanding. This combination of senses used in teaching deaf children is referred to as the multisensory approach to teaching language. The child can learn through his sense of hearing; through his sense of sight, which he will use for

" 'I Heard That!' Auditory Training At Home," Joan C. Rollins, *The Volta Review*, 1972.

lipreading; and through his sense of touch, with which he can feel many sounds—motors, appliances, musical instruments, and even speech if his hand is placed on the speaker's face.

I have heard many parents express their disappointment when a new hearing aid was first put on their child. They had expected some dramatic changes to result, and they eagerly watched for the child to light up with pleasure at the sound of the TV or of an airplane passing overhead. To their surprise and dismay the shiny, new, expensive hearing aid seemed to make no difference whatsoever. The child was as unaware of the sounds around him as he had been without the instrument. Auditory training was the missing ingredient; for until a child is taught to be aware of sounds and learns to attach some meaning to the sounds he hears, the hearing aid is of little use to him.

We know that most deaf children have some residual hearing, and that children who are amplified do get some feedback. Even the smallest amount of residual hearing can be very important in helping the deaf child become a communicating, oral adult. But how do we begin to train him to use this residual hearing in the most efficient way? There is a great deal of difference between hearing and listening. Listening requires some effort and training in order to understand and interpret what is heard. We must teach our deaf children to learn to listen, to be aware of sounds, and to realize that they *can* hear certain sounds. Next, we must help them to develop some understanding of these sounds. Later they will learn to distinguish between different sounds.

As the exposure to various sounds increases, the child will progress from the recognition of loud, easy-to-hear sounds, which we call gross sounds, to awareness of softer or higher pitched sounds that are more difficult to hear. Eventually, some children may be able to tell without looking when someone is speaking; and they may learn to detect changes in the pitch and rhythm of speech. They may even learn to discriminate, using only their hearing, between various spoken speech sounds, between some words, and between similar phrases or sentences.

Even though a child receives individual auditory training at school, parents should be helping the child every day to develop and use the sense of hearing. Some parents are afraid to attempt auditory training at home because they feel that the subject is too technical or that they need special training and expensive electronic equipment. That is not true at all. Parents can engage in auditory training at home. There are hundreds of activities which can form the basis for auditory training, using inexpensive materials that are on hand.

The child *does* need amplification of sound through a properly fitted hearing aid. Once he has become accustomed to his hearing aid, a child should be encouraged to wear it throughout the day, not just when he is having a lesson. Don't take the aid off when he comes home from school—listening should be an all-day job. This is the child's means of "picking up" information about the world around him. So, be sure that the hearing aid is kept in good working order and that the battery is fresh.

Auditory training at home can be accomplished in two ways: Parents can work informally with a child—taking advantage of any situation which happens to come up and using the normal sounds that occur in every home. Secondly, they can work with the child in regular lessons, using material and listening activities which have been carefully planned. But whether the occasion is a casual one or a formal lesson, one basic rule should always be observed: it is not necessary to shout; speak in a normal voice to avoid causing distortion of the sounds your child hears.

Opportunities for informal auditory training are numerous. You may be working in the kitchen, with your child playing nearby, when you accidently drop a pan on the floor. Call his attention to the noise and exclaim, "Oh, I heard that! It was loud." Point to your ears as you tell him about the loud sound, and don't be afraid to be dramatic. Dented pans are not too important. As your child watches, pick up the pan and drop it again. Again, call attention to the noise it made. Get into the habit of using the vocabulary that your child must understand in auditory training: *hear, listen, soft, loud.*

Suppose that someone comes in and slams the door. Point out the sound and make your child aware of it. Slam the door again as he watches. Let him use touch, too. He can put his hands on the wall near the door and feel the vibrations as he hears the sound. Make him aware of the sound of thunder. You can take him outside and tell him about the loud sound while he watches the storm approach. Point out the planes overhead and tell him you hear them. Better still, on a sunny day take a drive out to an airport and spend some time watching and listening to the planes as they take off and land.

Your child may not respond to any of these sounds at first. Beginning attempts at auditory training often seem useless and discouraging. But if you continue to work with him, eventually he will respond. Begin with some sounds he already hears. One mother says that her child can tell when a train is coming down the tracks near their house. Another told me that her little girl heard the toilet lid as it accidently banged down one day. Now the mother deliberately lets the lid fall from time to time and talks about the loud banging sound it makes. Of course, you do not want to be constantly startling the child with loud, unexpected noises; so watch for startle reactions such as eyeblinks and flinching, and then let him see the source of the sounds to which he has reacted.

If you have a piano or organ, you can use them for auditory training. Show your child how the high notes tinkle and how the low notes rumble. Again, combine sight, hearing, and touch. Be sure he knows that a car makes a sound; listen to the honking horn together. When you run the vacuum, take a few minutes to let him feel and hear it. Turn it on and off and talk about the sound it makes. *The important thing at first is to help him become aware of sounds and to teach him to listen for them.*

When he has a good awareness and understanding of these loud, easy-to-hear sounds, move on to the somewhat more difficult ones. Perhaps he can learn to hear your doorbell. You might say, "Oh, I hear the bell. Let's go to the door. Someone rang the bell. Open the door." Show him also that the telephone makes a noise. Talk about the dog barking to get in. Take the child to the door and let him see the dog. Begin now to call your child by name when you want him. If he fails to hear you, call his name again, in addition to using the other ways you have developed for attracting his attention. Build up from the sounds that are easy to hear to those which are more difficult. This is informal auditory training. It is casual, not a sit-down lesson, and is something you do whenever the opportunity arises.

You can also use auditory training in a regular, planned lesson. You can effectively teach a beginning child to respond to a gross sound without using elaborate equipment. Each of these items can be found in most homes: a large metal pan, a wooden spoon, clothespins

1. AUDITORY IMPAIRMENT

sprayed with bright colored paint, and a large plastic bleach bottle with the top cut off. Create the sound you want the child to hear by banging on the pan with the wooden spoon. Begin by letting him use three senses—sight, hearing, and touch. Place one of his hands on the side of the pan and strike the pan so that he can watch as well as listen. Put one of the clothespins in his other hand, and help him hold it to his ear as he listens. Create the sound by striking the pan, and help him make the response by putting the clothespin into the container. Repeat this activity a few more times, and then give him the opportunity to respond all by himself. Next, remove the sense of touch by taking his hand from the pan and letting him respond by using just sight and hearing. If he succeeds, remove one more sense—that of sight—by placing the pan where he can't see it. Now he responds by using hearing alone. Be careful that he cannot see any movement as you strike the pan, and make a special effort not to present the sounds in any rhythmical pattern.

When you use this activity, don't expect the child to accomplish all of this in one lesson; you will want to be sure that the child is able to succeed at each step of the procedure before you go on. Stay with the same sound until you are sure the child can respond to it, but vary the responses to keep the game interesting. You might use buttons in a jar, large beads in a coffee can, poker chips in a dish, and so on.

Everyone who has had the experience of straining to hear a speaker, a TV show, or a movie knows that listening can be hard work. So keep your auditory training activities short, and try to make them as much fun as possible.

Let's assume that a year has passed, and your child can now recognize many sounds in the house and outside and can tell if a sound is loud or soft. Now we are working on the ability to discriminate between words he hears. You know that he lipreads the words *airplane* and *boat,* so you might fasten a small boat on one piece of Styrofoam and a toy airplane on another piece. Now lay out eight fancy cocktail picks and demonstrate to him that he is to put a pick into the Styrofoam piece which holds the object he hears named. Since this is an auditory training activity, not lipreading practice, cover your face with a small piece of cardboard so that he will have to depend upon hearing alone to make the choice.

Another step in auditory training might be to have him discriminate between similar phrases such as *the big airplane* and *the little airplane.* Finally, if he is able, help him make very difficult discriminations between such similar sentences as: *The boy is running; The boy is crying.* The sentences are much alike, and he will have to listen very carefully to tell the difference. During this advanced auditory training, the child uses only his hearing since the speaker's lips are covered; but, of course, the final goal is for the child to learn to combine this trained sense of hearing with the sense of sight.

In conclusion, the following recommendations are useful for beginning an auditory training program at home: First, watch a news broadcast without sound, and then with just enough sound for you to barely hear it. See whether this "residual hearing" helps your understanding of speech. Second, listen to all the sounds which occur in your home and select the loudest sound which your deaf child does not seem to hear. Use the techniques which have been described to see if you can help your child develop an awareness of the sound you have chosen. Finally, make "I heard that!" a phrase you use often in working with your hearing impaired child.

Loop Auditory Training Systems For Preschool Hearing Impaired Children

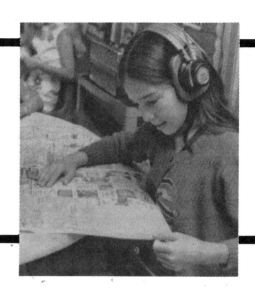

Mark Ross, Ph.D.

LOOP AUDITORY TRAINING SYSTEMS have been widely adopted for use with hearing impaired children. They are an outgrowth of conventional auditory training units which, because of the earphone cord, had the disadvantage of interfering with the children's mobility. On the contrary, the loop systems permit normal mobility thus giving the teacher greater flexibility in planning classroom activities. At first these systems were restricted to school-age children, but more recently their use has been extended to younger children in preschool settings. Since, however, the training situation for preschool and school-age children is different, an examination of the auditory consequences of this extension is relevant. In this paper, some of the problems of using loop systems with preschool children which have not been previously examined in the literature will be discussed.

TWO TYPES OF LOOP SYSTEMS

There are basically two different types of loop systems, one based on magnetic field induction and the other based on carrier wave transmission. Since some problems are unique to the type of system used, each of the systems will be described briefly. The interested reader is referred to the many excellent articles which describe the technical aspects of both types of loop systems and which evaluate the problems encountered when they are used with the school-age child.[1, 2, 4, 7, 11, 13, 14]

Inductance Loop Amplification (ILA). This type of loop system is the simplest and the oldest. It consists of a microphone, an amplifier, and, in the place of a loudspeaker, a coil of wire placed around the room. Sound waves which impinge upon the microphone are changed into alternating electrical current, amplified and then led to the coil of wire which emits a magnetic field in the room. This field crosses a tiny induction coil in the child's hearing aid—this is really the telephone attachment of the aid—and induces an electrical current in the coil. This current is then amplified and converted back into sound waves by the child's hearing aid receiver. To permit a child to hear his own voice, the hearing aid used by children in an ILA system is usually modified to provide simultaneous activation of the microphone and the telephone attachment (the M/T switch position).

Carrier Wave Transmission. Superficially, a carrier wave system is quite similar to an ILA system. The teacher's voice is picked up by a microphone, amplified, and also delivered to a coil of wire placed around the room. The difference is that the carrier wave system does not emit a magnetic field, but transmits a very high frequency carrier wave which is modulated by the audio signal either by means of frequency (FM) or amplitude (AM) modulation. The child wears a special receiver * which detects the carrier wave, separates this from the modulation, and then leads the amplified modulation to the child's ear either through earphones or through hearing aid receivers.

SPECIFIC PROBLEMS

Classroom Situation. When using any type of loop system, it is important to remember that the teacher's voice is being delivered to each child in the room, no matter where he is and no matter what he is doing. With older children, this usually presents no problem since the teacher almost always desires group communication even when addressing her remarks to one particular child. The auditory signal that these children receive relates to the ongoing activity, and so the all-important association between the auditory event and the experiential event is preserved. With preschool children, however, the training situation is quite different. Group communication may comprise less than half the total classroom time; the rest of the time is usually spent in free play or individual work. The younger the children, the more time in free play and the less time in group communicative activities. If a teacher is not fully familiar with the limitations of loop systems, the following kinds of situations can occur:

1. With the children scattered in free play, or in separate small-group activities, the teacher may intend to talk to just one or two children. If these children are only a few feet from the teacher, a direct communicative situation exists for them in which the other children are not apparently involved. If, however, the loop system is still operative, the magnetic field or the car-

rier wave permeates the entire room with nearly equal strength,** with the intensity of signal any child is receiving not dependent upon his proximity to the teacher. The other children will receive the teacher's voice as loudly as those to whom she intends to talk. An aide, parent, or another child may be attempting to talk to one of these other children through his personal microphone; what happens is that the child hears the teacher as loud as or louder than the person attempting direct communication with him. The association between the auditory event (what he hears), and the experiential event (what he is doing), is shattered.

If for example, the teacher talking with an active loop is telling one child to "make a cow sound" and an aide is telling another child to "pile up the blocks," this latter child hears "make a cow sound" to associate with the activity of piling up blocks. This situation is hardly conducive to meaningful language and auditory training. The problem could be avoided if the teacher de-activates the loop system as the children scatter in free play or in separate small group activities. This is an obvious precaution, but one that is easy to overlook in the hectic atmosphere generated by preschool children.

2. Some carrier wave systems provide several microphones in addition to the teacher's lavalier microphone. They may be affixed to the ceiling in the center of the room, placed on a table near where the children are engaged in individual activities, or attached to a stand near the amplifier/transmitter. With school-age children some centers may find that these additional microphones can serve some useful purposes; with preschool children, however, it is hard to conceive of any but the most limited positive functions, with major problems occurring when the additional microphones are used uncritically. All the auditory signals arriving at each of these microphones are amplified and transmitted to each child in the room, no matter where he is or what he is doing.

Furthermore, each child is also provided with a personal microphone which not only enables a child to moni-

tor his own voice, but also detects sounds in the vicinity. With all of these active microphones delivering auditory stimuli to the child's ear, the kind of signal a child hears is a composite of all of the direct sounds and all of the reflected sounds of all of the auditory stimuli being produced in the room at the time.

To give an example of what can occur, the author once fitted a child's unit to himself and attempted conversation with the teacher standing a few feet away, who was talking to him through a lavalier microphone hung around her neck. It was impossible to understand her. About 40 feet from them, four or five children were sitting at a table engaged in moderately noisy play. Superficially, the activity of these children appeared irrelevant to the conversation between the teacher and the author. However, the noise they were generating was picked up by an active microphone suspended above their heads and delivered to the author's ears at a loudness level equal to the teacher's voice. The additional activated microphone effectively precluded any auditory foreground; that is, there was no clearly distinguishable auditory signal which could be separated from the auditory background and which could be clearly related to the ongoing activity.

An adult who has normal knowledge of the language can attempt to select the desired auditory configurations and suppress the undesired ones, and thus function in moderately noisy circumstances. A child learning the language, however, has not yet learned to distinguish the desired from the undesired sounds. He cannot select the appropriate auditory configuration from either equally intense random noises or from equally intense conflicting auditory configurations.***

Language learning through the auditory channel will never be optimally successful unless this foreground/background requirement is consistently and frequently accomplished.

Electro-Acoustic Modifications.
There is general recognition of the need for a child to monitor his own vocal utterances if his speech and voice quality are to approximate normalcy. Recognition of this fact has led to the inclusion of a microphone/telephone switch on some hearing aids. This permits the child to hear both the loop transmission and the air-borne sound waves using the same external hearing aid adjustment. Without this modification, a child can only hear the sound impinging upon the microphone of the loop system and cannot hear his own voice or the voices of individuals attempting direct communication with him.

In compensating for this problem with ILA systems, that is, by providing for both an active telephone coil and microphone input into the amplifier of the hearing aid, electro-acoustic changes were introduced into the system. One such change is the frequency response, which is different for signals received through the telephone coil and through the microphone.[13] Another such change is the power loss of six dB when a hearing aid is switched from the microphone to microphone telephone. In a personal communication, Bellefleur[3] indicates that this drop can be compensated for by the manufacturer. Still an unanswered question, however, is the effect these changes have upon the intelligibility of a speech signal when it is detected at slightly different times and intensities by both the loop microphone and the child's microphone.

Another problem which is essentially unique to preschoolers using carrier wave loop systems is the frequent conversion from headphones to hearing aid receivers while using the unit. Carrier wave systems are supplied with headphones and the acoustic characteristics of the unit are usually described in terms of these headphones. Because of the size of the headphones compared to the average preschooler's head, many programs switch from using headphones to using hearing aid receivers with these children. Unfortunately, consequent changes in the acoustic characteristics of the system are frequently not described in the specifications nor considered for their possible effect upon the children. For example, the use of hearing aid receivers in place of headphones will usually

---

** There are many exceptions to this, some quite significant,[1,16] but rather than invalidating the argument these exceptions make the training situation even more variable and uncontrolled.

*** A complicating factor is the fact that the child learning language through a loop system is functioning essentially as a monaural listener, although with modifications depending upon number and location of the various microphones. The ability of the two-eared listener to suppress the auditory background is a long established and well-recognized clinical and experimental fact.

narrow the frequency range, increase distortion, and increase the maximum acoustic output. Each of these changes can have adverse effects upon the child:

1. By narrowing the frequency range, the child may be deprived of much desirable acoustic information at both the lower and upper ends. We know from the work of Ling and others [5, 6, 12] that, at least for the child with residual hearing concentrated only in the low frequencies, the lower frequency range can provide valuable auditory information and assist both in the perception and production of speech. We also know that a great deal of speech energy, particularly in the sibilant and fricative sounds, lies above the upper frequency range of the usual hearing aid receiver and that when this information is provided it can improve a child's discrimination for speech.[8, 18]

2. Evidence is accumulating in the hearing aid literature [9, 10, 15] relating decrements in speech intelligibility to increased distortion in hearing aids. If speech discrimination is reduced with increased distortion, what must be the effect of distortion upon the development of verbal language? While we have no direct evidence to answer this question, inferentially it seems clear that the effect of increased distortion would be at least as negative upon the development of language as it is upon the recognition of known words.

3. In some units with which the author is familiar, the change from headphones to hearing aid receivers increases the maximum output by 10 or 15 dB. If the unit is rated at 130 dB SPL output with headphones, then the maximum output with hearing aid receivers would be 140–145 dB. This latter level exceeds the threshold of pain and may, though the evidence is far from conclusive, be responsible for a further decrement in the child's hearing acuity.[17] Not having adequate verbal facility, the preschool child cannot report this painful experience. He can only refuse to tolerate the earphones or, if forced to wear them, develop unpleasant or inhibiting associations for the auditory sensation accompanying the painful experience.

It is not suggested that hearing aid receivers should never be substituted for headphones. As indicated earlier, for preschool children there frequently is no alternative. It is recommended that when such a substitution is made,

teachers be aware of the negative changes they have wrought in the acoustical situation. It is conceivable that the advantages presumably attendant to the use of auditory training systems, i.e., a high-fidelity, broadband acoustic system, may be completely obviated by the improper substitution of hearing aid receivers for headphones. In this instance, it would be less expensive and less cumbersome for a child to wear his individual hearing aid rather than the loop auditory training system.

DISCUSSION

This paper is concerned with some problems which can occur when loop auditory training systems, either ILA or carrier wave, are uncritically used with preschool age children. Many problems inherent in the use of loop systems are not unique to preschool age children. Some of these problems, all of which are covered in the cited literature, deal with magnetic field variations and overspill in ILA systems, with the orientation of the telephone coil in the hearing aid, with the acoustic changes wrought by different systems, and with the necessity of good microphone technique regardless of the system used. The focus in this paper has been those problems unique to preschool children and which have not been previously discussed in the literature.

The use of loop systems with preschool children may have a great deal of merit, though there do not appear to be any published investigations concerning results of use with any population, but we will never realize this merit if these systems are used with little knowledge of the variables involved.

The author has on many occasions visited programs for preschool and school-age hearing impaired children and has observed repeated instances of poor management of all types of auditory training systems. One significant factor in these observations appeared to be the teachers or therapists who are insecure with anything remotely "technical." Switches, batteries, VU meters, patchcords, earmolds, etc., are considered to be the province of the audiologist and are scrupulously avoided.

It is not, however, the audiologist who is the most responsible profes-

sional concerned with the education of preschool hearing impaired children; it is the teacher/therapist, and until she develops a realistic appreciation of the beneficial potential of auditory training systems, and the skill to manipulate them, the full exploitation of residual hearing will remain an unattainable goal.

Loop auditory training systems hold great promise as a significant tool in the education of hearing impaired children. The problems discussed above and in the cited literature should not discourage the utilization of this tool, but should motivate teachers, therapists, and audiologists to investigate the means by which this tool can be most effectively employed. A great deal of creative clinical research must be accomplished.

One promising development, not discussed above, is the recent advent of the wireless microphone/transmitter. This unit obviates the need for a great deal of bulky equipment and a loop around the room. The teacher suspends the microphone around her neck—helping to ensure good microphone technique—and the child wears a receiver unit around his neck. Some of the units are supplied with two internal microphones, which provide the child with capability to hear his own voice and environmental sound stimuli separately or simultaneously with the teacher's transmission. A number of transmitting frequencies are provided, thus precluding spill-over problems. Technically, we are in an era of many such rapidly changing possibilities; our responsibility as professionals requires us to keep abreast of these possibilities and not become fixated to any one particular approach.

BIBLIOGRAPHY

1. BELLEFLEUR, P. A., AND S. B. MCMEN-AMIN. "Problems of Induction Loop Amplification," *The Volta Review,* 67, pp. 559–563, 1965.
2. BELLEFLEUR, P. A., "Induction Loop Amplification—Its Adaptation to Television for the Deaf," *The Volta Review,* 68, pp. 561–565, 1966.
3. BELLEFLEUR, P. A., Personal communication, 1967.
4. BORRILD, K., "Electro-Acoustic Aids Applied in the Training of Deaf and Hard of Hearing Children," *Proceedings of the 1967 International Congress on Oral Education of the Deaf,* pp. 564–576.

Auditory Dysfunction Accompanying Noise-induced Hearing Loss

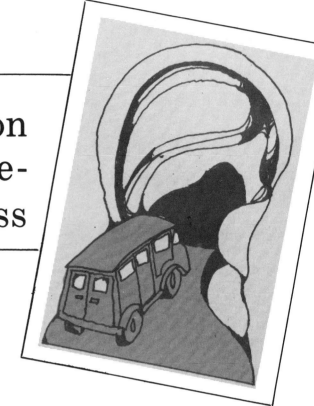

Robert C. Findlay

University of Pittsburgh, Pennsylvania

Two groups of 16 young male subjects with normal low- and midfrequency hearing were compared on a series of audiometric measures. One group was composed of subjects with 12- to 24-month histories of noise exposure and hearing loss at 4000 Hz greater than 40 dB; the other group was composed of normal-hearing subjects with no history of unusual noise exposure. On fixed-frequency Bekesy audiometry at 2000 Hz, 12 of the noise-exposed subjects demonstrated separation of 5 dB or more between pulsed- and continuous-tone tracings; similar separation occurred for only one of the non-noise-exposed subjects. Significant between-group differences also occurred on three tests of speech discrimination: PB-50 word lists and CID W-22 lists presented with two forms of competing noise.

Recent reports based on animal studies (Carder and Miller, 1972; Mills and Tato, 1972; Melnick, Migliore, and Lim, 1972; Henderson, Hamernic, and Sitler, 1972) have indicated that damage to cochlear structures as a result of exposure to high noise levels is not invariably accompanied by permanent auditory threshold shifts. These reports suggest that injury to the human cochlea may not always be detected by standard pure-tone threshold audiometry.

More sensitive audiological test procedures might indicate cochlear dysfunction not apparent from the results of the basic audiometric battery. Findlay and Patterson (1973) studied threshold adaptation in a group of 10 young listeners with noise-induced hearing loss centered at 4000 Hz. In each case Bekesy sweep-frequency audiometry through 2000 Hz indicated normal hearing. Fixed-frequency tracings at 2000 Hz for eight of the 10 subjects demonstrated 5 dB or more consistent separation between the midpoints of the tracings for pulsed- and continuous-tone stimuli, the continuous-tone stimulus indicating higher thresholds.

The present study was undertaken to consider further possible differences in auditory function between noise-exposed and normal listeners not apparent from the results of the basic test battery. Using fixed-frequency Bekesy audiometry, we made a comparison of tracings between the two groups of listeners at octave frequencies from 500 to 4000 Hz. Results of the two groups on the SISI test at 2000 Hz were also compared. In addition, in view of the reports of noise-exposed subjects that they experience considerable difficulty understanding speech in noise, a comparison was made of the abilities of normal and noise-exposed subjects to discriminate speech stimuli presented under adverse listening conditions.

TEST PROCEDURES

Subjects

Audiometric data were obtained from 32 males, aged 18–29 years, in good health and with no history of psychiatric or otologic pathology. Each subject was administered a preliminary test battery consisting of pure-tone air- and bone-conduction audiometry, SRTs (in decibels of hearing level, ANSI, 1969), and speech discrimination using CID W-22 Lists 1 and 2. One ear of each subject was selected for special testing according to the criteria described below. Pure-tone thresholds in the test ear were no poorer than 20 dB HL (ISO, 1964) at octave frequencies from 250 through 2000 Hz. Subjects were divided into two groups.

The noise-exposed group consisted of 16 subjects with histories of almost daily exposure to noise over periods from 12 to 24 months. The noise was commonly of small arms, armor, or jet engine origin. Pure-tone threshold sensitivity at 4000 Hz in the test ear was 40 dB HL or poorer. Six subjects were studied in the right ear and 10 in the left. Mean test ear thresholds and speech discrimination scores are presented in Table 1.

TABLE 1. Means and standard deviations of pure-tone threshold (decibels of hearing level, ISO, 1964) SRT (decibels of hearing level, ANSI, 1969) and speech discrimination scores for noise-exposed and normal subjects.

Subjects	Frequency (Hz)							SRT	CID W-22 (%)
	250	500	1000	2000	3000	4000	8000		
Noise-Exposed									
Mean	15.0	10.6	7.8	9.7	41.9	60.3	48.7	2.6	91.1
SD	5.6	4.3	4.7	4.1	14.9	12.2	11.4	2.9	5.5
Normal									
Mean	8.4	6.6	4.7	5.0	9.4	8.8	9.3	−1.1	95.9
SD	2.9	3.4	4.5	5.6	3.9	4.5	4.6	3.9	2.1

The normal-hearing subject group consisted of 16 subjects with no history of prolonged noise exposure. Pure-tone thresholds were no worse than 20 dB HL at 4000 Hz. In order to match the ears tested of noise-exposed subjects six right and 10 left ears were tested. Mean thresholds and speech discrimination scores are presented in Table 1.

Testing

Testing took place in a two-chamber IAC sound suite. Following the preliminary test battery the tests described below were administered in randomized order among subjects.

Bekesy Fixed-Frequency Audiometry

Fixed-frequency audiometry was administered with a Grason-Stadler Bekesy audiometer Model E-800-4 equipped with TDH-39 headphones. Threshold tracings were recorded for pulsed- (250 msec on–250 msec off) and continuous-tone stimuli for two minutes at each of four frequencies (500, 1000, 2000, and 4000 Hz). The rate of stimulus attenuation was 2.5 dB/sec. Test frequency presentation order was counterbalanced among subjects.

1. AUDITORY IMPAIRMENT

SISI Test

SISI testing at 2000 Hz was administered with a SISI adapter (Gordon-Stowe, Model 1259) connected through a Beltone 15C audiometer to TDH-39 earphones. Baseline presentation was 30 dB SL, after the recommendation of Harford (1966) that sensation level greater than 20 dB be used in cases of mild hearing loss. Test increments were 1 dB every five seconds.

Speech Tests

Speech stimuli were presented from phonograph recordings (Technisonic Studios) played on the turntable of a Grason-Stadler Model 162 speech audiometer to TDH-39 earphones. Before each presentation, the record was calibrated by adjusting the 1000-Hz carrier tone on the record to 0 dB on the VU meter.

Eight subjects of each group listened to PB-50 word List 7-B and eight listened to List 8-B, presented at a level 40 dB above SRT. CID W-22 word Lists 3-A and 4-A were presented at 30 dB above SRT, each accompanied by one of two competing background noises: a speech spectrum noise, obtained from the Grason-Stadler audiometer, and a "cocktail party" noise, obtained by recording three males and three females reading aloud simultaneously. The acoustic spectrum of the "cocktail party" noise in the present study was measured by a one-tenth octave band General Radio sound and vibration analyzer, Model 1564-A, in conjunction with a General Radio graphic level recorder, Model 1523. It rose 10 dB per octave between 100 and 150 Hz, remained relatively flat to 500 Hz, then declined at 10 dB per octave. The amplitude variability of the noise was approximately 5 dB. The "cocktail party" noise was presented from a Sony TC-580 tape recorder. The background noises were calibrated prior to presentation by adjusting a prerecorded 1000-Hz tone with reference to 0 dB on the VU meter.

The speech spectrum noise was presented with a CID W-22 word list at 0 dB speech-to-noise ratio, and the "cocktail party" noise with a second CID W-22 word list at −4 dB speech-to-noise ratio. Based on earlier pilot work and the results of Findlay and Patterson (1973), the speech-to-noise levels selected were those at which normal listeners score slightly below 100%. The subjects wrote responses to all speech stimuli.

RESULTS

Bekesy Fixed-Frequency Audiometry

The criterion for Bekesy audiometry analysis was based on the amount of separation of continuous- and pulsed-threshold tracings, the continuous tracing indicating higher threshold. The tracings were divided into those with less than 5 dB separation between the midpoints of the pulsed- and continuous-tone tracings during at least 60 of the final 90 seconds of recording, and those with 5 dB or more separation. The 5 dB minimum value was considered appropriate in view of the modal values of tracing width which were between 5 and 7 dB. Figure 1 presents the frequency of occurrence of adaptation of 5 dB or more among the subjects of the two groups at each test frequency. At 500 Hz three subjects in the noise-exposed group demonstrated separation between tracing midpoints by values from 5 to 10 dB. None of the normal listeners, the group with normal hearing, showed as much as 5 dB separation at 500 Hz. At 1000 Hz four noise-exposed subjects demonstrated 5 dB or more separation of the tracing midpoints; complete separation of the tracings occurred in one case. Only one normal subject demonstrated more than 5 dB separation at 1000 Hz. Twelve noise-exposed subjects demonstrated separation of 5 dB or more at

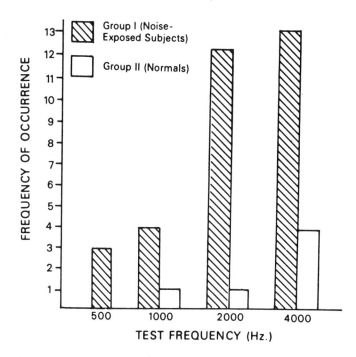

Figure 1. Frequency histogram showing number of subjects in each group who presented 5 dB or more consistent separation between midpoints of Bekesy fixed-frequency pulsed- and continuous-threshold tracings at four test frequencies.

2000 Hz, with two of those subjects showing separation greater than 10 dB. Eight of the 12 subjects demonstrated complete separation between tracings. Only one normal subject demonstrated 5 dB midpoint separation at 2000 Hz. At 4000 Hz 13 noise-exposed subjects showed 5 dB or more separation between the tracing midpoints, with complete separation of the tracings in four cases. Four normal subjects demonstrated 5 dB or more separation between tracings with total separation in three of four cases. In each case in which separation of 5 dB or more occurred at a lower frequency it was followed by separation at the next octave higher.

SISI Test

The score for the noise-exposed subjects ranged from 0 to 45% (mean = 20.94, SD = 14.60). Scores for normal listeners ranged between 0 and 60% (mean = 21.88, SD = 20.83). A t test indicated no significant difference between scores for the two groups (t = 0.14, df = 30, p > 0.05).

Speech Discrimination Tests

Mean scores for the PAL PB-50 test were 62.88% for noise-exposed listeners and 69.00% for normal listeners. Standard deviations were 9.51 and 4.53% respectively. Student's t test for paired subjects (Hays, 1963) indicated a significant difference between the two groups beyond the 5% level of confidence (t = 2.25, df = 30, p < 0.05). There was considerable overlap in the distribution of scores for the two groups.

Mean scores for the W-22 word lists in competing speech spectrum noise were: noise-exposed subjects, 49.25%, and normal listeners, 58.13%. Standard deviations were 9.07 and 6.50% respectively. A t test indicated a significant difference between the two groups beyond the 1% level of confidence (t = 3.08,

1. AUDITORY IMPAIRMENT

$df = 30$, $p < 0.01$). Again there was considerable overlap in the distribution of scores for the two groups.

Mean scores for W-22 word lists with competing "cocktail party" noise were 56.75% for noise-exposed subjects, with a standard deviation of 12.04%, and 75.38% for normal listeners, with a standard deviation of 9.30%. A t test indicated a significant difference between groups beyond the 1% level of confidence ($t = 4.92$, $df = 30$, $p < 0.01$). There was little overlap in distribution of scores for the two groups on this test condition; three noise-exposed subjects and 14 normal subjects had scores of 70% or above.

In summary, among the special tests of the present battery, Bekesy fixed-frequency audiometry and the W-22 test presented with competing "cocktail party" noise were most consistent in indicating differences between subjects of the two groups. Although the W-22 lists presented with competing speech noise and the PB-50 lists demonstrated significant intergroup differences, there was considerable overlap of scores among the subjects of the two groups. The SISI test failed to indicate differences between the groups.

DISCUSSION

Komovic (1973) studied auditory functions in 18 young male listeners who had normal auditory thresholds through 2000 Hz but hearing sensitivity worse than 40 dB HL (re ISO, 1964) at 4000 Hz apparently because of noise exposure. He found that at 2000 Hz compressed temporal integration functions and tone decay results were consistent with cochlear involvement in 12 subjects. Findlay and Patterson (1973) found consistent separation of Bekesy fixed-frequency tracings at 2000 Hz for eight of the 10 noise-exposed subjects with normal hearing through 2000 Hz. The results of the present study demonstrated a similar incidence of fixed-frequency tracing separation among noise-exposed subjects at 2000 Hz, although not at 500 or 1000 Hz. It may be noted that despite differences between thresholds obtained at 2000 and 4000 Hz among our noise-exposed subjects, the incidence and magnitude of threshold adaptation were approximately equal at both frequencies. It appears that changes in adaptation may precede significant permanent threshold shifts. Together, the results of these studies suggest that traditional pure-tone audiometry may fail to identify certain frequency regions for which auditory function is abnormal and may minimize estimate of damage to the cochlea resulting from noise exposure.

Speech discrimination test scores for the two groups indicated that before significant hearing loss is apparent at the mid-frequencies, listeners may begin to experience undue speech perception difficulties under conditions of competing speech and noise. This finding agrees with frequent complaints by younger noise-exposed listeners that they encounter difficulties in complex verbal communication situations such as conversations in groups, or listening in noisy environments. The results for the CID W-22 lists presented with competing "cocktail party" noise are in agreement with the report by Lovrinic, Burgi, and Curry (1968) that the distribution of listeners' W-22 scores in "cocktail party" noise correlated with the presence of auditory impairment better than any other speech test condition.

Decreased speech discrimination performance among listeners with noise-induced hearing loss apparent above 2000 Hz is often attributed to reduced high-frequency responsivity. However, from the Bekesy fixed-frequency tracing results we have observed, auditory dysfunction may occur at 2000 Hz or below and may account in part for decreased speech intelligibility. A comparison of performances of two groups of subjects, similar to those of the present study, for the CID W-22 lists presented with competing "cocktail party" noise, but with the signal low-pass filtered at 2000 Hz could determine whether auditory dysfunction involving frequencies below 2000 Hz contributed to speech discrimination difficulties among noise-exposed listeners.

In conclusion, tests of the basic audiometric battery may not indicate the full extent of auditory dysfunction, or hearing handicap, related to noise-induced hearing loss. Auditory changes may be reflected more accurately by other tests, including tests of adaptation and discrimination of speech under adverse listening conditions. It may be of interest to determine whether special tests may also indicate more fully the extent of hearing dysfunction associated with other cochlear disorders.

ACKNOWLEDGMENT

Requests for reprints should be addressed to the author, Department of Speech, 1117 Cathedral of Learning, University of Pittsburgh, Pittsburgh, Pennsylvania 15260.

REFERENCES

CARDER, H. M., and MILLER, J. D., Temporary threshold shifts from prolonged exposure to noise. *J. Speech Hearing Res.*, 15, 603–623 (1972).

FINDLAY, R. C., and PATTERSON, M. D., Effects of noise exposure upon low- and mid-frequency hearing. Paper presented at the Annual Convention of the American Speech and Hearing Association, Detroit (1973).

HARFORD, E., The SISI test. *Maico Audiological Library Service,* Vol. 4, Report 9 (1966).

HAYS, W. L., *Statistics for Psychologists.* New York: Holt, Rinehart and Winston (1963).

HENDERSON, D., HAMERNIC, R. P., and SITLER, R. W., A comparison between hair cell losses and permanent threshold shift produced by three levels of impulse noise. Paper presented at the 83rd Annual Meeting of the Acoustical Society of America, Buffalo, N.Y. (1972).

KOMOVIC, J., Auditory temporal integration in subjects with cochlear pathology due to noise exposure. Master's thesis, Univ. of Pittsburgh (1973).

LOVRINIC, J. H., BURGI, E. J., and CURRY, E. T., A comparative evaluation of five speech discrimination measures. *J. Speech Hearing Res.*, 11, 372–381 (1968).

MELNICK, W., MIGLIORE, M., and LIM, D., Asymptotic TTS in chinchillas. Paper presented at the 83rd Annual Meeting of Acoustical Society of America, Buffalo, N.Y. (1972).

MILLS, J. H., and TATO, S. A., Temporary threshold shifts produced by exposure to high-frequency noise. *J. Speech Hearing Res.*, 15, 624–631 (1972).

The Fine Art of Auditory Training, or Is Anyone Listening?

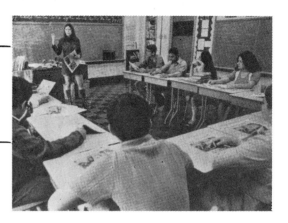

Frank B. Withrow, Ph.D.

Dr. Withrow is Executive Secretary of the National Advisory Committee on the Handicapped, U.S. Department of Health, Education, and Welfare. Presently he is on leave as a Battell Institute Fellow in Columbus, Ohio. He will be doing research in psycholinguistic development among handicapped children during this fellowship year.

The sense of hearing is used for both safety and communication. Through auditory training, the hearing impaired child should learn to use his residual hearing 1) to identify noises which mean possible danger, and 2) to distinguish frequencies, patterns, rhythms, and elements of speech. The development of the child's residual hearing should be a foremost component of any educational program for the hearing impaired.

Hearing as one of the distant senses has two major purposes: safety and communication. The first has become so second-nature to the hearing person that he is seldom aware of its importance. Hearing functions as an early warning system, alerting the person to his physical environment and providing feedback as to the status of the world. Even during sleep it acts as an alerting or guard system which awakens the sleeper when danger may be near. For the mother of young children, hearing serves as a guardian of their well-being, setting the limits of where they may play and providing a steady stream of information that allows the mother to know the children are playing in safety. The absence of this stimuli alerts the mother to check on the whereabouts and activities of her children.

There are constant auditory feedback signals that provide information with respect to the well-being and stability of our environment. We know we have turned off the water faucet if we do not hear it flowing or dripping; we know various machines serving us are functioning properly by the auditory stimuli they produce; we know the house door and the car door are properly shut by the click of their latch. The sounds of traffic guide us when we drive, and warning sirens are the mark of our emergencies. This constant sea of background noise so engulfs us that we use it automatically. It is so much a part of our environment that it seldom rises to our consciousness.

The most common and conscious use of the sense of hearing is in

"The Fine Art of Auditory Training, or Is Anyone Listening?" Frank B. Withrow, Ph.D., *The Volta Review*, Vol. 76 No. 7, 1974. ©1974 The Alexander Graham Bell Association for the Deaf, Inc.

communication. Human communication probably developed via the auditory pathway because it could be superimposed over the primary function of hearing—i.e., warning and localization of environmental dangers—with a minimum of interference with other physical actions of the human being. In our modern complex society, hearing is an ideal sensory mode for communication. The pilot of an airplane can perform the needed tasks to maneuver the airliner while he is communicating with the ground control. Similarly, in many instances of our daily lives communication through speech and hearing enhances our physical performance.

From a functional standpoint, the sense of hearing is an ideal receiver of communication. The stimuli may be detected from any direction with almost the same degree of accuracy. Meaningful signals can be selected from background noises. Obviously, sound signals are not dependent upon light sources, so they are available to us 24 hours a day. Once the signal has been detected and the listener begins to perceive it as a message, meaning can be associated with the intensity (loudness), frequency (pitch), inflection, and rhythm of the stimuli.

auditory training to enhance hearing for safety and communication

Auditory training for an individual deaf or hard of hearing child will vary depending on the degree and severity of the hearing loss, the nature of the speech signal, the age of the child, and his ability to synthesize language codes. Generally, however, there are three major objectives in auditory training which can be matched to the needs and requirements of each hearing impaired child.

1. Through the use of amplification devices, the child will learn to detect environmental auditory cues which can provide warning and alerting information.

1.1 The child will detect warning signals such as sirens, bells, horns, etc., and will develop appropriate adaptive, adjustive, and/or avoidance behavior.

1.2 He will detect and identify low frequency environmental noises.

1.3 He will identify traffic noises such as trucks, buses, trains, etc., and will develop appropriate responses.

1.4 He will detect the presence of speech within his environment and will learn visual searching techniques to identify the speaker.

2. The child will be able to distinguish among various frequencies, stress patterns, and rhythmic beats in speech.

2.1 He will be able to distinguish between the presence and absence of sound.

2.2 He will be able to distinguish between high and low pitched sounds and their order of occurrence in time; i.e., whether the high or low pitched sound occurs first.

2.3 He will be able to distinguish between loud and soft sounds and their order of occurrence.

2.4 He will be able to detect the affective tone of the speaker's voice and positive and negative attitudes expressed by the speaker.

2.5 He will be able to distinguish among various monosyllables when presented with as many as ten words.

2.6 He will be able to distinguish stress and rhythmic patterns in sentences and to choose a specified sentence from among several possibilities.

2.7 He will be able to distinguish stress and rhythmic patterns in questions and to choose a specified question from a number of possibilities.

1. AUDITORY IMPAIRMENT

3. Using his amplified residual hearing, the child will be able to distinguish certain speech elements within the range of his usable hearing.

3.1 He will be able to distinguish consonant and vowel combinations.

3.2 He will be able to distinguish words, phrases, and sentences that are developed to exercise and maximize the use of his residual hearing.

3.3 He will be able to answer questions about material he has heard or read.

3.4 He will be able to carry on a dialogue through the synergetic use of sound and sight.

maximizing residual hearing

Many educators over the years have realized and emphasized the importance of using residual hearing. Max Goldstein's acoustic method (1939), developed prior to the time of modern electronic hearing aids, used a mechanical means of amplification. He designed a set of stethoscope-like tubes which were used to amplify speech sounds for deaf children. The teacher spoke directly into the mouth of the hearing tube, which provided 80 to 90dB of amplified sound at the ear. Teachers using such a system were able to modify and adapt the amplification to maximize the effects of their auditory training.

The Association Method developed by Mildred McGinnis (1963) also contributed to our knowledge of auditory training. Miss McGinnis believed that speech should be spoken directly into the ear without electronic or mechanical amplification. This would provide an acoustical signal at close enough proximity that it could be used by the learner. She insisted that all parts of the sensory system be constantly associated so that, together, they formed a synergetic whole. Speech production, reading, and writing were all related to audition. Her techniques utilized incremental steps and patterns based upon discrete discrimination tasks within very narrowly defined boundaries. The child was expected to select from among a few very different stimuli within a prescribed universe of stimuli which was gradually increased to represent the world at large. Great emphasis was placed on a child's ability to generalize his learned knowledge. After he had learned to discriminate a phoneme, word, or phrase, he was expected to be able to do so in an infinite variety of circumstances. In effect, communication was broken up into its smallest units—phonemes and/or graphemes—and these were gradually put together into words, phrases, and sentences.

Working with very young deaf children, Erik Wedenberg (1951) has charted the residual hearing of the infant and matched it with a vocabulary that the infant is most likely to hear. The child's father—with his relatively low pitched voice—is instructed to speak samples of this vocabulary into the ear of the child. In recent years, the utilization of residual hearing has been further sophisticated by Wedenberg by transposing energy in the speech signal to give a maximum signal in the lower frequencies, which are the ones most likely to be perceived by the child. Although the transposed signal may sound peculiar to a person with normal hearing, the assumption is that the deaf child with his hearing aid will have a wider range of information from the available speech signal to use with his residual hearing.

Wedenberg believes that the sequencing aspect of audition, i.e., the temporal patterning of the auditory signal, is a basic component of the psycho-linguistic set from which symbols are developed and symbolic and conceptual thought grows. As the base for a symbolic code, the aural stimulus is irreversible in time, nonspatial, and sequential in nature. It is like a rapidly moving stream of informational bits which change over time. The very nature of the sensory stimuli partly dictates the organization of the thought structure of the individual. Thus, Wedenberg believes that this flow of aural language structures the cognitive organization of the learner, and he advises that the use of audition be tailored around the hearing of the infant as the *primary* signal of early communication.

audition as the foundation for language and communication

Many professionals involved in the development of early education programs for the hearing impaired have emphasized the importance of audition as an early foundation for language and communication (Simmons-Martin, 1968; Pollack, 1970; Northcott, 1972). Dr. Simmons-Martin has recognized the desirability of combining sight and sound as the basis of an initial mode of receptive communication and has emphasized the blending of auditory training and lipreading to provide the basic symbolic code association required to develop language. She stresses that these skills develop best in an atmosphere free from conflict and totally accepting of the child.

Schlesinger and Meadow (1971) suggest the synergetic relation between sight and sound as a foundation for language, emphasizing the need for mutual reinforcement of the two sensory systems. Great importance is placed on the affective domain of the child's experience. Acceptance of the child and of all modes of communication without overemphasis on either sight or sound is important. Harmony within the family and a positive relationship with the deaf infant, they feel, is the foundation for the development not only of an effective and exoteric communication system, but also of a mentally healthy and inquisitive personality. The deaf child ultimately may function as a bilingual person, conversant in speech and lipreading as well as in the language of signs. This bilingualism, they feel, enhances both systems and serves as an asset to the child in the modern world.

summary: a goal for future efforts

Every effort must be made to remedy the medical problems associated with hearing loss. Once all remedial medical action has been taken, amplification should be prescribed and used as soon as the hearing loss is identified. Early auditory training must be practiced, both by the father and the mother, on a daily basis. Prior to the use of electronic amplification, the father as well as the mother should speak directly into the young child's ear.

The objective of early infant auditory training is to build the foundation for communication via the cybernetic loop of self-stimulation through babbling to word association. This foundation will provide for the genesis of natural language and thought processes. Once this loop is established, a synergetic association of sight and sound elements of language may be developed.

The use of residual hearing allows the deaf child to 1) use his hearing as a warning and alerting system; 2) be aware of speech; 3) discriminate stress and temporal patterns in speech; and 4) discriminate words and/or parts of words and phrases and attach meaning to them. Not all deaf persons can achieve all the objectives, but each deaf child is entitled to the opportunity to learn to use his residual hearing to the best of his ability. Audition is the foundation for the world's communication systems—it is not the only system, but it decides the rules of the game called language.

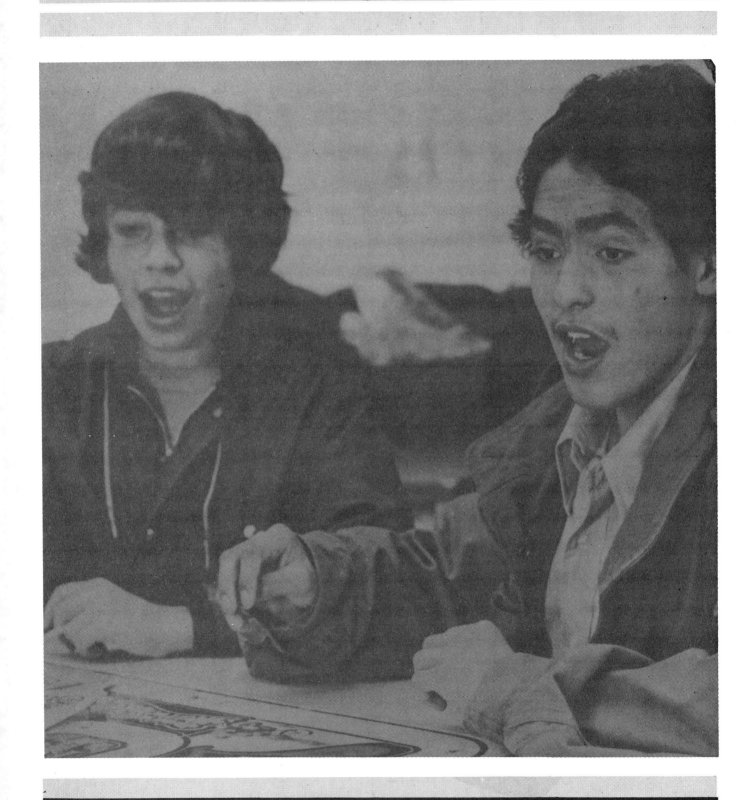

Speech Disorders: Pathology and Classification

A speech disorder can be defined as a situation in which a person's speech presents such a problem as when listeners pay as much attention or more, as to how one speaks as to what one is saying. This is a defect or an impairment of speech.

Pathologically speaking, impairment can be related to a number of factors, such as incorrect pronounciation, personality maladjustment, mental subnormality, improper grammar, or in association with one or more of these conditions. In children, organic disorders may be found, such as cleft palate and cerebral palsy. In retarded children, speech defects are the most dificult to diagnose and present the largest single challenge to speech pathology, primarily due to the fact that causes may be individual to each child and his environment, thus producing both extrinsic and intrinsic causes for delayed speech.

Hearing impairment has been recognized for centuries to be a congenital affliction of the inability to talk as a result of deafness. Other pathological classifications include, motor difficulties, failure to speak due to difficulty in tongue control, the palate, the lips or other structures of the body which aid speech and which may have been affected at birth due to brain injuries. Environmental causes of motivation and stimulation must also be considered; emotional shock from a harrowing experience can also enter into pathological classification.

Aspects of stuttering, problems of speech fluency, articulation, distortions, disorders of the voice are all included in this section, so that we might address the student, the speech therapist, the teacher, the social worker, the psychologist, the parent . . . to increase understanding of the whys and the wherefores of human behavior of this handicapping condition.

Tongue Thrust:

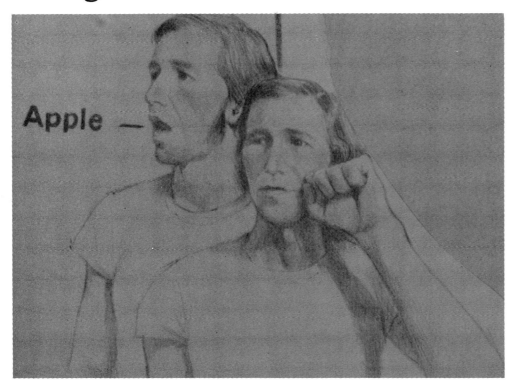

Apple —

A Point of View

Marvin L. Hanson

In recent years a number of articles have appeared in professional journals which have tended to deny the value of therapy for tongue thrust or to recommend limiting its application to the postadolescent patient. (Brader, 1972; Mason and Proffit, 1974; Subtelny and Subtelny, 1973; Worms, Meskin, and Isaacson, 1971). The Joint Committee on Dentistry and Speech Pathology (1973) has issued a statement questioning the validity of such therapy.

The progress of therapy for oral myofunctional disorders has paralleled that of other fields involved in changing human behavior. Whereas, ideally, scientific experimentation should precede clinical application of a procedure or program, traditionally the clinical approach has had to prove itself to be of some worth before anyone was willing to invest the time to test it scientifically. The research completed up to the present time has only provided fuel for the controversies. Much of it has suffered from poor design or from limitations due to heterogeneity of subjects. What is more, the researchers and their readers have generalized liberally in applying results to the general population.

The purpose of the present article is to present evidence supporting the validity of therapy for tongue thrust. More specifically, the following hypotheses will be discussed:

1. There is a relationship between tongue thrust and malocclusion, and it is probably a reciprocal one.
2. Tongue thrust may yield spontaneously to nonthrusting patterns.
3. If tongue thrust does not yield spontaneously to nonthrusting patterns, some form of treatment should be considered.

"Tongue Thrust: A Point of View," Marvin L. Hanson, *Journal of Speech and Hearing Research*, Vol. 41 No. 2, May 1976. ©1976 Journal of Speech and Hearing Research.

4. If myofunctional therapy is the treatment of choice, its timing with respect to patient age, developmental factors, and orthodontic treatment should be an individual matter.

The author admits to being limited by the same inadequacies of research that he finds in the literature purporting to disprove the value of myofunctional therapy. Nevertheless, what little knowledge we do have is at least sufficient to preclude closing the topic to further research.

DEFINITION

In order for research on this behavior to be valid, investigators need to agree on a definition of tongue thrust. It has been described as (1) a syndrome and (2) lingual contact against the teeth during swallowing. Neither description is adequate.

Tongue Thrust as a Syndrome. Most of the literature over the past two decades has described tongue thrust as a symptom pattern, involving tongue protrusion during swallowing, lack of molar occlusion, hypercontraction of the circumoral muscles, a diminished gag reflex, and various other features. This concept of a consistent set of symptoms has proven untenable. Research by Subtelny (1970), Hedges, McLean, and Thompson (1965), and Long (1963) has shown that many of these characteristics are present in normal swallowing as well as in tongue thrusting, and that the only criterion which can be used to differentiate tongue thrust from normal swallowing is the presence or degree of tongue contact against or between the anterior dentition.

Tongue Thrust as Lingual Contact with the Teeth. Research has found that in normal swallowers with normal occlusion, the tongue may rest and push against the molars and bicuspids, and even against the lingual surfaces of the cuspids and incisors near the gingival margin (Subtelny and Subtelny, 1962; Hedges et al., 1965). It would seem prudent, for research purposes, to label lingual behavior as thrusting only when it involves contact of greater than normal areas of the teeth, or contact of greater than normal frequency or force.

If tongue thrust is to be studied objectively, it should be measurable. Quantification of lingual pressures has proven to be a very difficult task. Pressure research has been done, but difficulties in eliminating the artifact of transducers make the validity of such measures questionable. Another approach to quantification is through the use of cinefluorography. In the writer's research, involving a total of 890 cineradiographic studies of 178 children, the determination of presence or absence of tongue thrust in most of the films was found to be extremely difficult. In lateral view, unless the teeth were not occluded during swallowing or an open bite was present, the precise location of the anterior border of the tongue was obscured by the teeth. Furthermore, no well-defined tongue-tip was evident in any of the films. The reliability of judgments made by independent, sophisticated viewers of these films was so low as to preclude their use as a diagnostic tool for research purposes.

Independent judgments made by the same persons based on direct observation of swallowing behavior were consistently in agreement (above 90%). Until more objective procedures are devised to measure tongue activity, it seems advisable to define tongue thrust as a behavior identifiable through direct visual observations.

Proposed Definition. The writer offers the following definition hesitatingly:

When, in resting position, the anterior or lateral portions of the tongue contact more than half the surface area of either the upper or lower incisors, cuspids, or biscuspids, or protrude between them; or when, during the swallow of any two of the three media (liquids, solids, and saliva) there is a visibly observable increase of (1) force, (2) degree of protrusion, or (3) amount of surface area of the teeth contacted by the tongue, there is a tongue thrust.

Once researchers accept a common definition of the problem and determine to conduct well-controlled investigations into the area of swallowing and malocclusion, some of the controversies may begin to be resolved. In the meantime, hypotheses such as those presented in the remainder of this article must be formulated based on the scant work that has been done. The hypotheses will be listed for two purposes: (1) to reply to those who would discourage the continuation of therapy for tongue thrust on the grounds that there is no evidence to support the validity of such treatment; (2) to encourage better, more extensive research.

RELATIONSHIPS BETWEEN TONGUE THRUST AND MALOCCLUSION

Tongue thrust and malocclusion sometimes occur together. Rix (1946) studied 93 children between the ages of seven and 12 years. Sixty-one were found to be swallowing with the teeth together. Of this group, 36% had "deviant dentition." Twenty-seven swallowed with teeth apart. Eighty-one percent of this group had "deviate dentition." (In the 1940s and 1950s the "teeth apart" swallows were equated with tongue thrust and the "teeth occluded" swallows with normal behavior).

Werlich (1962) studied 640 elementary and secondary school children, and found that 30.4% were tongue thrusters. Of those who had Class II, Division I malocclusions, 50.7% swallowed with a tongue thrust. Of the children with open bite, 98.5% were thrusters. He also found, in children in two younger age groups (mean ages, 6.6 and 11.5 years), a significant relationship between tongue thrust and posterior crossbite.

Rogers (1961) compared a group of orthodontic patients with a group of children from the public schools, some of whom had orthodontic problems. The incidence of tongue thrust was high in both groups, 56.9% in the schoolchildren and 62.8% in the patients. It was particularly high among subjects with deep overbite (79.7 and 62.8% in the two respective groups). Subjects with open bites demonstrated a great tendency toward tongue thrust. Among the schoolchildren with open bite the incidence was 98.2%, and 92.8% of the orthodontic patients with open bite were tongue thrusters.

Intra- and Extraoral Muscular Forces

Some kind of balance exists between intra- and extraoral muscular forces against the teeth. Mason and Proffit (1974, p. 121) state, "It has been observed that there is no balance of pressure against the teeth. The expansive forces of the tongue are never balanced by the containing forces of the lips, even when prolonged periods of time are considered."

The word *balanced* is important and deserves consideration. The word *never* is also important and always a little dangerous to use. People who treat tongue thrust are primarily concerned with the anterior dentition and sometimes with the bicuspids. Most of the patients present overjets, usually involving maxillary incisors and canines. It is true that lingual pressures as measured by several researchers nearly always exceed labial and buccal pressures. If *balance* means *equal*, then the forces rarely balance. If *balance* is considered a transitive verb, and the direct object is the teeth, it acquires a different meaning. A 200-pound man and a 100-pound boy can balance a seesaw, if they sit in the right places. Dentition, especially the anterior maxillary dentition can be balanced by unequal intra- and extraoral forces.

One reason teeth normally remain straight may be found in the architecture of the dentition and its supporting structures. Brader (1972) discussed the geometry of the dental arches and the effects of opposing muscular forces upon those arches. He theorized that the teeth are in equilibrium between the forces of the tongue musculature and the labiobuccal musculature. Strang and Thompson (1958) explain that the bone of the alveolar process is designed to give to the teeth the greatest support with the least possible bulk. Where there is an increase in bulk it is to meet some special force.

Bone is most dense, they explain, but least in bulk on the side against which developmental forces have been exerted, and less dense but greater in bulk on the sides from which the forces have come. If this is true, we would expect to find the bones more dense, but having less bulk, on the labial and buccal sides of the teeth, and less dense but with more bulk on the lingual aspect. This is indeed the case.

Normally, the greater bulk in the bone on the lingual aspect, at the root of the tooth, helps keep the incisor in balance even though the lingual pressures are greater than the labial pressures. This difference in bulk between the labial and lingual aspects of the alveolar process supporting the central incisor can be seen in Figure 1, an illustration from Sicher and DuBrul (1970).

This difference between amounts of bulk of bone tissue is not seen in sections of the corresponding mandibular teeth. A characteristic of many tongue thrusters with overjet is that the maxillary incisors are tipped labially. If it is normal for lingual pressures to exceed labial pressures in people with normal occlusion, the question arises, do even greater differences between lingual and labial pressure occur in people with tongue thrust, malocclusion, or both? This hypothesis has not been adequately tested experimentally. However, Mendel (1962) compared labial and lingual pressures of five teenaged females whose

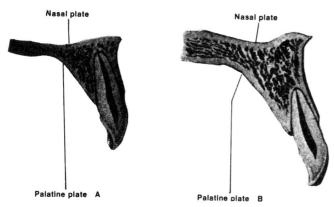

Figure 1. Labiolingual sections through the upper first incisor (Sicher and DuBrul, 1970, p. 386).

corrected open bites had remained stable for at least one year after the retention phase of treatment with those of six females of similar ages who had relapsed into an anterior open bite and who exhibited a tongue thrust. The mean tongue pressure for all swallows of the open-bite cases was 285 g/cm² as opposed to 128 g/cm² for the control samples. The mean upper-lip pressure of the open-bite sample was 45 g/cm² while the closed-bite sample had a mean pressure of 70 g/cm². The ratio of tongue to lip pressure in the relapse group was 6.3 to 1.0; and in the group with stable dentition, 1.7 to 1.0.

Unfortunately, much more attention is given in the literature to tongue thrust as related to open bite than to relationships between tongue thrust and overjet, a condition much more frequently seen by oral myofunctional therapists. An analysis of 220 patients on whom the present writer had kept sufficiently complete records to permit a study of changes in malocclusions during treatment found only 8.6% had open bite as their primary orthodontic problem. Eighty-four percent had overjet as the primary problem, and the remaining 5% had miscellaneous other types of occlusions. A study similar to Mendel's, carried out with subjects who relapsed to an overjet, would be helpful.

2. SPEECH DISORDERS

Lear and Moorrees (1969) studied lingual and buccal pressure in seven adult males with normal occlusion. Strain gauges were placed lingual and buccal to the premolars, and measures were taken during speech, mastication, deglutition, and with the oral musculature in a state of rest. The amount of time apportioned daily to each type of oral function was recorded with automatic equipment in the subjects' homes. Pressure was recorded in terms of gram minutes of force. General conclusions from the analysis of the data are given pertaining to their group of seven subjects, but specific data are included for only subject Number 4. With the exception of subject Number 2, lingual forces were found to exceed those of the cheek by factors varying from one and one-half to almost four. Subject Number 4, then, was not one in whom lingual and buccal forces were described as being in balance.

When mandibular and maxillary totals for subject Number 4 are combined, an imbalance is evident, but not when only the maxillary pressures are considered. Since the great majority of tongue thrusters seen for therapy have maxillary overjets, it is important to examine the maxillary data separately. For this adult male, there was a close counterbalance between lingual and buccal forces in the maxillary arch. The total lingual to buccal pressure ratio was 0.9 to 1.0. Total pressures, expressed in gram minutes, against the transducer placed lingual to the left maxillary premolar, were 1628. Buccal pressures near the same tooth totaled 1705 gram minutes. Similarly, lingual totals for the right maxillary premolar were 1537 gram minutes, compared to 1660 for the buccal totals. On both sides of the mouth, then, at the level of the maxillary premolars, total buccal pressures were greater than total lingual pressures.

The authors do not state why they selected subject Number 4 on whom to give complete data. The breakdown of maxillary and mandibular data is not presented for the other six subjects. The data for this one normal adult subject, nevertheless, indicate that lingual forces may be balanced by labial forces.

Lingual Pressure

Lingual pressure may be capable of moving teeth. Weinstein (1967, p. 892) reviewed a series of investigations of the effects of light constant pressures on tooth position, and concluded, "Muscle forces of such low values as 1.68 gm. above the resting force, if acting over a sufficient time, are capable of moving teeth." In one of the experiments reported by Weinstein, a premolar in a child moved nearly 1 mm in eight weeks because of a gold onlay secured to the buccal surface of that tooth. The onlay increased the buccal pressure on the premolar by only 1.68 g/cm^2.

Lingual resting pressure may be an important factor in malocclusion. If the tongue rests continuously against the anterior maxillary teeth, the light constant pressure might affect the incisors, which move more easily than do the premolars, in a manner similar to the movement of the premolar in the research described by Weinstein.

Very little research has been reported concerning lingual resting pressures. The Lear and Moorrees study (1969), involving seven adult males with normal occlusion, included measurement of lingual and buccal resting pressures at the premolar level, but the data for the total group were presented in bar graph form only. From these graphs the present author has taken the following estimates: total lingual resting pressure for all seven subjects, 10,000 gram minutes; total buccal resting pressure, 7500 gram minutes; total resting time, 1283 minutes; mean constant lingual resting pressure, 1.11 grams; mean constant buccal resting pressure, 0.81 grams.

Ideally, similar data would be collected from patients with various types of malocclusions and oral habit disorders. Preferably, pressures would be measured lingual to the incisors, rather than the premolars. It does seem conceivable, though, comparing the findings of Lear and Moorrees with those of Weinstein, that the anterior teeth might either be tipped labially or hindered in their eruption by such light constant pressures aided by stronger intermittent pressures during swallowing. This would seem plausible especially if the equilibrium discussed by Brader were upset in some way, resulting in an increased ratio of tongue to lip pressure. Furthermore, once the tipping process began, or the open bite began to develop, whatever their cause, the constancy of the labial or buccal pressure would be likely to diminish, because of the increasing difficulty of keeping the lips closed at rest.

Form and Function

Form and function probably affect each other reciprocally. Very few cause-and-effect studies are reported in the literature. At times inferences are drawn regarding cause and effect from research not designed to determine such relationships.

Subtelny (1970) posed the question:

> If there is an abnormal oral or dental environment and a concomitant abnormal pattern of muscle activity did the muscular structures create the abnormal environment or are the muscular structures adapting to the environment? (p. 170)

His answer: ". . . the indications are that functional movements of orofacial muscular structures adapt to the variables of the form of the oral environment" (p. 170). This conclusion is not warranted by his research, which was not designed to determine cause-and-effect relationships. Subtelny's paper reports various phases of research concerning relationships between lip and tongue habits and occlusion. A portion of his report describes cineradiographic observations of the swallowing patterns of six subjects with Class II, Division I malocclusions before and after orthodontic treatment. Marked improvement or complete correction in tongue or lip habits was observed in all six subjects; however, no control group was included in the research.

The present author objects not only to Subtelny's conclusion, but to the dichotomous nature of the question, ". . . did the muscular structures create the abnormal environment or are the muscular structures adapting to the environment?" Observations indicating the possibility of cause and effect in one direction do not in any way rule out that same possibility in the other direction.

The only research designed to test the hypothesis that function has an effect on form is a pilot study done by Harvold, Vargervik, and Chierici (1973), and a study on rats by Negri and Croce (1965). Harvold et al.'s research involved the insertion of an acrylic block in the posterior palates of the monkeys, forcing the tongue forward. Open bites were created during the nine months of the experiment, as well as changes in arch width. Negri and Croce performed total glossectomies on 10 rats. Three months after surgery the diameters of both jaws in the experimental rats were found to be significantly smaller than those of a group of control rats.

Need for More Research. The only way to demonstrate the relative effects of form and function upon each other would be to conduct longitudinal research, preferably with three groups of subjects. Group I would have normal occlusion and no tongue thrust, and would receive no treatment of any kind. Group II would have a malocclusion, preferably Class II, Division I, along with a tongue thrust, and would receive orthodontic treatment but no therapy for tongue thrust. Group III would also have a Class II, Division I, and would receive therapy for tongue thrust. The groups should be followed from the age of eight through 15 years, to allow for all orthodontic treatment to be accomplished and a retention period to occur. Variables to be studied should in-

2. SPEECH DISORDERS

clude: tongue size, degree of malocclusion, age, allergy, and airway obstruction.

Ideally, even more groups would be included, representing other types of malocclusions and therapy involving dental cribs. The difficulties of conducting such research are apparent, but unless carefully controlled research is done, the literature will continue to abound with inferences and suppositions.

SPONTANEOUS MODIFICATION

Effect of Age

The incidence of abnormal swallowing declines with age. Research at the University of Utah has agreed with that of Fletcher, Casteel, and Bradley (1961), Andersen (1963), and Werlich (1962), in finding an apparent spontaneous modification in swallowing patterns through the mixed dentition period. Percentages of children with tongue thrust found by Hanson and Cohen (1973) in 178 subjects were: four years, nine months, 57.9%; five years, eight months, 43.8%; six years, seven months, 51.7%; and eight years, two months, 35.4%. When 92 of their original 178 subjects were reexamined at 12 years of age, however, instead of finding a continuing decrease in incidence, the investigators found the incidence had increased to 48.9% (Hanson and Hanson, 1975).

The incidence expected by the researchers was much lower than this figure. Twenty-one of those found to be tongue thrusting were protruding the tongue into spaces created by missing maxillary cuspids. If these 21 were judged to be possible transitional thrusters and subtracted from the total of 45 tongue thrusters, the remaining 24 would constitute 26.1% of the total group.

Thirty-one of the 92 subjects had been diagnosed as tongue thrusters at the age of eight years, two months. Four years later, excluding the possible transitional thrusters, 24 were still demonstrating abnormal swallows. Had these children been seen by orthodontists at the age of eight, and a decision been made to postpone therapy until during or after adolescence, only seven of the 31 would have changed to normal swallowing patterns over the four-year period.

Nonlongitudinal studies should be viewed with caution. Worms et al. (1971) found a smaller incidence of simple open bite in older Navajo children than in younger ones, hence warn against giving credit to therapy for what may well be spontaneous remission of open bite. They report that, in children with simple open bites, the incidence of simple open bite among 148 seven-to-nine year olds was 12.8%, while incidence among 240 10-to-12 years olds was only 2.5%. However, when children with all types of open bite were included, the decline in incidence was less dramatic: from 36.4% at seven to nine years to 17.8% at 19–21 years. Depending on how the data were viewed, a reader could conclude either that 80% of the children who had open bites at seven to nine years would experience a spontaneous modification to normal occlusion between the ages of 10 and 12, or that only approximately half of the children at seven to nine would lose their open-bite malocclusion by the age of 21. Neither conclusion, of course, is justified by nonlongitudinal data.

Retention of Tongue Thrust

Certain factors are associated with the retention of tongue thrust and contribute to prognosis. The Hanson-Cohen research (1973) which followed 178 four and one-half year olds through the age of eight years two months found several such factors to be significantly related to the retention of tongue thrust.

When compared to children who were tongue thrusters during the initial examination but changed to a normal swallowing pattern at some time during the five-year period (transitional thrusters), those children who retained a thrusting pattern at eight years two months (1) contracted the masseter muscle less forcefully during swallows; (2) contracted circumoral muscles more during swallows; (3) dentalized linguoalveolar consonants more frequently; (4) had larger tonsils; (5) had higher, narrower palates; (6) had fewer allergies; (7) did more digit-sucking; (8) did more mouth breathing; (9) had less buccal crossbite; (10) had greater maxillary arch circumference; and (11) had less anteroposterior maxillary arch depth at the level of Point A on lateral head films (p. 76). The level of significance on these factors varied from 0.01 to 0.05.

It should be emphasized that none of the criteria listed was consistently found to be related to the persistence of tongue thrust during all the years of research.

PROPOSED TREATMENT

If tongue thrust does not alter spontaneously, some form of treatment should be considered. Four alternatives have been proposed: (1) surgical or orthodontic modification of the oral environment, (2) mechanical restraints or reminders, (3) speech therapy, and (4) oral myofunctional therapy.

Surgical or Orthodontic Modification of Oral Environment

Partial glossectomies, tonsillectomies, and labial and lingual frenectomies are performed to produce more favorable spatial relationships or to improve mobility of structures. The orthodontist can create more space for the tongue by expanding the maxillary arch. He repositions teeth to produce more normal arch configurations and occlusions, which, in turn, facilitate non-thrusting resting positions and swallowing patterns. In cases of extreme over-jet, orthodontics can foster better lip and tongue resting postures by moving the maxillary incisors posteriorly. Nose breathing will be encouraged because lip closure is made easier.

Mechanical Restraints or Reminders

In some areas of the country, dentists persist in using devices. The only controlled research (Subtelny and Sakuda, 1964) found the effects on tongue thrust to be only temporary. When the appliances were removed, the tongue thrust returned. The "cribs" cause the wearer discomfort, but apparently, according to some clinical reports, work for some dentists.

Speech Therapy

Mason and Proffit (1974) contend that when abnormal speech and tongue thrusting occur together in a child, articulation therapy will promote proper positioning of the tongue at rest as well as for the initiation of speaking and swallowing tasks in young children. In most cases, they state, the tongue-thrust swallow will correct itself with additional maturity (p. 126).

The experience of the present author differs from that of these writers. There is no research in the literature to support either the contention that articulation therapy promotes proper lingual rest positions or lingual positioning for swallowing. Nor are there any textbooks or published approaches to articulation therapy that pay any attention to habitual tongue resting postures in ordinary therapy for articulation problems.

The only speech problem referred to specifically by Mason and Proffit is lisping. It is undoubtedly possible to correct frontal lisp when tongue thrusting is present without giving any attention to the tongue thrust. However, if speech therapy is to be included in the total treatment of a child with tongue thrust and malocclusions, it is important to treat not only the very easily heard /s/ distortion, but also the more subtle, but often present, dentalization of the /l/, /t/, /d/, and /n/ sounds. These other consonants, according to research of McGlone, Proffit, and Christiansen (1967), are produced with greater lingual pressures than the /s/.

Oral Myofunctional Therapy

The efficacy of therapy for tongue thrust needs to be tested with strict controls before definitive statements regarding its role in total dental treatment can be made. There are several studies which indicate that swallowing patterns can be modified, but most have been poorly designed or controlled.

Short-term changes were measured by Case (1968) palatographically. Judges were able to differentiate consistently palatographs of 20 children with corrected tongue-thrust patterns from those of 20 children with tongue-thrust patterns.

Stansell (1969) studied three groups of 18 subjects each, aged nine and one-half to 14 years, all of whom had tongue thrust, sigmatism, and overjet. Group I received swallowing training only; Group II received only speech therapy for the lisp; and Group III received no training of any kind. Before and after dental impressions and lateral head X rays were taken, and measures were repeated three months posttreatment. Speech training alone was found to result in a significant decrease in overjet, and tongue-thrust therapy alone prevented an increase in overjet. Several of the control group subjects showed an increase in overjet during the treatment time.

Overstake (1970) gave therapy for swallowing to 28 of 48 children manifesting tongue thrust and lisps. The other 20 received therapy for tongue thrust and for the lisp. Both subgroups changed their swallowing patterns significantly in the direction of a normal pattern. After nine months of swallowing therapy only, 24 of the 28 children were using normal /s/ patterns in unguarded conversational speech. In the total group of 48 children, 39 (81%) were judged by orthodontists to have manifested positive changes toward more normal occlusion after swallowing therapy.

INDIVIDUALIZED MYOFUNCTIONAL THERAPY

If myotherapy is administered, treatment timing should be individualized. In the absence of research to compare relative effectiveness of various approaches to treatment timing, we must rely on clinical experience. Therapy for tongue thrust may precede, accompany, or follow orthodontic treatment.

There are certain advantages to completing therapy before orthodontic appliances are attached. The patient who has been told by his orthodontist that he must correct his abnormal oral habits before orthodontic work begins is relatively easy to motivate. The progress reports the orthodontist receives from the clinician help him to know what kind of cooperation he can expect from the patient and his parents. Many orthodontists report that it is easier to work on patients who have learned to rest their tongue back further into the mouth. Others report that movement of teeth progresses more rapidly when the swallowing has been corrected. When the therapy is successful, the orthodontist can proceed with his work with greater confidence, not having to gamble on whether the patient would actually see a clinician for treatment when orthodontics was completed, or on whether the tongue thrust therapy might fail after all the orthodontic work was done. Finally, therapy preceding orthodontics can promote proper tongue posturing and movements without concern that the patient might be using wires and bands as cues. A habit even partially dependent upon cues which are only temporary may not be as stable as one learned without such cues.

Some clinicians prefer that tongue-thrust therapy and orthodontics be

52

carried out concurrently. This is advantageous especially when the therapy is administered in the orthodontist's office. One visit can serve two purposes for the patient. In addition, the orthodontist can assist the clinician in his efforts to motivate the patient. The early stages of tooth movement often involve the use of a headgear. This usually does not interfere with oral myotherapy, except for some difficulty in achieving habitual lip closure at rest. When the patient is initially seen at an age when the bands should already be applied, concurrent treatment allows for the immediate commencement of orthodontics.

When orthodontic treatment is completed before therapy is administered, whatever maturational modifications in swallowing and resting postures that might occur are given time to do so, obviating therapy that would not have been necessary. The patient is also provided with a more normal oral environment in which the tongue may function. If swallowing patterns do not modify spontaneously, the task of therapy may be facilitated. This last advantage, however, may not always be present. The majority of patients seen by oral myologists have an overjet. Ordinarily, the result of orthodontics is to reduce the overjet, which decreases the anteroposterior space available to the tongue and possibly facilitates unwanted linguadental contact.

Until research provides us with more definitive data concerning treatment timing, it would seem wise to make determinations on an individual basis, considering anatomical factors, age of patient, nature of orthodontics to be done, developmental criteria, and other prognostic factors referred to earlier in this article.

CONCLUSIONS

Research has determined that open bite, overjet, and overbite occur concomitantly with tongue thrust to a statistically significant degree. Whether a cause-and-effect relationship exists between malocclusions and abnormal oral habits has not been demonstrated conclusively. There is enough evidence to suggest the possibility that dental abnormalities and tongue habits may affect each other reciprocally. This hypothesis needs to be tested through well controlled longitudinal research.

There are advantages to providing oral myofunctional therapy at various stages in the total treatment program of the child with malocclusions, depending on individual developmental and orthodontic considerations. Rather than accept a blanket recommendation that therapy always be carried out either in conjunction with, or following, orthodontic work, or that it always be postponed until after adolescence, the clinician is urged to consider advantages and disadvantages of various alternatives. For many patients, correction of abnormal oral habits prior to the initiation of orthodontics is advisable.

Effect of Vicarious Punishment on Stuttering Frequency

RICHARD MARTIN *and* SAMUEL HAROLDSON

University of Minnesota, Minneapolis

This investigation explored the effect of vicarious response-contingent stimulation on the frequency of stuttering. Twenty adult stutterers spoke for 20 minutes, then observed a speaker on a videotape for 10 minutes, and then spoke for an additional 20 minutes. In one condition the speaker on the videotape was a severe stutterer who experienced a dramatic reduction in stuttering under a contingent time-out procedure. In a second condition, the videotape speaker was a severe stutterer who received no experimental manipulations. In the third condition, the videotape speaker was a normal talker who received no experimental manipulations. All subjects participated in all three conditions. Twenty of the stutterers experienced a significant decrease in stuttering as a result of watching the videotape model who received contingent time-out. The subjects did not exhibit significant changes in stuttering after watching the severe stutterer who received no treatment or the normal talker.

Most learning theorists agree that a concept of vicarious learning is necessary to explain some important human and animal behaviors. One paradigm for vicarious experience involves a model who performs and is reinforced or punished, and an observer who simply watches the procedure. The effect of the vicarious procedure is determined by the extent to which the frequency of some criterion behavior of the observer changes as a result of his watching the reinforced or punished model.

There is considerable literature to indicate that, under certain conditions, human subjects increase their frequency of responding after observing other subjects being reinforced contingently for emitting similar responses. For example, Kanfer and Marston (1963) and Marston and Kanfer (1963) found that subjects emitted significantly more human nouns after listening to tape recordings in which models were told "good" contingent upon a human noun. Barnwell and Sechrest (1965) reported that first-grade children chose one of two games more or less frequently depending upon whether a paired partner (model) previously was reinforced or punished for choosing that game. Marston and Smith (1968) demonstrated that when subjects were placed in a self-reinforcement, word-association task, the frequency of self-reinforced responding was dependent partly upon the number of reinforcements received by a model.

Recently, considerable experimental and clinical evidence has been published indicating that for certain stutterers under certain conditions, the frequency

"Effect of Vicarious Punishment on Stuttering Frequency," Richard Martin, Samuel Haroldson, *Journal of Speech and Hearing Research*, Vol. 20 No. 1, March 1977. ©1977 Journal of Speech and Hearing Research.

of stuttering can be reduced through response-contingent stimulation (for example, Martin and Ingham, 1973). Many researchers, clinicians, and theorists believe that the observed decrease in stuttering which accompanies response-contingent stimulation supports the view that stuttering is an operant behavior.

As indicated earlier, considerable evidence is available suggesting that a variety of operant behaviors are susceptible to manipulation through vicarious response-contingent stimulation. It seems appropriate, therefore, to determine the extent to which stuttering is modifiable as a result of vicariously experienced consequences. Such a determination has potential significance both for theoretical and therapeutic considerations of stuttering. The present experiment was designed to determine the extent to which stuttering frequency changes as a function of vicarious response-contingent stimulation.

METHOD

Subjects and Conditions

The subjects were 20 adult stutterers enrolled in the University of Minnesota Speech and Hearing Clinic. Each subject participated in three 50-minute sessions separated by at least one week. Each subject was exposed to a different experimental condition each session. The order in which a subject was assigned to experimental conditions was random. The number of subjects assigned randomly to each possible experimental order was as follows: normal speaker condition–stutterer not timed-out condition–stutterer timed-out condition (NORM-SNTO-STO), 3; SNTO-STO-NORM, 3; STO-NORM-SNTO, 4; SNTO-NORM-STO, 3; NORM-STO-SNTO, 4; and STO-SNTO-NORM, 3.

The first 20 minutes and the last 20 minutes of all conditions were the same; the subject simply spoke spontaneously. After the first 20 minutes of speaking, subjects in the stutterer timed-out condition (STO) stopped talking and watched a videotape for 10 minutes. The videotape showed a stutterer being exposed to a "time-out" (TO) procedure and experienced a marked reduction in stuttering. At the end of the 10 minutes of viewing, the subject again spoke spontaneously for another 20 minutes. In the stutterer not timed-out condition (SNTO), the subject followed the same procedures as in the STO Condition, except that the 10-minute videotape showed a stutterer speaking spontaneously, but without receiving TO. Procedures in the normal speaker condition (NORM) were identical with those of the other two conditions, except that the 10-minute videotape showed a normal talker speaking spontaneously.

Videotapes

The videotape that subjects viewed in the STO condition was prepared as follows. An adult male stutterer was instructed to speak spontaneously. He was told that at some point a red jewel light on a panel in front of him would illuminate and a chime would sound each time he stuttered. He was instructed to wait until the light was extinguished (five seconds), and then begin speaking again from the point where he was interrupted. The speaker was allowed to speak for five minutes, after which the TO procedure was initiated and continued for the remaining five minutes. The speaker experienced a marked reduction in stuttering frequency during the TO procedure. During the first five minutes the talker spoke an average of 79 words per minute and stuttered on 26% of those words. During the last five minutes, the subject spoke an average of 102 words per minute and stuttered on 2% of those words.

The videotape employed in the SNTO condition showed an adult male stutterer speaking spontaneously for 10 minutes during which time no TO procedures were utilized. The subject spoke an average of 49 words per minute and stuttered on 30% of the words spoken. There was no systematic increase or

2. SPEECH DISORDERS

decrease in words spoken or words stuttered across the 10 minutes. The percent words stuttered per minute was 22, 29, 25, 30, 25, 31, 41, 31, 35, and 28 for minutes one through 10, respectively. The videotape used in the NORM condition contained the spontaneous speech of an adult male normal (nonstuttering) speaker. No TO procedures were introduced. The videotapes employed in all conditions presented a front view of the speaker's head and upper body.

Procedure

Each subject was seated in an experimental room and instructed to speak spontaneously until told to stop. The subject was provided with a stack of word cards and told to use the cards to help him think of things to talk about if necessary. The subject was told that at some point a speaker would appear on the television monitor located on a table in front of him. The subject was instructed to stop talking, and to listen to and watch the speaker until the image disappeared. The subject was told that when the image disappeared he was to resume talking.

In the control room the experimenter monitored the subject through a one-way mirror and intercom system. After 20 minutes elapsed the experimenter activated the videotape playback (Sony, Model AV 3600) connected to the monitor on the subject's table. At the end of the next 10 minutes the experimenter stopped the videotape playback, after which the subject spoke for an additional 20 minutes.

All sessions were tape recorded. The number of words spoken and the number of words perceived to be stuttered were determined for each tape recording.

Reliability

A one-minute segment was chosen randomly from among the 40 one-minute segments of speech for each of the 20 subjects. These 20 one-minute segments were dubbed, in random order, onto a master reliability tape. Word-for-word protocols were prepared for each sample on the reliability master tape. Separately, the experimenter and an independent observer unfamiliar with the experiment underlined each stuttered word on the protocol. Their task was simply to "mark each time you think the person stutters." The percent agreement for stuttered words between the independent observer and the experimenter was computed as follows: number of words underlined by both experimenter and observer divided by total number of different words underlined, multiplied by 100. The percent agreement between the observer and the experimenter for all 20 samples on the reliability master tape was 92%.

RESULTS AND DISCUSSION

The mean numbers of words spoken per minute by all 20 subjects in the first 20-minute segment (prevideotape) and the last 20-minute segment (postvideotape) of each experimental condition were as follows: NORM-pre, 90.0; NORM-post, 87.2; SNTO-pre, 92.8; SNTO-post, 89.0; STO-pre, 86.7; STO-post, 90.7. These data were submitted to an analysis of variance in which segments (prevideotape, postvideotape), conditions (NORM, SNTO, STO), and the segments-by-conditions interaction all were within-subjects factors. Neither the segments nor the conditions factor was significant, but the segments-by-conditions interaction was significant ($F = 3.38$; $df = 2, 38$; $p < 0.05$). The differences among the six means were tested for significance using the Neuman-Keuls procedure (Winer, 1971). None of the comparisons among the means was significant at the 0.05 level. Inspection of the data suggests that the significant segments-by-conditions interaction probably was due to the fact that observed mean word outputs in two conditions (NORM, SNTO) were slightly lower in the pre than in the post segments. The results of these analyses suggest that the small changes in word output probably were a function of chance.

Table 1 shows, by subject, the percent of words stuttered during the first and second 20-minute segments of each experimental condition. The data in Table 1 were submitted to a segments (prevideotape, postvideotape) by conditions (NORM, SNTO, STO) analysis of variance similar to that utilized with the word output data. The segments factor was significant ($F = 5.67$; $df = 1, 19$; $p < 0.05$), the conditions factor was not significant ($F = 1.05$; $df = 2, 38$; $p > 0.05$), and the segments-by-condition interaction was significant ($F = 9.44$; $df = 2, 38$; $p < 0.01$). Results of the analysis of variance suggest that whether or not the percent of stuttered words differed in the prevideo and postvideo segments depended upon the experimental condition.

The differences among means for the six segments were tested for significance using the Newman-Keuls procedure. The results indicated that subjects stuttered significantly less, at the 0.01 level of confidence, in the posttreatment segment of the STO condition than in any of the other five segments. None of the other comparisons among means was significant at the 0.05 level. The various statistical analyses indicate that only after subjects observed the videotape of a stutterer speaking under contingent TO did percent words stuttered decrease. Observing the videotape of a normal speaker or of a stutterer not receiving contingent TO, had little effect on stuttering.

TABLE 1. Percent words stuttered, by subject, during the pre- and postsegments of the NORM, SNTO, and STO conditions.

	Words Stuttered (%)					
	NORM		SNTO		STO	
Subject	Pre	Post	Pre	Post	Pre	Post
1	4.5	5.5	4.3	3.9	3.9	3.2
2	5.3	6.0	3.7	5.1	7.1	3.1
3	3.2	4.0	1.5	2.8	2.9	1.8
4	4.6	5.8	3.5	4.5	5.1	2.0
5	7.6	5.1	6.3	7.9	20.8	16.3
6	3.9	4.9	2.3	1.9	2.5	1.9
7	24.4	21.4	5.7	4.4	17.4	13.1
8	1.6	1.5	0.9	0.5	0.7	0.4
9	41.0	40.3	40.5	48.4	50.8	41.3
10	51.4	54.1	53.0	64.2	57.7	50.4
11	3.3	3.4	4.7	4.2	3.1	1.3
12	4.6	4.3	5.0	5.6	2.8	3.0
13	2.1	2.7	0.9	0.9	2.6	2.1
14	3.6	2.6	4.5	6.2	4.8	2.5
15	24.9	26.2	29.7	33.0	29.6	19.9
16	23.6	26.9	27.3	20.6	17.8	13.9
17	38.1	39.3	57.2	45.0	29.4	18.1
18	5.2	6.1	6.7	3.8	8.1	3.6
19	8.1	8.1	5.4	5.7	4.3	4.5
20	17.1	19.3	23.8	26.6	19.5	10.2
Mean	13.9	14.4	14.3	14.8	14.5	10.6

The finding in the present study that only the vicarious situation involving response-contingent stimulation resulted in a change in stuttering frequency is consonant with the notion that stuttering is an operant behavior. On the other hand, it is possible to account for this reduction in stuttering in the same way suggested by Martin et al. (1975) for stutterers who receive direct response-contingent stimulation; namely, that the response-contingent stimulation, whether experienced directly or vicariously, served to call a speaker's attention to his stuttering in a systematic manner, and thereby occasioned a reduction in stuttering.

Results of the present study suggest some interesting, but tentative, implications for treatment. The results suggest that a client may realize some reduction in stuttering frequency simply by observing another client responding dramatically to a treatment procedure. Whether or not the model's marked reduction in stuttering must be occasioned by a response-contingent procedure, as it was in the present study, needs to be determined experimentally.

Listeners' Impressions of Speakers With Lateral Lisps

Ellen-Marie Silverman

Marquette University, Milwaukee, Wisconsin

This paper reports research conducted to determine whether the lateral lisp is a speech defect. The specific purpose of this research was to determine whether the lateral lisp calls adverse attention to the speaker. Two groups of broadcast communication students rated the concept "The Person Speaking" on a 49-scale semantic differential. One group performed the task after listening to a tape recording of a young woman reading contextual material with a simulated lateral lisp. The other group performed the task after listening to a recording of the same woman reading the material in a normal manner. Analyses of the scale values computed for the two conditions indicated that the lateral lisp called adverse attention to the speaker. A systematic replication was undertaken to assess the generality of this finding. The procedures of the original investigation were followed except that business administration students served as judges. The results replicated those of the original investigation. These data indicate that the lateral lisp is probably a speech defect and suggest that the practice of eliminating school speech services for children whose only speech difference is a lateral lisp should be reconsidered.

Most speech pathologists are in agreement that every speech difference is not a speech defect. A speech deviation is not considered a speech disorder unless it interferes with communication, calls adverse attention to the speaker, or causes the speaker to become self-conscious or maladjusted (Van Riper, 1972). For some speech deviations, such as stuttering, dysarthria, and aphasia, there is sufficient documentation to conclude that they are speech disorders as well. However, for other speech deviations, such as the misarticulation of one or two phonemes, documentation is lacking to conclude whether they are also speech disorders (Emerick and Hatten, 1974). Because of this, clinicians must rely upon their own value judgments to decide whether such differences are disorders. This paper will report research conducted to determine whether one such deviation, the lateral lisp, is a speech disorder. This research was designed to determine whether the lateral lisp calls adverse attention to the speaker. The general plan involved having two groups of judges rate the concept "The Person Speaking" on a 49-scale semantic differential (Osgood, Suci, and Tannenbaum, 1957). One group was to perform the task after listening to a tape recording of a young woman reading contextual material with a simu-

2. SPEECH DISORDERS

lated lateral lisp. The other group was to perform the task after being presented with a tape recording of the same woman reading the material in a normal manner. A less favorable evaluation of the speaker when she lisped than when she spoke normally would be considered evidence that the lisp had called adverse attention to the speaker.

METHOD

Preparation of Stimuli

A 21-year-old graduate student in speech pathology who demonstrated normal vocal and articulatory behavior and who spoke with a general American dialect served as the speaker. She attended a different university than the one the judges attended and was, therefore, unknown to the judges.

She read Fairbank's (1959) "The Rainbow Passage" twice, once in a normal manner and once while simulating a lateral lisp. She had been instructed to lisp in a "natural" manner, that is, to lisp only when it seemed comfortable. In other words, she was not instructed to lisp on every occurrence of a siblant since a characteristic of misarticulation is inconsistency (Spriestersbach and Curtis, 1951). She also was instructed to try to make the two readings identical, with the exception of the lisp. The readings were tape-recorded in a sound-treated room using an Ar'tik recorder.

Analyses of the recording involving the lisp indicated that only /s/ and /z/ were misarticulated. /s/ and /z/ were laterally emitted 40 and 34 times, respectively, or 90.0% and 79.0%, respectively, of their occurrences in the passage. The general impression upon listening to this recording was one of spontaneity. There appeared to be no suggestion of unnaturalness or awkwardness. In fact, colleagues commented that the lisp seemed representative of actual lateral lisps.

In order to assess the severity of the lisp and, more importantly, whether the only apparent difference between the two recordings was that the speaker spoke with a lateral lisp during one of them, three colleagues who possessed the certificate of clinical competency in speech pathology and who had no knowledge of the experiment evaluated the recordings. They were asked to indicate for each recording whether they believed the speaker had lisped. If they thought she had, they were then to indicate whether they had perceived an interdental lisp or a lateral lisp and to rate its severity on a 5-point scale, where *1* represented least and *5* most severe. Finally, they were requested to state the essential way(s) in which they believed the two recordings differed.

All three speech pathologists reported that the speaker spoke with a lateral lisp during the reading in which she had simulated it but she had not spoken with a lisp during the other reading. Furthermore, each rated the severity of the lisp as *3*, or moderate, and stated that the only apparent difference between the two recordings was the lisp.

Rating Task

The judges for this experiment were 48 students enrolled in two junior-level broadcast communication courses. It was assumed that broadcast communication students would be critical judges of speaking behavior yet, presumably, without the biases concerning speech differences that students majoring in speech pathology might be expected to have.

The judges rated the concept "The Person Speaking" on a 49-scale semantic differential that had been constructed in the usual manner. That is, the 49 bipolar, adjectival scales (for example, congenial-quarrelsome) selected from Osgood et al. (1957) were randomly ordered and the "positive" members of the adjective pairs were randomly assigned left-right placement on the page. The scales were 7-point scales.

The scales comprising the semantic differential were substantial-insubstantial; intelligent-unintelligent; interesting-boring; conventional-eccentric; important-unimportant; usual-unusual; motivated-aimless; respectful-disrespectful; intelligible-unintelligible; active-passive; good-bad; wise-foolish; calm-excitable; sophisticated-naive; brave-cowardly; direct-circuitous; serious-humorous; resolute-irresolute; congenial-quarrelsome; aggressive-defensive; reputable-disreputable; happy-sad; sane-insane; sensitive-insensitive; sociable-unsociable; witty-dull; attracting-repelling; mature-youthful; fortunate-unfortunate; educated-ignorant; perfect-imperfect; extrovert-introvert; honest-dishonest; concise-diffuse; colorful-colorless; feminine-masculine; influential-uninfluential; strong-weak; refined-vulgar; leading-following; urban-rural; smooth-rough; famous-obscure; non-handicapped-handicapped; careful-careless; skillful-bungling; deliberate-impulsive; successful-unsuccessful; and rational-intuitive.

The ratings were performed in the students' classrooms so that the recordings could be evaluated under ordinary listening conditions. One class of 28 students (22 males and six females) rated the lisp recording, another 20 students (17 males and three females) rated the nonlisp recording. If a student happened to be enrolled in both classes, he served as a judge only once, the first time he had the opportunity.

The recordings were presented free-field in the classrooms using the external speaker for the Ar'tik tape recorder. They were played once in their entirety following the instructions for performing the task.

RESULTS

The mean scale values for each condition were computed. When determining the values for these 7-point scales, the numeral *1* was assigned the extreme scale point corresponding to the negative adjective while the numeral *7* was assigned the extreme scale point corresponding to the positive adjective. Thus, for example, a value of 3.8 under the nonlisp condition and a value of 3.0 under the lisp condition for a given scale would indicate that on that scale the speaker had been evaluated more negatively, or less favorably, when she lisped.

The judges evaluated the speaker less favorably when she lisped. When she lisped, they rated her more negatively on 37 of the 49 scales comprising the semantic differential. This tendency to rate her more negatively when she lisped was statistically significant at the 0.01 level of confidence (normal curve approximation for the sign test, Siegel, 1956). Moreover, the scale for which there was the largest difference between the two conditions was the nonhandicapped-handicapped scale. When she lisped, the judges rated her handicapped.

She was rated more positively on 10 of the remaining 12 scales when she lisped. These scales were motivated-aimless; interesting-boring; active-passive; brave-cowardly; congenial-quarrelsome; sensitive-insensitive; witty-dull; attracting-repelling; colorful-colorless; and refined-vulgar. The judges rated her identically under the two conditions on two scales, important-unimportant and aggressive-defensive.

The results of this investigation indicate that the lateral lisp called adverse attention to the speaker. This conclusion is based on the findings that the speaker was rated more negatively on the majority of scales when she lisped and that the largest difference between the two conditions occurred on the nonhandicapped-handicapped scale. The fact that she was evaluated more positively on some scales when she lisped is not inconsistent with this conclusion, since people tend to attribute certain positive traits such as sensitivity to individuals they consider handicapped (Wright, 1960, p. 57).

How typical these broadcast communication undergraduates' evaluation of the speaker may have been, however, is uncertain since they may have been

2. SPEECH DISORDERS

more critical of speaking behavior than the majority of people. It was, therefore, decided to evaluate the generality of this finding by systematically replicating (Sidman, 1960, p. 110) the investigation using business administration undergraduates as judges. It was assumed, based on vocational choice, that business administration students would neither be exceptionally interested in nor critical of speaking behavior.

SYSTEMATIC REPLICATION

The same procedures followed in the original investigation were followed here. Two groups of business administration undergraduates rated the concept "The Person Speaking" on the same 49-scale semantic differential used in the first investigation. One group of 37 students (32 males and five females) performed the task after listening to the lisp recording. The other group of 48 students (40 males and eight females) performed the task after listening to the nonlisp recording. As before, the recordings were presented freefield and in their entirety in the students' classrooms.

The findings of this study replicated those of the original investigation. That is, the judges evaluated the speaker less favorably when she lisped, rating her more negatively on 33 of the 49 scales comprising the semantic differential. The probability of this outcome being due to chance was less than 0.01 (normal curve approximation for the sign test, Siegel, 1956). As before, the largest difference between the two conditions was associated with the nonhandicapped-handicapped scale. When she lisped, the judges rated her handicapped.

She was rated more positively on 12 of the remaining 16 scales when she lisped. These scales included five on which the broadcast communication students had also evaluated her more positively when she lisped. These scales were motivated-aimless; active-passive; congenial-quarrelsome; witty-dull; and sensitive-insensitive. The seven additional scales on which the judges rated the speaker more positively when she lisped were conventional-eccentric; important-unimportant; respectful-disrespectful; resolute-irresolute; extrovert-introvert; urban-rural; and deliberate-impulsive. The judges rated her identically under the two conditions on four scales: usual-unusual; reputable-disreputable; happy-sad; and honest-dishonest.

CONCLUSION AND IMPLICATIONS

The findings of the two studies reported here provide evidence that a lateral lisp calls adverse attention to a speaker. In fact, the findings of these two studies indicate that, on the basis of an initial encounter, an adult with a lateral lisp is likely to be evaluated by peers as handicapped. This suggests, then, that the lateral lisp is probably a speech disorder since, in at least some instances, it meets one of the three criteria suggested by Van Riper (1972) for determining whether a speech deviation is also a disorder, namely that of calling adverse attention to the speaker.

Assuming that the findings of these studies are replicated, they would have definite implications for clinical practice with both children and adults. Shriberg (1975, p. 92) stated that there has been a trend over the past several years to reduce or eliminate school speech services for children who misarticulate only one or two phonemes. He attributed this trend to the assumption that such errors are not handicapping. The findings of the studies reported here indicate that this assumption is not accurate for the lateral lisp and suggest that therapy should be provided for children with this speech deviation. This recommendation would be appropriate whether or not children with lateral lisps would be evaluated as handicapped. There is evidence that the lateral lisp is a deviation which is unlikely to improve with maturation (Krueger and Schmidt, 1968), and since adults with lateral lisps may be considered handicapped the condition should be treated as soon as possible.

Word Frequency and Stuttering: The Relationship to Sentence Structure

IRWIN RONSON

Bronx Community College of CUNY, New York

This experiment was designed to determine the relationship between word-frequency level and stuttering within the context of three selected sentence types: simple-active-affirmative-declarative, negative, and passive. Sixteen adult stutterers, rated into three groups of mild, moderate, and severe, read aloud 36 test sentences which were controlled for other linguistic factors known to affect stuttering. The results indicated that when the group rating was severe and the sentence type was either simple-active-affirmative-declarative or negative, stuttering increased significantly as word-frequency level decreased; no relationship was discerned between stuttering and word-frequency level within the passive sentence structure. It is suggested that stuttering in relation to word-frequency level is a differential response that is subject to variables of sentence type and severity rating of stuttering.

An inspection of the written lexicon reveals that not all words are used with the same frequency. The pioneer work investigating word-frequency distribution in English was done by Thorndike and Lorge (1944), and researchers have used their data to explore relationships between stuttering and word-frequency levels.

A number of experiments have shown that stuttering is more likely to occur on words that appear less frequently in the language, but most of those studies were based primarily on the reading of word lists aloud. The larger syntactic unit—the sentence—was not considered as an independent variable. Thus, Hejna (1963), Schlesinger, Melkman, and Levy (1966), Soderberg (1966), and Wingate (1967) all used word lists as their stimulus material. In only one study (Schlesinger et al., 1965) were the data derived from words in sentences, and that study involved an oral reading task from a third-grade Hebrew primer with no attempt being made to control sentence type or sentence length. It is significant to note here that Bloodstein (1974) has recently considered the sentence as an important unit in accounting for the kinds of words stuttered by young children.

The importance of the sentence unit is supported by the theory of transformational grammar proposed by Chomsky (1957, 1965) and the subsequent psycholinguistic research concerned with differential responses to sentences of varying syntactic structure. As DeVito (1971, p. 24) states it, "syntactic structure is not merely some abstract creation of the linguist but rather . . . it has a

2. SPEECH DISORDERS

psychological reality; it influences such psychological processes as comprehension, memory, and perception." The purpose of this experiment, therefore, was to investigate the relationship between word-frequency level and stuttering within the context of the selected sentence types: SAAD (simple, active, affirmative, declarative), negative, and passive.

METHOD

Subjects

The subjects were 16 adult male stutterers whose ages ranged from 19 to 29 years with a mean of 21.8 years. Each subject was rated for severity by the experimenter and the subject's speech clinician, if he currently had one, according to the 7-point scale described in the Scale for Rating Severity of Stuttering (Johnson, Darley, and Spriestersbach, 1963, p. 291). Twelve of the subjects were rated by the experimenter and their own speech clinician; four subjects were rated by the experimenter in consultation with another speech clinician. The ratings were based on tape-recorded conversation and reading material, and observation.

Table 1 shows the number of subjects at each severity level and how the

TABLE 1. The number and grouping of 16 subjects according to severity of stuttering. Group I = mild, Group II = moderate, and Group III = severe.

Severity Rating	Subjects	Group
1. Very mild	0	–
2. Mild	2	I
3. Mild to Moderate	3	I
4. Moderate	4	II
5. Moderate to Severe	2	II
6. Severe	3	III
7. Very Severe	2	III

subjects were divided into three groups on the basis of severity. Five subjects were rated as mild, six as moderate, and five as severe in these categories adapted from the Scale for Rating Severity of Stuttering. The adaptation was as follows: Scale numbers 2 and 3 (mild—mild to moderate) were combined to mild; 4 and 5 (moderate—moderate to severe) were combined to moderate; and 6 and 7 (severe—very severe) were combined to severe.

Test Material

The oral reading material was 36 test sentences constructed to represent three transformational sentence types: 12 SAAD, 12 negative, and 12 passive. Each sentence type was constructed from simple noun phrase and verb phrase combinations to which adjective modifiers were added in balanced form, similar to a technique used by Schuckers, Shriner, and Daniloff (1973). For example, a SAAD form of one of the test sentences was *The kind gentle teacher helped the seven new children*; its negative sentence form was *The kind gentle teacher didn't help the seven new children*; and its passive form was *The seven new children were helped by the kind gentle teacher*.

The test sentences were controlled for linguistic factors known to influence stuttering (Brown, 1945; Taylor, 1966; Bloodstein, 1969, pp. 184-189). All the words in every sentence began with a consonant, and the grammatical parts of speech were identical for all sentences within each sentence type. Other linguistic factors controlled in the sentence construction were transitive main verb type (Thomas, 1965), type-token ratio (Felstein, 1950, Carroll, 1964), case relationship (Fillmore, 1968), selectional and strict subcategorization restrictions (Chomsky, 1965), and sentence length within each sentence type as measured by number of phonemes and number of words.

Word Frequency Level

Each of the three sentence types was constructed from lexical items of three word-frequency levels[1] (Thorndike and Lorge, 1944). More explicitly, four SAAD sentences were composed from AA-frequency content words, four from A-frequency content words, and four from (1-49)-frequency content words. Their negative and passive counterparts were constructed from the same words.

Procedure

Each sentence was typed on a 5 × 8 card and was presented in a random order. To avoid the possibility of a direct adaptation effect, a further stipulation was that no two transformations of the same sentence should occur back to back. The subjects were instructed to read each sentence silently first to insure perception of its syntactic structure before reading it aloud. Besozzi and Adams (1969) and Robbins (1971) found that repeated silent readings of the same material did not create a reduction in stuttering. All responses were tape recorded for later analysis.

Identification of moments of stuttering was made according to the criteria listed by Williams, Silverman, and Kools (1968) and included part-word repetitions, word repetitions, phrase repetitions, interjections of sounds and syllables, revisions, tense pauses (tension), and disrhythmic phonations. Following a procedure used by Frank and Bloodstein (1971), segments of the tape of each subject were listened to on two occasions. The experimenter's reliability was determined by comparing two successive markings of stuttering separated in time by at least three weeks. The samples used to compute the reliability indexes were markings of the tenth and thirtieth recorded test sentences for each of the 16 subjects. An additional speech pathologist listened independently and marked the same samples in order to determine interexaminer agreement; the second listener did not know the purpose or design of the experiment. Intraexaminer reliability was estimated utilizing a product-moment correlation coefficient (Chase, 1967, p. 99) and was 0.98; interexaminer agreement was 0.95.

RESULTS

Word-Frequency Level and Sentence Type

The mean frequency as well as the standard deviation of stuttering on each word-frequency level for each sentence type, averaged over all subjects, is shown in Table 2. Three separate analyses of variance (Edwards, 1967, pp. 293-

TABLE 2. Mean frequency of stuttering on three word-frequency levels for 16 stutterers reading three sentence types: SAAD, negative, and passive.

| | Word-Frequency Level | | | | | |
| | AA | | A | | (1-49) | |
Sentence Type	Mean	SD	Mean	SD	Mean	SD
SAAD	1.75	2.02	1.89	2.02	2.25	2.13
Negative	1.92	2.03	2.19	2.29	2.44	2.30
Passive	2.06	2.33	2.25	2.58	2.50	2.69

322) were performed comparing the three word-frequency level means of stuttering within each sentence type. Statistical significance was found for the SAAD ($F = 6.18$; df 2,30; $p < 0.01$) and the negative ($F = 5.63$; df 2,30; $p < 0.01$) sentence types. There were no significant differences across the word-

frequency level means of stuttering for the passive sentences. For each significant F of the SAAD and negative sentence types, a post hoc Scheffe procedure was performed to investigate pairwise contrasts of the three word-frequency level stuttering means. The Scheffe analysis for the SAAD sentences showed that stuttering frequency increased significantly between the AA- and the (1-49)-word-frequency levels ($F = 5.82$; df 2,30; $p < 0.01$). The Scheffe analysis for the negative sentences also showed that stuttering frequency increased significantly only between the AA- and the (1-49)-word-frequency levels ($F = 5.73$; df 2,30; $p < 0.01$).

Word-Frequency Level, Group Severity, and Sentence Type

Table 3 shows the mean frequency as well as the standard deviation of stuttering on each word-frequency level for each group of stutterers (mild, moderate, severe) and each sentence type (SAAD, negative, passive). Nine separate analyses of variance were performed comparing the three-word-frequency

TABLE 3. Mean frequency of stuttering on three word-frequency levels for mild, moderate, and severe stutterers reading three sentence types: SAAD, negative, and passive.

Sentence Type	Group Severity° Rating of Stuttering	Word-Frequency Level					
		AA		A		(1-49)	
		Mean	SD	Mean	SD	Mean	SD
SAAD	Mild	0.50	0.50	0.80	0.65	1.00	0.81
	Moderate	1.35	0.74	1.70	0.78	1.65	0.95
	Severe	3.50	2.90	3.35	3.15	4.35	2.67
Negative	Mild	0.65	0.38	0.80	0.86	1.15	0.80
	Moderate	1.55	1.05	1.70	0.76	1.70	1.14
	Severe	3.65	2.86	4.10	3.34	4.45	3.19
Passive	Mild	0.60	0.45	0.75	0.85	0.80	0.69
	Moderate	1.75	1.35	1.75	1.20	2.15	1.29
	Severe	4.00	3.27	4.35	3.74	4.75	3.83

°N = five subjects in each group. One subject from the total number of six in the moderate group was randomly excluded in order to balance the totals for each of the three groups.

level stuttering means for each of the three sentence types and each of the three groups of stutterers. Statistical significance was only found for the severe group of stutterers in the SAAD ($F = 11.08$; df 2,8; $p < 0.01$) and the negative ($F = 5.25$; df 2,8; $p < 0.05$) sentence types. There was no significant relationship found between stuttering and word-frequency level within the passive sentence type.

For each significant F of the severe group for the SAAD and negative sentence types, the Scheffe post hoc procedure was performed to investigate pairwise contrasts of the three word-frequency level stuttering means. The Scheffe analysis of the SAAD sentences for the severe group showed that stuttering frequency increased significantly between the AA- and the (1-49)-word-frequency levels ($F = 6.88$; df 2,8; $p < 0.05$) and the A- and (1-49)-word-frequency levels ($F = 9.52$; df 2,8; $p < 0.01$). The Scheffe analysis for the negative sentences for the severe group showed that stuttering frequency increased significantly only between the AA- and the (1-49)-word-frequency levels ($F = 5.22$; df 2,8; $p < 0.05$).

DISCUSSION

A positive relationship between stuttering and word-frequency level has previously been reported by researchers such as Hejna (1963), Soderberg (1966), and Schlesinger et al. (1965). But, when the results of stuttering were averaged over the 16 subjects studied in this experiment, a statistically significant relationship between stuttering and word-frequency level was corroborated only within the linguistic context of the sentence types SAAD and negative, and that result possibly is attributable to the performance of the severe stutterers. The fact that the stuttering did not significantly increase in frequency as word-frequency level decreased in the context of the passive sentence structure is all the more remarkable since the same content words were used for the passive sentences as for the SAAD and negative counterparts.

One other report containing inconsistency of response in regard to the effect of word-frequency level on stuttering is cited in the literature, but on a different linguistic level. Wingate (1967) found that word-frequency level was only significantly related to the stutterings of his subjects when they read a shorter one-syllable word list as compared to a two-syllable word list. Wingate's (1967, p. 150) comment was that "the presumed demands posed by word length and unfamiliarity are not additive." The results of the present study suggest that the presumed demands on motor planning posed by the more complex passive syntactic structure and unfamiliarity (low word-frequency level) are not additive either. It is assumed that the passive is more syntactically complex than the SAAD and negative, (Slobins 1966, McNeill, 1970).

In addition, when the stutterers were divided into groups of mild, moderate, and severe, a statistically significant relationship between stuttering and word-frequency level only held for those stutterers rated severe. Significant experimental findings, not considered by previous investigations of stuttering and word-frequency level, were therefore found for sentence type and grouping of stutterers according to severity rating.

It should also be noted that the word-frequency level contrasts between AA and (1-49) are those that appear to be more significantly related to a respective increase in stuttering frequency. For example, in the present study, the Scheffe analysis showed no significant pairwise contrasts between the AA- and A-word-frequency levels, and only one between A and (1-49). These results support the findings of Soderberg (1966) who used comparable word-frequency levels and found that only the differences between high (AA) and low (1-26)[2] were significant when considering word-frequency levels and their relationship to stuttering.

In summary, the relationship between word-frequency level and stuttering has been shown to be subject to variables such as sentence type and severity rating of stuttering. The present investigation suggests that the word-frequency effect not be considered as a general characteristic of the stuttering response; strict linguistic contextual qualifications, careful description of subjects according to severity rating of stuttering, and specific word-frequency level usage appear to be indicated. Further research relating linguistic factors to stuttering is recommended in which sentence type is considered along with other linguistic cues which have been demonstrated to be associated with stuttering. Moreover, there would seem to be a need for much more investigation of the relationship between stuttering and sentence type for inferences to be made concerning the concept that there is a psychological reality to transformational processing of sentences that affects stuttering.

---

[2]Soderberg chose the range of (1-26) for his low word-frequency level, based on the Thorndike and Lorge word-frequency count. The actual average low word-frequency level used in the present experiment was 22.75—falling within the (1-26) range of Soderberg's choice of low frequency words.

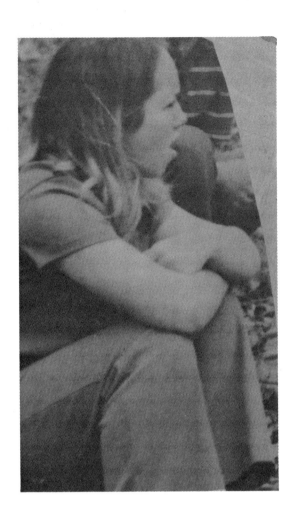

Stuttering:

Discoordination of Phonation With Articulation and Respiration

WILLIAM PERKINS, JOANNA RUDAS,

LINDA JOHNSON, *and* JODY BELL

Rational analysis, clinical investigation, and systematic research are lending support to an old suspicion: many of the abnormal disfluencies judged as stuttering involve problems of smooth coordination of phonation[1] with articulation and respiration (Travis, 1931). After reviewing the vast literature of stuttering, Van Riper (1971) concluded that the core of the disorder is a disruption of timing of the motor sequences of sound, syllable, and word production. He suggested that the marked reduction of stuttering during whispering and its elimination during pantomimed speech could be attributed to the high degree of conscious articulation at slower speech rates that permit synchronization. He also proposed the alternative that this puzzling reduction of stuttering "could be accounted for on the basis of a simplified synergy (the absence of voice and/or airflow) . . ."

Adams (1974) has offered a physiologic and aerodynamic analysis of stuttering and fluency. He proposed that fluency is dependent on smooth coordination of activities of the respiratory, phonatory, and articulatory systems. He suggested "that the muscles and forces that promote control, and coordinate subglottic pressure, glottal resistance, and supraglottal pressure are the major determinants of both fluency and stuttering." Discoordination of these elements would be manifested as difficulty in achieving transglottic pressures that would

[1]Phonation is used in a generic sense in this report to identify any laryngeal adjustments made to coordinate the breath stream with utterance of syllables. Hence, it will refer to whispered as well as voiced speech. For convenience, we will use the term articulation to identify supraglottal processes, even though phonation also includes an articulatory function. Respiration will refer to subglottic processes. Thus, phonation will be used to differentiate laryngeal from subglottic and supraglottic activities.

"Stuttering: Discoordination of Phonation With Articulation and Respiration," William Perkins, Joanna Rudas, Linda Johnson, Jody Bell, *Journal of Speech and Hearing Research*, Vol. 19 No. 3, September 1976. ©1976 Journal of Speech and Hearing Research.

promote the precisely timed glottal airflow and vocalization required to facilitate smoothly articulated speech. Thus, discoordination of elements of speech does not cause stuttering, it is the stuttering.

Because evidence of disrupted motor timing can be found during stuttering at all levels of the speaking system, the possibility exists that each level could serve as a focus of difficulty that triggers discoordinations with other levels of the system (Adams, 1974). In other words, respiratory mistimings could disrupt phonatory and articulatory processes, and conversely oral articulatory or phonatory mistimings could impair the smooth management of subglottic, transglottic, and supraglottic pressures required for fluent speech.

SELECTION OF PHONATION AS THE INDEPENDENT VARIABLE

Simplification of the phonatory process was selected as the independent variable in this experiment for several reasons. A practical consideration was that the complexity of phonatory valving required for generating a breath-stream that can be modulated for speech can be systematically altered. Intelligible speech can be produced not only with a normally voiced and voiceless breathstream, but also with a whispered breathstream or, for viewers who can lip-read, with oral articulatory movements produced without breathstream management for speech. Neither vocal tract articulatory processes nor subglottic respiratory processes permit equally as systematic alterations as those that can be made in the phonatory system. Admittedly, respiration for maintaining alveolar pressure can be achieved with a variety of muscular activities (Hixon, 1973). Similarly, variation is permissable in articulatory adjustments provided they remain within limits of producing intelligible speech. Such respiratory and articulatory alterations, however, do not appear to be easily varied systematically.

An extension of this argument is that the phonatory process appears to be the only one that permits progressive simplification of motor coordinations, either in rate or number of adjustments to be coordinated. Speech normally flows at roughly 14 ± 2 phonemes per second, about twice the speed at which individual articulators can be controlled (Lenneberg, 1967; Stetson, 1951; Miller, 1951; Hudgins and Stetson, 1937). Hence, the necessity of coarticulatory overlapping of vocal tract movements to achieve such rates. No alteration in articulation would conceivably simplify the complexity of these coordinations. The rate at which they would have to be made and the number of distinctive features that would have to be controlled would presumably remain constant regardless of articulatory adjustment. The same reasoning would seem to apply to respiration. The necessity of maintaining sufficient alveolar pressure to produce a typical average of five to seven syllables per second along with various prosodic stresses within a phrase would also appear to be relatively constant irrespective of respiratory adjustment (Lenneberg, 1967; Daniloff, 1973).

Complexity of phonatory coordinations, on the other hand, is progressively simplified by changing from normal voicing to whispering to articulating silently, as shown in Figure 1. Normal speech requires that the vocal folds be abducted and adducted for voiceless and voiced sounds, respectively. Voiced and voiceless sounds are often produced alternately, as in the nonsense phrase, *put it off a ketchup*. Thus, glottal openings and closings can occur at the same rate as articulatory movements. Moreover, prosodically appropriate pitch and loudness adjustments must be made for each voiced sound. These adjustments require precise adduction and vocal fold adjustments of effective mass, elasticity, and viscosity.

With whispering, both number and rate of adjustments are simplified. For a loud whisper, the tips of the arytenoids are firmly approximated while the posterior borders are separated, thereby creating a glottal chink. The vocal folds are adducted tightly enough to prevent vibration; any adjustment in which cord resistance exceeds subglottal pressure is sufficient (Pressman, 1942; Perkins, 1971b). Softer whispers can involve sufficient adduction of the cords to generate turbulence from airflow through the glottis, but not sufficient for the cords to be set into vibration (Broad, 1973). Spectral pitch and loudness are probably determined by respiratory adjustments of subglottal pressure or by adjustments of the glottal chink, or both. They can occur, potentially, as rapidly as from syllable to syllable. Because only a voiceless breathstream is generated through the glottis, no adductory/abductory movements are needed between phrase initiation and termination.

With silent articulatory movements (lipped speech), further phonatory simplification along with respiratory simplification is achieved. The breath-stream is managed independently of speech needs. Whether the vocal folds are abducted or adducted, or are tense or lax is immaterial; prosodic and voiced/voiceless requirements are eliminated. Phonation and respiration need not be coordinated with articulation.

Rational analysis provides another reason for studying effects of simplifying phonation. Logically, laryngeal valving would seem to be the most complex process to coordinate for fluent speech. That voiced/voiceless phonatory co-ordinations are more complex than subglottic respiratory and supraglottic articulatory adjustments seems reasonable. Whereas normal high-speed supra-glottal articulation can be achieved by overlapping movements of a variety of vocal tract structures at slower speeds, phonatory abductory/adductory move-ments must be capable of occurring at high-speed articulatory rates. No alternative laryngeal mechanism exists for opening and closing the glottis, so movements of these structures cannot be overlapped at slower speeds to achieve high speeds; presumably, they must be capable of moving at about twice the speed of articulatory structures. Moreover, the small size of laryngeal structures suggests that they must be controlled with greater precision than supraglottal structures.

Too, the dynamic interrelations among muscular and aerodynamic forces for managing glottal vibratory characteristics would seem to be much more intricate than the pharyngeal, labial, lingual, and velar constrictions, occlusions, and cavity shapings used to modulate the breathstream. For these adjustments, the essential requirement is to position the structures in the vocal tract. By contrast, vocal fold vibrations are dependent on effective vocal fold mass, elasticity, and viscosity adjustments that must be coordinated with subglottal and supraglottal pressures to maintain the precise transglottal pressure that will produce the desired pitch and loudness of each syllable (Adams, 1974; Moore, 1968; Perkins, 1971a).

As for a comparison of phonatory with respiratory complexity, the contrast would seem to be even greater. Both in precision and rate of control, the dif-ference seems sharp. Thoracic structures are large. Their speech task is to maintain a breathstream for the duration of each phrase. Presumably, the fastest adjustments that might have to be made are for loudness from syllable to syllable, a rate less than half that of phonetic articulation. Timing of respiratory muscle contraction is apparently a relatively slow process that has to do primarily with maintaining steady alveolar pressure against a background of declining relaxation pressure (Draper, Ladefoged, and Whitteridge, 1959; Hixon, 1973; Netsell, 1973). Thus, respiratory processes seem to be less com-plex to coordinate than supraglottal articulatory processes and certainly than phonatory processes.

Finally, a growing body of evidence points to laryngeal functions as being crucial in stuttering. Wingate (1969) concluded from his review of the litera-ture that stuttering is reduced by "artificial" fluency because "the stutterer is induced, in one way or another, to do something with his voice that he does not ordinarily do." Adams and Reis (1971, 1974) demonstrated that difficulty

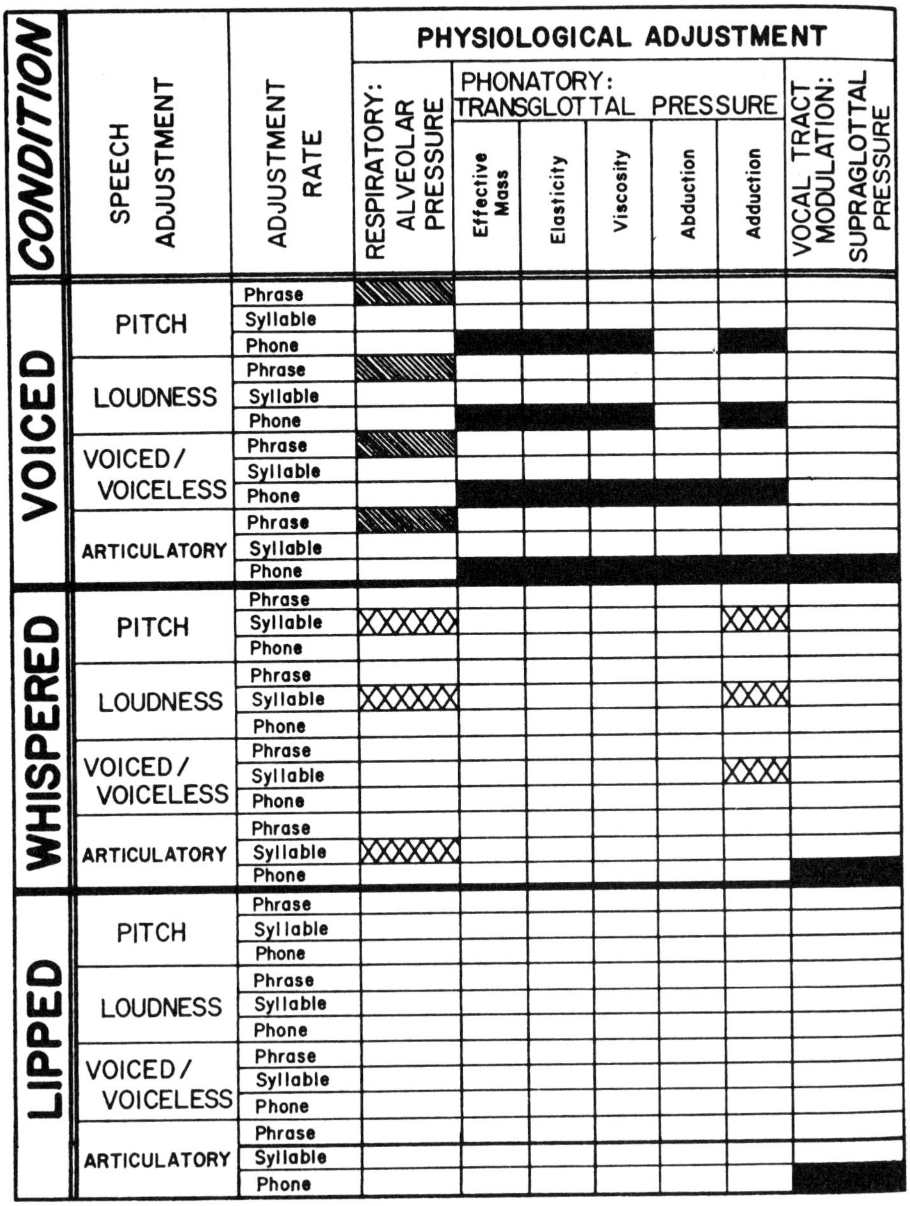

PHYSIOLOGICAL ADJUSTMENT

CONDITION	SPEECH ADJUSTMENT	ADJUSTMENT RATE	RESPIRATORY: ALVEOLAR PRESSURE	PHONATORY: TRANSGLOTTAL PRESSURE — Effective Mass	Elasticity	Viscosity	Abduction	Adduction	VOCAL TRACT MODULATION: SUPRAGLOTTAL PRESSURE
VOICED	PITCH	Phrase	▨						
		Syllable							
		Phone		█			█		
	LOUDNESS	Phrase	▨						
		Syllable							
		Phone		█		█			
	VOICED/VOICELESS	Phrase	▨						
		Syllable							
		Phone		█	█	█	█	█	
	ARTICULATORY	Phrase	▨						
		Syllable							
		Phone		█	█	█	█	█	
WHISPERED	PITCH	Phrase							
		Syllable	▩					▩	
		Phone							
	LOUDNESS	Phrase							
		Syllable	▩					▩	
		Phone							
	VOICED/VOICELESS	Phrase							
		Syllable						▩	
		Phone							
	ARTICULATORY	Phrase							
		Syllable	▩						
		Phone							█
LIPPED	PITCH	Phrase							
		Syllable							
		Phone							
	LOUDNESS	Phrase							
		Syllable							
		Phone							
	VOICED/VOICELESS	Phrase							
		Syllable							
		Phone							
	ARTICULATORY	Phrase							
		Syllable							
		Phone							█

FIGURE 1. Number and rate of physiological adjustments involved in speaking aloud (voiced), whispering, and articulating silently (lipped). The slowest adjustments are from phrase to phrase ▨▨▨▨▨▨, the most rapid are from phone to phone ██████ (about 14 ± 2 per second) and in between are syllable to syllable adjustments ▩▩▩▩▩▩ (about 6 ± 2 per second).

initiating phonation is "an important predictor of stuttering—certainly more powerful than such variables as word length and grammatical class." Brenner, Perkins, and Soderberg (1972) found that neither silent rehearsal with articulatory movements nor whispered rehearsal reduced stuttering in normal speech as much as aloud rehearsal. They suspected that the differences were due to complexity of the phonatory processes rehearsed in each condition. Most recently, Adams and Hayden (1976) showed that stutterers are slower than normal speakers in a nonspeech task of initiating and terminating phonation. They thereby supported their alternate explanation that the direction of causation of stuttering disfluencies is from phonation to articulation, not vice versa. Direct evidence of phonatory involvement has been provided by Freeman and Ushijima's (1975) demonstration that abductor/adductor reciprocity is disrupted during moments of stuttering.

2. SPEECH DISORDERS

THE PROBLEM

This experiment was undertaken to determine the effects on stuttering and speech rate of systematically simplifying the complexity of phonatory and respiratory coordinations for speech. The foregoing analysis led us to suspect that complexity of phonatory adjustments can trigger discoordinations of the activities seen in the prolongations, repetitions, and hesitations of stuttering. Although these motor discoordinations occur at a physiological level, they can best be observed at a behavioral level (Perkins and Curlee, 1969; Perkins, 1971a). Prolongations and hesitations are identified by listener judgments of inappropriate durations of phonetic elements. Physiological correlates of these judgments have not yet been determined, so no criteria yet exist for recognizing phonetic discoordinations physiologically. The purpose of this study was not to reveal biological details of motor discoordinations in the speech system directly, but rather it was to determine by observing speech behavior if the discoordinations of stuttering were affected by alterations in phonation and respiration. Efficient research strategy dictated determining first if the general outline of our suspicions was defensible before pursuing this lead in detail.

We reasoned that if laryngeal adjustments were progressively simplified without systematically varying articulatory targets,[2] we should be able to determine whether or not complexity of the phonatory process is related to stuttering. If it is not, then stuttering should not be affected from one treatment condition to another. If it is, then frequency of stuttering should be reduced during whispering and eliminated during silent articulation without phonation.

An explanation for reduction of stuttering with reduced phonatory complexity could be inferred from speech rate. If Van Riper's (1971) suggested explanation is accurate that whispering and silent articulation require greater concentration, then speech rate should be retarded, as he suspects, and coordinations would thereby be facilitated. If his alternate explanation is accurate that simplification of phonatory complexity facilitates synergic coordinations of the speaking system, then speech rate should at least be maintained if not increased.

METHOD

Subjects

Twenty-five male and five female subjects who stuttered when whispering were used to determine the effects on frequency of stuttering during reading under three speaking conditions: voiced, whispered, and articulated without phonation. The subjects consisted of stutterers awaiting initiation of treatment at the University of Southern California Center for the Study of Communicative Disorders at the time of the study. They ranged in age from 14 to 67 and represented a wide range of educational, ethnic, and socioeconomic backgrounds. In general, they appeared to constitute a representative sample of stutterers found in a large metropolitan area.

We had determined from a pilot study of 15 subjects that in four of them whispering consistently reduced stuttering to zero. Without exception for these subjects, stuttering remained at zero when articulating without phonation. Because the effects of reducing "off-on" phonatory adjustments as is accomplished in whispering could be inferred from the effects of all-voiced

---

[2]We assumed that the speaking system functions as a dynamically integrated unit in which a change in glottal resistance alters the balance of subglottic, supraglottic, and transglottic pressures. Thus, respiratory and articulatory adjustments could presumably accompany experimental manipulations of phonation. Speech disfluency would, therefore, reflect physiological discoordinations in the whole speaking system, not just in the isolated phonatory portion of the system that would be systematically varied. The fact that articulatory targets were held constant would not imply that the same vocal tract adjustments would necessarily be made to produce target sounds from one experimental condition to another.

passages used by Adams and Reis (1971, 1974), the crux of this experiment was to ascertain the effects of further simplification of phonatory and respiratory complexity by articulating without phonation. Obviously, a determination of the effects of this condition in comparison with the condition of whispering could not be made in subjects who did not stutter when whispering. Accordingly, stuttering during whispering was a subject selection requirement for this investigation. Other requirements were that subjects be free of neuro- or laryngeal pathology, that they meet criteria for speaking under the three treatment conditions, and that they not attempt to use syllable prolongation procedures.

Procedures

Each subject read three 130-131 syllable excerpts from the "Rainbow Passage," a different one under each treatment condition. Conditions were systematically rotated across passages as the data were gathered originally. We selected the first 30 subjects who qualified for the experiment. This rotational arrangement was thereby somewhat imbalanced; seven were accepted from the voiced-lipped-whispered (V-L-W) order, 11 from L-W-V, and 12 from W-V-L. The fact that a Friedman two-way analysis of variance of percent syllables stuttered revealed no significant order effect ($p < 0.05$) in a pilot study of these procedures suggests that the experimental results were not seriously confounded.

Three judges made independent measures from frontal head and chest video recordings (without sound) for 10 subjects each. The resulting 90 passages were analyzed to obtain measures of stuttering and rate. Stuttering was defined as any syllable disfluency–prolongation, repetition, hesitation, or interjection. The measure of stuttering used was percent syllables disfluent, and the measure of rate was syllables per minute.

Reliability among judges was determined in advance of the experiment by having them measure 30 passages in common, 10 voiced, 10 whispered, and 10 articulated without phonation. Because the counts were made using video without sound, the judges were never certain of which condition was being viewed. To test ability to lip-read a wide range of types of speech and stuttering, each passage was from a different subject. The intraclass correlations among these judges were 0.99 for both syllables per minute and percent syllables disfluent.

The reason for using video measures only was to obtain comparable measures of the voiced and whispered conditions with the silent condition of articulation without phonation. To ascertain whether or not stuttering and rate could be judged validly by visual stimuli alone, another set of measures, video with sound, was used to determine the relationship of visual with audiovisual measures. Comparing these two sets of measures, Pearson product-moment coefficients for both percent syllables disfluent and syllables per minute were higher than 0.98 for both whispered and voiced conditions. These correlations were high enough to give us confidence that visual cues were sufficient to approximate the audiovisual information normally used to judge stuttering.

The rate measure of syllables per minute can be deceptive as a description of articulatory rate. A typical method of measurement is to record time at the beginning and end of speaking and count the number of syllables spoken. The problem with this method is that the resulting measure can be so strongly affected by duration of stuttering and pauses between phrases that variations in articulatory rate can be obscured. Because syllable prolongation is a powerful means of reducing stuttering (Curlee and Perkins, 1969), a slight prolongation could reduce the severity or frequency of prolongations and hesitations enough to increase the rate measure considerably. The result, paradoxi-

2. SPEECH DISORDERS

TABLE 1. Percent syllables disfluent of subjects under three treatment conditions arranged in order of voiced condition severity.

Subject	Voiced	Whispered	Lipped
DH	5.4	1.6	0.0
AI	6.9	3.1	1.6
LZ	7.5	6.0	4.7
RH	8.2	9.0	0.0
LF	10.5	2.3	1.6
TM	12.9	13.2	0.7
BW	13.2	5.4	2.3
AS	13.9	3.7	0.0
CM	14.2	11.8	0.0
CM	15.6	16.9	3.1
TR	16.0	6.9	0.0
JM	18.1	1.5	0.0
JH	20.0	10.0	0.0
RB	20.2	12.3	1.5
FM	21.9	10.9	0.0
RP	22.1	4.6	1.5
LD	23.5	12.5	0.0
SS	24.2	15.8	0.0
RD	24.4	3.0	0.7
DP	25.6	3.8	0.0
MK	29.4	7.6	0.0
FH	29.7	19.8	2.8
JS	29.8	4.7	3.1
RP	29.9	7.5	0.0
MW	37.4	9.7	0.8
LL	38.9	25.4	0.0
LB	39.7	16.3	0.0
KS	42.9	1.6	0.0
CB	61.2	55.4	0.8
RH	70.5	7.6	0.0

cally, would be that an increase in syllables per minute would have been accomplished by a retarded articulatory rate.

To meet this objection, a measure of syllables per minute was computed from the elapsed speaking time for the total number of syllables in the passage. Speaking time was measured by manually activating an electric timer with a telegraph key that was depressed for the duration of each syllable. An instance of stuttering was counted as comparable to one fluent syllable regardless of the number of syllable repetitions or duration of moments of stuttering. The key was not depressed during pauses between phrases. The measured speaking rate thereby reflects the speed at which the stutterer was attempting to speak irrespective of time consumed by pauses and stuttering.

RESULTS

Inspection of subject performance in Table 1 shows unambiguously that syllable disfluencies were progressively reduced as the complexity of phonatory and respiratory coordinations was simplified. One-tailed t tests of the predicted differences between correlated means show that stuttering was reduced significantly ($p < 0.001$) from 24.6% syllables disfluent in the voiced condition to 10.3% in the whispered condition. In the silently articulated condition, stuttering was further reduced significantly ($p < 0.001$) to 0.8% syllables disfluent in comparison with the whispered condition. All subjects stuttered less without phonation than when whispering, and the three exceptions (CM, RH, and TM) to a reduction of stuttering from voice to whisper were slight.

The possibility that reduced stuttering might be attributed to a slower speaking rate was rejected. A randomized block design showed that significant ($p < 0.01$) differences did exist; speaking rate increased progressively with simplification of phonation. Dunn's multiple comparisons showed a significantly faster ($p < 0.01$) syllable rate during whispering (209.6 syllables per minute) in comparison with voiced speech (176.6 syllables per minute), and a rate (237.2 syllables per minute) while articulating without phonation that was significantly ($p < 0.01$) faster than the whispered rate.

DISCUSSION

The most striking feature of these results is that they are practically invariant. Twenty-seven of 30 subjects showed a reduction of stuttering from the voiced to whispered condition (the three exceptions differed by 1.3% syllables disfluent or less). All 30 without exception showed further reduction from whispering to silent articulation. Of these, 17 reduced syllable disfluency to zero; for the remainder, the highest frequency was 4.7 percent syllables disfluent. Even this measure was probably high because we used a strict criterion of syllable disfluency. As a result, many of these disfluencies would probably be judged as normal rather than stuttered.

Clearly, some condition existed during this experiment powerful enough to exert almost complete control of stuttering. Such other variables as influence abnormal disfluency must somehow exert their effects through that condition. Whatever the ultimate explanation, it must account for these results.

The explanation that seems to fit the evidence best is that stuttering is a function of complexity of phonatory coordinations with articulatory and respiratory processes. The fact that phonatory complexity was progressively simplified, as the independent variable, was demonstrably accomplished. All subjects met criteria for speaking under voiced, whispered, and silently articulated conditions which, of necessity, required the physiological simplifications of laryngeal adjustments discussed earlier. Because this was the only variable that was deliberately altered systematically, and because reductions of stuttering consistently followed these simplifications, the cause-and-effect relation seems likely.

Additional evidence that supports a discoordination hypothesis is revealed by a split-half analysis of the data in Table 1. Subjects were rank ordered according to percent syllables disfluent under the voiced condition. The mean for the least severe half was 13.6% syllables disfluent under the voiced condition, 7.6% during whispering, and 1.0% during silent articulation. The mean for the most severe half, on the other hand, was 35.3% during voicing, 12.7% during whispering, and 0.5% during silent articulation. The point to note is that silent articulation reduced syllable disfluency somewhat more effectively for the most severe than for the least severe. This inverse relation between voiced and lipped conditions is also seen in the slightly negative, but not significant, Spearman rho coorelation (-0.10). Such results suggest that discoordination is more likely to be at the core of severe than mild stuttering. To the extent that factors other than discoordination contribute to stuttering, they may play a proportionately larger role, and accordingly may be more apparent when complexity of speech coordinations is minimized, in mild than severe stutterers.

Effects of these simplifications in phonatory complexity cannot be easily explained as the result of increased conscious effort and deliberate articulation. If this had happened, the articulatory rate would have been retarded. Instead, it accelerated progressively from voiced to whispered and from whispered to silently articulated conditions. Subjects were given no instructions regarding rate, so they apparently spoke faster spontaneously as complexity of their phonatory adjustments was simplified. This fits with the explanation that the problem is one of coordinating phonation with articulation and respiration.

Whether complexity of articulatory or respiratory adjustments could also trigger discoordinations of the speaking system cannot be conclusively affirmed or denied by this study. The fact that oral articulatory and respiratory discoordinations disappeared when phonatory complexity was simplified sufficiently only demonstrates the possible causal role of phonation. It does not eliminate the alternative that articulatory and respiratory processes could serve the same role.

Adams and Hayden's (1976) work, which is supported by our results, does bear on this issue, however. They tested alternative explanations of stuttering being caused, as one possibility, "by excessive speech mechanism constriction and tension" that interferes with quick initiation of phonation, and as the other possibility, by delays in voicing that prompt "oral articulatory" repetitions and prolongations. They tested the alternatives by measuring "the time it took stutterers to initiate voicing while not stuttering." They were significantly slower than nonstutterers in initiating and terminating voicing. Adams and Hayden reasoned that this result should not occur if oral articulatory processes caused stuttering, because the experimental tests of voicing were conducted when subjects did not stutter. Their finding does not conclusively rule out the possibility that complexity of supraglottal articulatory processes could trigger stuttering, but they weigh heavily against it.

Because we had to rely on subject compliance with our instructions, the possibility that intervening variables produced the results obtained cannot be categorically excluded. One possibility, the distraction effect, seems unlikely, though, because silent articulation invariably reduced stuttering more than whispering, yet both are atypical methods of speaking. To make the case for distraction, one would have to argue that silent articulation was more distracting than whispering for all subjects, or that it was more deliberate and slower than whispering or voicing. The first argument seems implausible, and the second is contradicted by the evidence; speaking rate accelerated under this condition.

A somewhat more plausible alternative is that communicative responsibility was reduced. Other explanations may also be possible, but to be competitive they must account for highly consistent results. Unlike research trends that permit varying operation of innumerable conditions, invariant effects point strongly to consistently related causes. Admittedly, a variety of psychological variables, such as communicative responsibility, may have operated in our subjects' compliance with instructions. The possibility, however, that each subject had practically the same uncontrolled psychological reaction to each experimental condition, and that this reaction determined the frequency of stuttering hardly seems credible. Equally unlikely is the argument that a variety of reactions produced consistent effects on stuttering in all subjects. Still, further work is needed to determine definitively the relevance of such alternative explanations.

We favor viewing complexity of phonatory coordination with articulatory and respiratory processes as the determinant of our results because systematic alterations in this variable yielded remarkably consistent effects on stuttering. If this explanation is to be pursued, two major directions are pertinent. One is to determine why stutterers have more difficulty coordinating phonation with articulation and respiration than do nonstutterers. Have they simply never learned the coordinations of normal speech, are they merely at the low end of the normal distribution of endowments of skill in coordinating the speaking processes, or are they below normal limits for this skill? If poorly endowed, is this characteristic transmitted genetically? What are the neurological correlates? Does the problem resemble dysarthria or apraxia; is cerebral dominance involved; is Schwartz's (1974) analysis of the laryngeal reflex that he suspects is at the core of stuttering supported by evidence; is the auditory system involved, and if so, how? These only suggest the wealth of leads that are open.

The other major direction is to determine how other variables that affect stuttering are related to phonatory coordinations. Some of these relations seem reasonably apparent. The work of Adams and his colleagues (1971, 1974, 1976) on voicing initiation is supported by our results and fits readily within the general framework of phonatory discoordination with subglottal and supraglottal processes. Similarly, the possibility that adaptation is a rehearsal effect also fits within this framework. It was from the research of Brenner et al. (1972) that the lead for the current investigation was obtained. They suggested that the reason stuttering was significantly less with aloud than with whispered or silently articulated rehearsal was that speaking aloud permitted practice in coordinating phonatory with articulatory movements.

Somewhat more speculative is the possibility that delayed auditory feedback reduces stuttering by enforcing a slow enough articulatory rate to permit fluent coordination of speaking system movements. Although Adams et al. (1973) and Ingham, Martin, and Kuhl (1974) have studied the effectiveness of slow speaking rate in the reduction of stuttering, the method of testing rate in both studies differed critically from the clinical procedure used to establish fluency. Adams and his associates had stutterers speak one word per second, whereas Ingham and his colleagues set a slow target rate that stutterers matched. No instructions were reported in either investigation as to how these slow rates were to be achieved. Our clinical experience with over 200 stutterers with whom rate control procedures have been used is that most must be instructed in the desired technique of prolonging syllables as the method of slowing rate. With this technique, fluency as well as reduction of the disruptive effect of delayed auditory feedback (DAF) is virtually assured. Conversely, no other rate control technique we have observed has insured fluency. This impression is buttressed by some experimental evidence that stutterers who slow their rate of speech by pausing between syllables articulated at a normally rapid rate continue to stutter (Brenner, 1969). Each pause seems to provide a potential opportunity for discoordinated initiation of the breathstream at the beginning of each syllable. When articulatory rate within the syllable remains rapid, regardless of time between syllables, coordination of speaking system movements, in theory, would not be facilitated as much as they would be by prolonging duration of the syllables. A DAF retarded rate, then, may reduce stuttering to the extent that it facilitates phonatory synergy with articulatory and respiratory processes.

Our results are also congruent with Bloodstein's (1974) hypothesis that stuttering reflects tension and fragmentation in "executing the motor plan of some element of speech." We are proposing that phonatory coordinations especially are among these elements, and that the linguistic factors that Bloodstein has described are related to stuttering by virtue of motor planning difficulties in coordinating phonation with articulation and respiration.

Some of the most profitable leads may well come from Wingate's (1966, 1967, 1969) work on voice and prosody. He has demonstrated that prosody is functionally related to stuttering and has proposed that its effects, along with those of singing, "shadowing," and choral speaking can be attributed to something the stutterer does differently with his voice. All of these activities are noted for their powerful capacity for reducing stuttering. Details of how they are linked to voice remain to be investigated. That they somehow simplify the complex motor planning required for coordinating phonation with articulation and respiration is tempting to consider.

Verbal versus Tangible Reward for Children Who Stutter

Walter H. Manning

Candyce K. Shaw

Phyllis A. Trutna

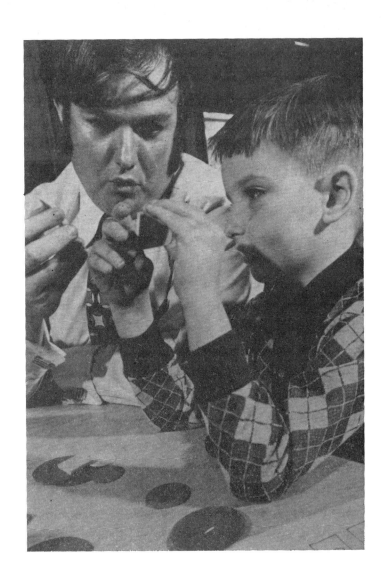

There is little question that one can influence the verbal behavior of most stutterers within the context of a behavior modification program. Clinicians working with both adults and children who stutter have demonstrated rather pronounced and obvious increases in fluency via the application of both response-contingent punishment (Flanagan, Goldiamond, and Azrin, 1958; Martin and Siegel, 1966; Quist and Martin, 1967) and reward (Rickard and Mundy, 1966; Nelson, 1968; Leach, 1969; Shaw and Shrum, 1972). While response-contingent reward appears to be more acceptable than punishment with this population (Nelson, 1968; Shaw and Shrum, 1972), there remains some question as to whether such rewards should be of a verbal or a tangible nature.

While not necessarily intending to do so, several authors have presented data that may lead clinicians to believe that rewards of a tangible nature are the most appropriate forms of reinforcement to employ when attempting to modify the verbal behavior of young stutterers. For example, Rickard and Mundy (1966) were able to elicit only insignificant increases in fluency when using verbal reinforcement. However, when tangible rewards were presented to the same subject, there was a continued increase in the number of fluent responses emitted. Further, Shaw and Shrum (1972), demonstrated a rather dramatic modification of both fluent and disfluent speech with three young stutterers us-

"Verbal versus Tangible Reward for Children Who Stutter," Walter H. Manning, Phyllis A. Trutna, Candyce K. Shaw, *Journal of Speech and Hearing Research*, Vol. 41 No. 1, February 1976. ©1976 Journal of Speech and Hearing Research.

ing tangible reinforcers. They attributed the successful modification of behavior to (1) subjects' awareness of the response-contingency; (2) reinforcement of easily identifiable behavior; and (3) selection of the reinforcers by the subjects.

While the above discussion supports the modification of stuttering behavior through the use of positive reinforcement, the relative effectiveness of tangible and verbal forms of reinforcement has not been investigated in a systematic manner. Thus, the purpose of this study was to investigate a possible difference in effectiveness of the two forms of reinforcement. It was hypothesized that there would be little or no difference between the effects of verbal and tangible forms of reinforcement on the fluency and disfluency of young stuttering subjects when the experimental sessions were preceded by instructions explaining the response contingency and when subjects selected their own verbal and tangible rewards.

PROCEDURES

Three children, aged 6-10, 8-11, and 9-1, were used as subjects. These children were receiving speech therapy in public schools. The only requirement was that each child display one or more types of observable stuttering behaviors such as interjections, repetitions, and prolongations. No stipulation was made as to degree of severity. A single or within-subject design was used since the purpose of this study was to modify individual stuttering behaviors.

The experimental material consisted of spontaneous connected speech in a traditional clinical setting. Thus, the subject and one of the authors (PT) were seated together in a room. Spontaneous speech was elicited by instructing the subject to discuss any topic he wished. Pictures and books were available for stimulation if the subject had difficulty finding topics of conversation.

Since it was not feasible to reinforce each fluently spoken word, time intervals during which the subjects remained continuously fluent were reinforced as suggested by Shaw and Shrum (1972). The length of each subject's fluent interval to be reinforced in the experimental sessions was determined by taking the average of the length of time each subject was able to remain fluent during the base rate session. A stopwatch was used to establish each subject's fluent interval and then to determine when the subjects had remained fluent for the required time. The stopwatch was reset at zero each time the subject stuttered and was not restarted until the disfluency was completed. The stopwatch was also reset at zero when the subject stopped talking and was started again when fluent speaking resumed. Thus, the fluent intervals recorded in the base rate and experimental sessions represented actual fluent speaking time, excluding the time during which the subjects were silent or disfluent.

Disfluencies were defined as interjections of sounds, syllables, words, and phrases; repetitions of part-words, words, and phrases; and, prolongations of sound or syllables. Disfluencies such as word and phrase interjections and repetitions are not necessarily thought of as stuttering. However, since the subjects in this study had been previously identified as stutterers, the terms *disfluency* and *stuttering* are used interchangeably. Individual characteristics of each subject's disfluencies are described in this study.

A Wollensak tape recorder and associated microphone were used to record each session. Each subject was seen for one 15-minute base rate session the first week, three 30-minute experimental sessions during three days of the second week, and one 15-minute carry-over session approximately two months later.

Base Rate Session

During the base rate session, no attempt was made to manipulate the subject's verbal behaviors. The subjects were given instructions to talk about anything they wished. No attempt was made to establish a stable base rate.

2. SPEECH DISORDERS

Rather, a sample of each subject's spontaneous connected speech during a 15-minute period was obtained. The number and duration of fluent intervals and number of disfluencies were counted for later experimental comparisons.

After the base rate session, the subjects were asked to choose the verbal and tangible reinforcers they would like to receive. Rather than the investigator assuming the reinforcing value of the rewards, the subjects were permitted to select their own reinforcements (Shaw and Shrum, 1972). For the verbal reward, subjects were asked to provide the experimenter with the statement they would like to have said to them for doing well on a task. For the tangible reward, the children were asked what kind of prizes they would like to receive for doing well. The children had no difficulty selecting either type of reward. If a child happened to select a relatively expensive tangible reward, he or she was asked to select other less expensive prizes which they also valued. The investigator subsequently provided the chosen reinforcers for use during the three experimental sessions.

Prior to Session I, the length of the fluent time interval necessary to receive reinforcement was determined for each subject based on the average length of time during which the subject was able to remain fluent during the base rate session.

Experimental Session I

Experimental Session I was divided into three 10-minute periods. During the first 10 minutes, the subject received a mark on a matrix composed of 36 squares for each fluent time interval. This 10-minute session was included in the design so that the relative effectiveness of the verbal and tangible reinforcements could be considered apart from the placing of the marks on the matrices by the experimenter.

The instructions preceding this first 10-minute period were:

Today I want you to talk to me again about anything you want. The pictures and books are here for you to get ideas from if you need them. This time we will do something a little bit differently. Sometimes when you talk you use your "hard" speech, don't you? [The investigator was informed that the subject's fluent and disfluent speaking behaviors were referred to as "easy" and "hard" speech respectively by their public school clinicians.] Can you show me how you talk when you use your "hard" speech? That's right, that's how I don't want you to talk. I don't want you to use your "hard speech." Can you show me how you talk when you use your "easy" speech? That's right, that's how I want you to talk. I'll place a mark in these squares when you use your "easy" speech. I want you to talk until I tell you to stop. I am going to use the tape recorder so that I can remember everything we say. Do you understand?

During the second 10-minute period of Session I, the subject also received a mark on the matrix for each fluent interval. Each subject was told that when he completed a matrix, he would be praised with his previously selected verbal reward.

During the last 10 minutes of Session I, the subject received the marks on the matrix, plus a tangible reward. The instructions preceding this session indicated to the subject that when he completed a matrix, he would receive one of his previously chosen tangible rewards. Subjects were able to complete (and receive rewards for) as many matrices as possible during each 10-minute session.

Experimental Session II

Disfluency rather than fluency was the chosen response to be reinforced in Session II. That is, while both number of fluent intervals and number of disfluencies were counted during this session, it was disfluent behavior which was rewarded. The purpose of this session was to determine if the subject's speaking behaviors were indeed under the operant control of the various reinforcers used. That is, an increase in stuttering should result if the reinforcements are operantly controlling the subject's verbal behaviors.

This session was also divided into three 10-minute periods and reinforcements were presented during each successive period as follows: (1) marks on a matrix alone; (2) marks plus verbal reinforcement for each filled matrix; and (3) marks plus tangible reinforcement for each filled matrix. The instructions given during Session II were similar to those given during Session I. The term "hard" speech, however, was described as the desired behavior.

Experimental Session III

Fluent intervals were again reinforced during this session using the same procedures and instructions as discussed under Session I. The types of reinforcements, however, were presented in reverse order. The order of presentation was arranged in the sequence of "marks plus a tangible reward," "marks plus a verbal reward," and "marks only." The purpose of this experimental session, like Session II, was to determine the extent of control the various reinforcers had on the subject's verbal behaviors. This reverse order was also used as a means of assessing possible adaptation and order effects. The instructions during Session III were the same as those in experimental Session I.

Carry-Over Session

During the carry-over session, as in the base rate session, no attempt was made to manipulate the subject's verbal behaviors. The results obtained during the carry-over session were compared with the base rate data to determine what, if any, long-term effect the experimental sessions had on the subject's speaking behavior. Instructions for this session were the same as the base rate session.

ANALYSIS OF THE SUBJECTS' RESPONSES

In order to determine the investigator's reliability in the judgment of fluent intervals and instances of stuttering, the investigator used the subjects' tape-recorded speech. A correlation coefficient from ungrouped data (Ferguson, 1971) was computed using the number of fluent intervals and instances of stuttering counted during the actual experiment and those counted as the recorded sessions were listened to approximately six weeks later. A correlation coefficient of 0.99 was obtained both for fluent intervals and instances of stuttering for all three subjects.

The number of fluent intervals and instances of stuttering per five minutes during the base rate and carry-over sessions and the average per five minutes for each of the 10-minute periods of Sessions I, II, and III were tabulated and graphically displayed for each subject.

Subject SK

During the base rate session, this six-year 10-month-old boy displayed stuttering behaviors consisting of repetitions of syllables, words, or phrases; infrequent prolongations; and infrequent interjections of "umm" and "uh." The fluent interval selected for SK was two and one-half seconds. He chose "That's very good talking" as his verbal reward. The tangible rewards he selected and subsequently received (one after each filled matrix) were army posters, army equipment, and models.

The number of fluent intervals and instances of stuttering per five minutes for Subject SK are shown in Figures 1 and 2. From Figure 1 it may be seen that there was an increase in the number of fluent intervals from the base rate to Sessions I and III and the carry-over session. The "reversal" used in

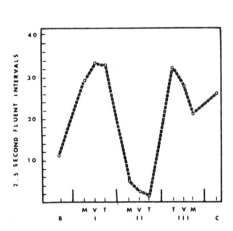

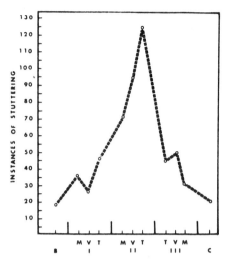

Figure 1. Subject SK. The number of fluent intervals per five minutes during the base rate (B) and carry-over (C) sessions and the average per five minutes for each of the 10-minute periods of experimental Sessions I, II, and III. The symbol M stands for marks only, V for marks plus verbal reward, and T for marks plus tangible reward.

Figure 2. Subject SK. The number of instances of stuttering per five minutes during the base rate (B) and carry-over (C) sessions and the average per five minutes for each of the 10-minute periods of experimental Sessions I, II, and III.

Session II resulted in a decrease in fluent intervals from the base rate session. Across all the experimental sessions, the verbal and tangible rewards were about equally effective in manipulating SK's speaking behavior, whereas the marks in the matrix alone were slightly less effective.

In Figure 2 it can be seen that there were fewer instances of stuttering during the base rate session than during the other four sessions. When Figures 1 and 2 are compared, it can be seen that although disfluencies increased during Sessions I, III, and carry-over, the number of fluent intervals also increased. This would indicate that the number of disfluencies actually decreased in proportion to the number of words spoken. This was shown to be the case as a tabulation of this subject's spoken words during base rate, Session I, III, and carry-over revealed average word per minute counts of 35.7, 73.6, 72.5, and 57.5 words respectively. There was no obvious order of effectiveness of the three types of reinforcement during experimental Sessions I and III.

As expected, the greatest increase in the number of instances of stuttering occurred during Session II when disfluencies were reinforced. There was a substantial increase in the number of disfluencies between each successive 10-minute period in this session with the tangible reinforcement schedule being the most effective.

Subject CR

Stuttering behaviors for this eight-year 11-month-old girl consisted of interjections of "umm," prolongations, and one to three repetitions of a sound, syllable, word, or phrase which were occasionally tense. The fluent interval chosen for CR was one and one-half seconds. She selected "good speech" for her verbal reward. The tangible rewards she chose and subsequently received during the three experimental sessions consisted of a soccer ball, dolls, chocolate candy, coloring books, and crayons.

The number of fluent intervals and instances of stuttering for Subject CR are displayed in Figures 3 and 4. As can be seen, there was an increase in the number of fluent intervals from the base rate session to Sessions I and III and the carry-over session. The 58.00 fluent intervals during the carry-over session more than doubled the base rate of 26.33 fluent intervals.

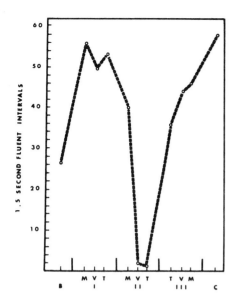

Figure 3. Subject CR. The number of fluent intervals per five minutes during the base rate (B) and carry-over (C) sessions and the average per five minutes for each of the 10-minute periods of experimental Sessions I, II, and III.

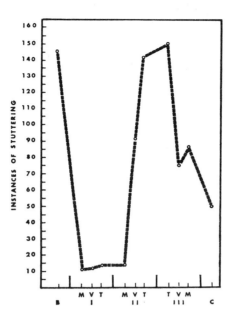

Figure 4. Subject CR. The number of instances of stuttering per five minutes during the base rate (B) and carry-over (C) sessions and the average per five minutes for each of the 10-minute periods of experimental Sessions I, II, and III.

During Sessions I and III, marks on a matrix alone were slightly more effective in increasing this subject's fluent intervals than either the verbal or tangible reinforcers. However, during the reversal session, verbal and tangible reinforcements were equally effective and considerably more effective than marks on the matrix alone.

It is evident from Figure 4 that there was a marked decrease in the mean number of instances of stuttering from the base rate session to the three 10-minute periods of Session I indicating equal effectiveness of the three reinforcement schedules. During Session III, the tangible reinforcement was not effective in decreasing the number of instances of stuttering, whereas the verbal and marks on a matrix reinforcers were again about equally effective.

There was a wide range of variation for the number of instances of stuttering during Session II. The marks on the matrix during the first 10-minute period of this reversal session resulted in 14.00 disfluencies which was well below that of the base rate session. However, there was a marked increase in disfluencies for both the second and third 10-minute periods of this session, with the tangible reinforcement schedule resulting in the most effective modification of CR's stuttering behavior.

Subject KW

The stuttering behaviors displayed by this nine-year one-month-old subject consisted of interjections of "umm" and "and umm," single-word repetitions, and infrequent prolongations and repetitions of a sound, syllable, or phrase. The fluent interval selected for this subject was two and one-half seconds. For her verbal reward KW wanted the investigator to say "You sounded real nice." The tangible reinforcers which she selected and subsequently received during the three experimental sessions consisted of dolls, stuffed animals, candy, and coloring books.

The number of fluent intervals and instances of stuttering per five minutes for Subject KW are displayed in Figures 5 and 6. It is evident from these data

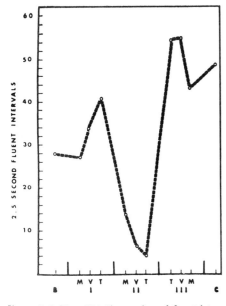

Figure 5. Subject KW. The number of fluent intervals per five minutes during the base rate (B) and carry-over (C) sessions and the average per five minutes for each of the 10-minute periods of experimental Sessions I, II, and III.

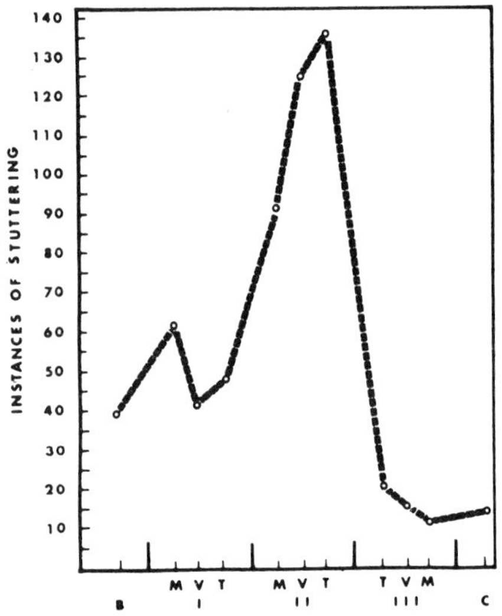

Figure 6. Subject KW. The number of instances of stuttering per five minutes during the base rate (B) and carry-over (C) sessions and the average per five minutes for each of the 10-minute periods of experimental Sessions I, II, and III.

that there was an overall increase in the number of fluent intervals from the base rate session to Sessions I and III and the carry-over session. More fluent intervals were elicited after the reversal session. The verbal and tangible reinforcers were consistently more effective in manipulating the number of fluent intervals than marks on the matrix alone. Except for Session II, the verbal and tangible rewards were equally effective.

Considering Subject KW's instances of stuttering as displayed in Figure 6, it may be seen that there was a slight increase in the number of disfluencies from the base rate session to Session I. As expected, there was a marked increase in the number of disfluencies from the base rate session to each successive 10-minute period of Session II with the tangible reinforcement schedule being the most effective in increasing KW's frequency of stuttering. Following the reversal session, Session III resulted in a decrease in the number of instances of stuttering below that of the base rate. And, the number of disfluencies during the carry-over session remained well below that of the base rate session.

DISCUSSION

As was hypothesized, there was no obvious difference in effectiveness of the two types of reinforcers on the modification of fluency for each of the three subjects. That is, the verbal and tangible reinforcers were about equally effective in increasing the subjects' fluent intervals during Sessions I and III. While the "marks alone" condition was slightly less effective than the verbal and tangible reinforcers in Sessions I and III for two of the subjects, Subject CR showed the greatest increase in fluent interval production when receiving marks only. Certainly it may be stated that application of all three types of reinforcers resulted in a rather obvious modification of the subjects' verbal behavior.

The findings of this investigation are considerably different than those of Rickard and Mundy (1966) who found that their subject achieved more fluency when receiving tangible rather than verbal rewards. Whether intended or not, the findings of Rickard and Mundy (1966), Leach (1969), and Shaw and Shrum (1972) might lead readers to think that tangible rewards are the most appropriate form of positive reinforcement to use when attempting to modify the fluency of young stutterers. The results of the present study indicate that verbal and tangible reinforcers are essentially equal in terms of eliciting an increase in the number of fluent intervals for each of the three young subjects. Thus it appears that factors other than the tangible or verbal nature of the particular reinforcement may be important in determining the extent to which the subjects' speaking behaviors can be modified within an operant conditioning paradigm.

The three variables proposed by Shaw and Shrum—(1) selection of the rewards by the subject, (2) reinforcement of easily identifiable behavior, and (3) subject awareness of the response contingency—although not studied here, appear to contribute to the effective modification of the young stutterer's speech. The fact that the actual verbal and tangible reinforcements were selected by the subjects probably contributed to the effective modification of their speaking behaviors in the present investigation. All of the subjects responded with enthusiasm when told that they were going to receive one of the previously chosen reinforcements. They also watched with eagerness as the investigator entered the marks on the matrix. A statement by Subject CR may help to illustrate the extent to which these reinforcements were controlling the modification of speaking behaviors. During the first 10-minute period of the reversal session she said "The reason I'm not gonna use my hard speech is because I don't do it right. I can't do it. It's too hard to do." However, during the second and third 10-minute periods of this reversal session when she received the verbal and tangible rewards respectively, Subject CR's disfluencies increased and it appeared that she was trying to stutter.

A second factor that may have contributed to the successful modification of speaking behaviors was the response chosen to be reinforced (fluent intervals). The present investigators found, as did Shaw and Shrum (1972), that rewarding each fluent interval resulted in more rapid and effective achievement of fluency than Nelson's (1968) reinforcement of approximations to fluent speech and Rickard and Mundy's (1966) and Ryan's (1971) reinforcement of progressively more difficult units of speech production. Perhaps fluent intervals are more easily identifiable responses. A possible problem with the present study may be the rather short fluent intervals (1.5–2.5 seconds) used. Although fluency was successfully manipulated with these intervals, there might have been an even more obvious demonstration of modification if the intervals had been somewhat longer.

A third factor which may have influenced the effectiveness of this conditioning was the subjects' awareness concerning the response to be manipulated and the manner in which these responses would be reinforced. As in the study by Shaw and Shrum (1972), the achievement of fluency was much more rapid following instructions than when subjects had to infer the response contingency (Rickard and Mundy, 1966; Leach, 1969; and Ryan, 1971).

Thus, as with Shaw and Shrum's (1972) study, it was probably a combination of these three factors which accounted for the effectiveness of this conditioning process. Since these same factors were also major variables in Shaw and Shrum's (1972) design which employed tangible rewards, it may be that these factors are more critical in the manipulation of speaking behaviors than whether or not the positive reinforcement takes the form of a verbal or tangible reward.

Acquisition of Esophageal Speech Subsequent to Learning Pharyngeal Speech: an Unusual Case Study

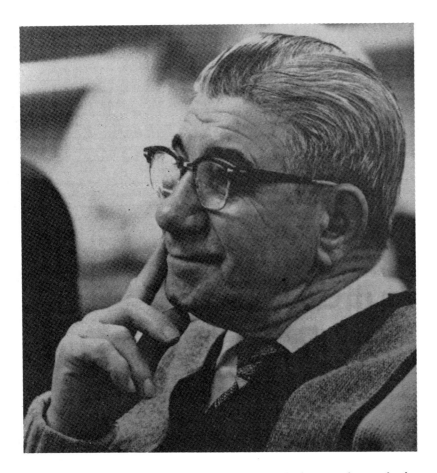

Pharyngeal speech represents an aberrant form of alaryngeal speech; its use as a primary means of communication is rare. According to Moolinaar-Bijl (1953) and Damste (1958) this form of alaryngeal speech may occur during the initial process of training an individual to inject air, when the patient is making his initial adjustments of the tongue and pharynx.

Damste (1958) feels that if the pharyngeal voice can be changed to esophageal voice it should be referred to as a temporary pharyngeal voice, but if it cannot be changed through therapy it should be considered pathological. According to Gardner (1971), in order to eliminate the pharyngeal voice and obtain esophageal voice, appropriate measures must be taken to assist the patient in getting air into the esophagus. He suggests the use of water or carbonated liquids to attempt to provide the individual with the initial sensation of inflation and expulsion of air from the esophagus. In addition, Gardner points out that the clinician may attempt to teach an inhalation technique whereby the patient sniffs air through the nose simultaneously with pulmonary inhalation.

Berlin (1964) indicates that clinical application of the inhalation method

John K. Torgerson

Daniel E. Martin

"Acquisition of Esophageal Speech Subsequent to Learning Pharyngeal Speech: An Unusual Case Study," John T. Togerson, Daniel E. Martin, *Journal of Speech and Hearing Research,* Vol. 41 No. 2, May 1976. © 1976 Journal of Speech and Hearing Research.

of air intake might be the method of choice for patients with a palatal paresis resulting from postsurgical complications and for individuals with palatal weakness that may be associated with advancing age. These patients are unable to generate sufficient intraoral pressure for the injection of air into the esophagus. Berlin suggests that concentrating on injection methods with these individuals might well impede their acquisition of esophageal speech. In reviewing the literature, one is convinced that the inhalation method of air intake has definite clinical application for certain laryngectomees.

PATIENT PRESENTATION

Patient GR was a 67-year-old male laryngectomee who developed and used pharyngeal speech as his primary method of communication for two years prior to enrolling in esophageal speech classes. Speech referral had been delayed due to complications involving a pharyngeal fistula.

During the initial intake evaluation, when it was first observed that the patient was using an aberrant form of alaryngeal speech, he was given instruction in the use of a neck-type electrolarynx (Western Electric, Type 5A). It was believed that this would be an acceptable substitute means of communication that would also reduce the continuous use of what was assumed to be pharyngeal speech.

In attempts to elicit esophageal sound, the patient was given specific instruction in the use of two types of air injection: the glossal press and consonant injection. Although both types of air injection proved successful initially in eliciting esophageal sound, it soon became apparent that the patient's pharyngeal sound production was gradually reappearing and being used more often than the esophageal sound production. With this turn of events, the clinical sessions became extremely frustrating for the patient as well as for the clinician.

The tongue is active in both the glossal press and consonant injection methods of esophageal air intake, and it serves as a part of the neoglottis in pharyngeal speech. Observation of the patient suggested to the clinician that the tongue movements in glossal press and consonant injection tended to trigger the well-established pharyngeal speech.

To test the assumption that this patient was producing a pharyngeal type of alaryngeal voice, radiographic observations were made using videofluoroscopy with synchronous sound. Sixteen-mm films with synchronous sound were produced from the videotape. The sites of the neoglottis and air reservoir were determined for the aberrant form of alaryngeal voice production and for the esophageal voice production. Tracings were made of representative frames of both forms of phonation.

Figure 1 shows that the site of the neoglottis in this patient's aberrant form of sound production is between the tongue and velum. An occasional frame was observed in which there appeared to be involvement of the posterior pharyngeal wall as well. The esophagus is closed and the only apparent air reservoir is located in the pharynx. This type of alaryngeal sound production would be considered pharyngeal, because as suggested by Diedrich and Youngstrom (1966), in pharyngeal voice the neoglottis may be formed by the tongue being approximated against the hard and soft palate, the faucial pillars, or posterior pharyngeal wall, with the air reservoir located in the hypopharynx. Figure 2 shows that in his production of esophageal sound, the site of the neoglottis is located in the area of the seventh cervical vertebra. It can be seen that the air reservoir is below this point, as evidenced by the column of air in the esophagus.

CLINICAL TECHNIQUE

It became evident that in order to change the pharyngeal voice to consistent esophageal voice a method of air intake demanding the least amount of

2. SPEECH DISORDERS

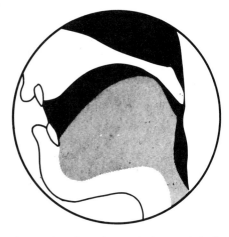

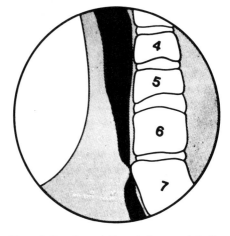

Figure 1. Site of neoglottis and air reservoir in the patient's pharyngeal voice production.

Figure 2. Site of neoglottis and air reservoir in the patient's esophageal voice production.

tongue involvement would have to be used. As pointed out by Gardner (1971), when the patient inhales air directly into the esophagus, the tongue remains immobile to permit a free flow of air. With this in mind, the inhalation method of air intake was introduced into therapy.

The patient was instructed to attempt a quick sniff through his nose simultaneously with inhalation through the stoma and to follow this immediately with an attempt at producing the vowel /ɑ/ in an easy, relaxed manner. This proved successful in eliciting esophageal sound on the second attempt. Within one week (four sessions) following the introduction of the inhalation method, the patient was able to produce most vowels consistently and with ease. With this accomplished, he was then instructed to precede the vowel with either the plosive /p/ or /t/ following initial inhalation. These consonants were employed early in therapy in an attempt to combine plosive injection with the inhalation method of air intake in order to facilitate insufflation of the esophagus. The /k/ sound was also attempted but was confusing to the patient because it resulted in an occasional pharyngeal sound rather than the desired esophageal sound. After the third week (12 sessions), further attempts at preceding a vowel with the /k/ sound proved successful without the occasional recurrence of pharyngeal sound. The patient then made a fairly rapid progression from monosyllabic words to bisyllabic words and short phrases. For two months following the initiation of the inhalation method the patient practiced his esophageal voice production a designated amount of time at home but continued to use the electrolarynx as a primary means of communication. His use of the electrolarynx was gradually decreased to use only for telephone conversations.

INTELLIGIBILITY AND FUNDAMENTAL FREQUENCY

Intelligibility. Determination of the overall intelligibility of the two different methods of speech was made using equivalent 50-word multiple-choice discrimination lists from the Multiple Choice Discrimination Test (MCDT), as described by Schultz and Schubert (1969) and recommended by them for use with laryngectomees. Fifteen unsophisticated listeners were used for the listening task. A mean intelligibility score of 59% was obtained for the patient's esophageal speech production. This is substantially higher than the mean intelligibility score of 45% obtained for his pharyngeal speech production. The difference of 14 percentage points in overall intelligibility scores between the two methods of speech, although not as large as one might have anticipated, is perhaps related to the patient's prolonged use of pharyngeal speech as compared to the esophageal speech. That is, he had used pharyngeal speech for two years and esophageal speech for approximately four months prior to the intelligibility determination. Intelligibility of pharyngeal speech is thought to be poor because the tongue postures associated with its production might interfere with the accuracy of articulation. Weinberg and Westerhouse (1973) observed this phenomenon in their study of pharyngeal speech.

Fundamental Frequency. Visicorder analysis of the acoustical data showed a fundamental frequency of 66 Hz for this patient's esophageal voice production. For his pharyngeal voice production, a fundamental frequency of 202 Hz was determined.

CLINICAL IMPLICATIONS

Alteration of pharyngeal voice to esophageal voice can be an extremely difficult task for the clinician. The purpose of this paper was to present a clinical technique that was successful in changing pharyngeal voice production to esophageal voice production with one patient in our clinic. It is presented as another possible method and lends support to the suggestion made by Gardner (1971) regarding the clinical application of the inhalation method of air intake to alter pharyngeal speech.

FOCUS...

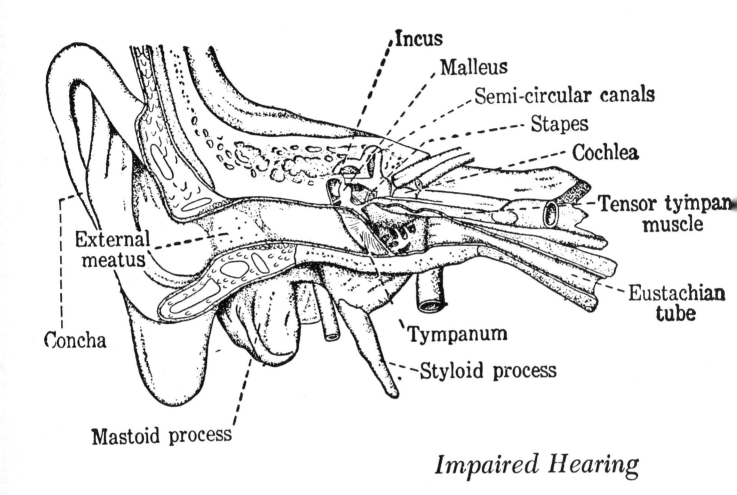

Incus

Malleus

Semi-circular canals

Stapes

Cochlea

Tensor tympani muscle

Eustachian tube

Tympanum

Styloid process

External meatus

Concha

Mastoid process

Impaired Hearing

The External Ear and the Middle Ear

The external ear is composed of the appendage on the side of the head that children learn to call "the ear," together with a canal lined with skin, at the inner end of which is the eardrum.

On the inner side of the eardrum is a small cavity, which is the second of the three parts of the organ and known as the middle ear. Inside the middle ear are three tiny bones. One is attached to the eardrum and one connects with the inner ear. The third or middle one forms a bridge between these two. Since the little bones are attached by means of ligaments and tiny muscles, they move when sound waves impinge upon the eardrum, and thus they carry the vibrations across the middle ear to the inner ear, which contains the sensitive endings of the nerve of hearing. It is interesting to note that the little bones in the middle ear are fully grown at birth and are the smallest bones in the body. Diagrams of the middle ear may give a false impression of the size of the cavity. It helps to remember that ten drops of water will fill it.

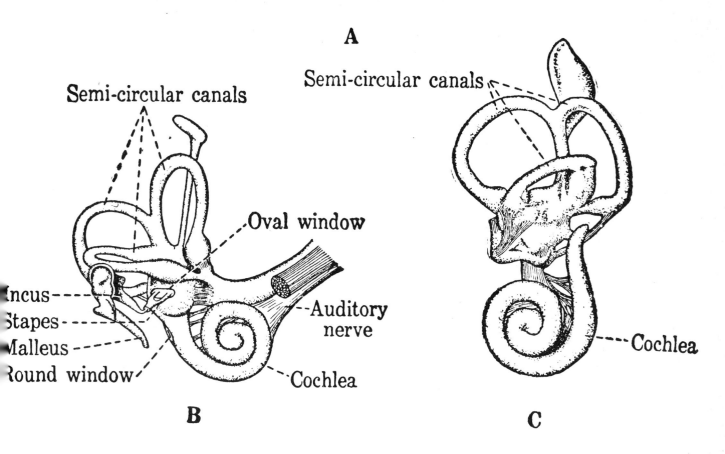

A

Semi-circular canals

Semi-circular canals

Oval window

Incus

Stapes

Malleus

Round window

Auditory nerve

Cochlea

Cochlea

B

C

Diagram of the ear, showing the inner ear. (From Gray and Wise, *The Bases of Speech*, rev. ed., Harper & Brothers; after Sobotta.)

The inner ear is composed essentially of three parts: (1) the three semicircular canals which are thought to be concerned only with the sense of equilibrium or balance; (2) the snail-shaped structure called the cochlea, which contains the sensitive endings of the auditory nerve; and (3) the part known as the vestibule, which connects the semicircular canals with the cochlea. One of the little bones in the middle ear fits into an opening in the wall of the middle ear known as the oval window, which lies between the vestibule and the middle ear. When the little bone is moved by sound vibrations this sets up corresponding movement of the fluid that fills the vestibule and this in turn excites the nerve endings in the cochlea and causes the sensation known as hearing.

The Inner Ear

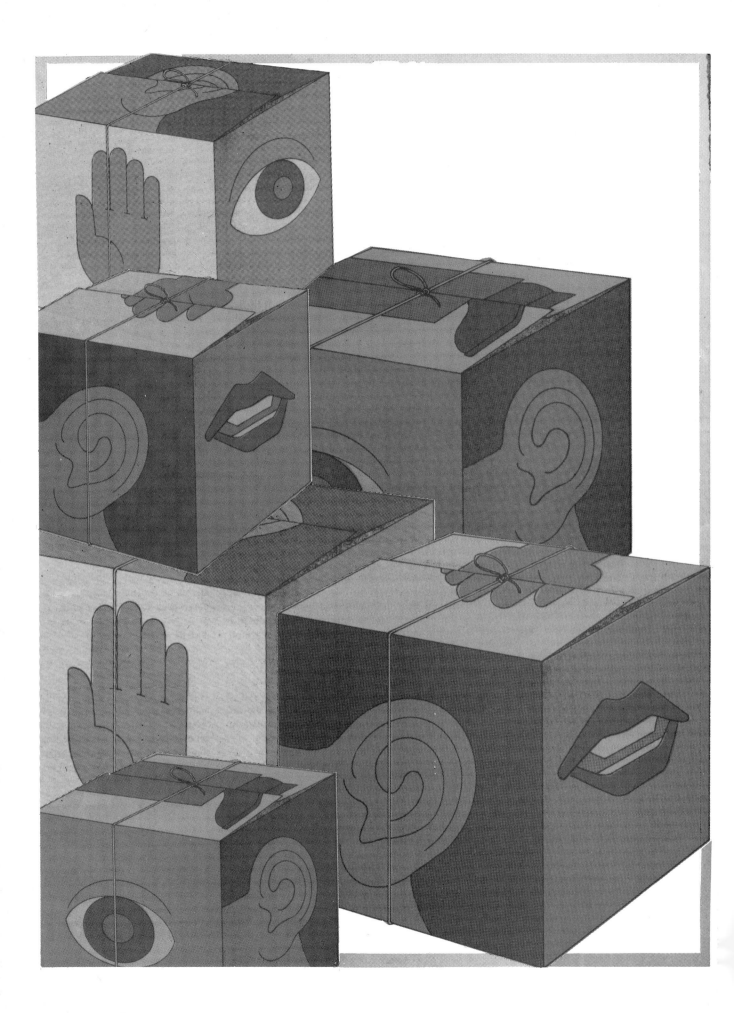

Linguistic Development

The process of learning to talk has been of interest to teachers, parents, and professionals for centuries due to the fact that children are our only link to the empirical facts of language acquisition.

Language development is the active process of hypothesis formation and hypothesis testing about the rules of heard language and self-construction of speech through utterance. Similarities of languages of the world are now being recognized . . . innate knowledge of these aspects may be present as the child approaches language acquisition. The first words are most crucial in phonetic form, meaning, and ways in which they are used . . . thus we have observable speech.

Up to this point we have concerned ourselves with linguistic development in normal children, as the most important and valuable research has been gained through them in the normal course of advancement. For some children, the process of learning language is very difficult, if not next to impossible. As a result, normative information is the actual basis of retarded speech development.

Speech pathology is given further difficulty by the fact that confusion exists as to the different causes of developmental delay of speech. The most common cause is mental retardation, or mental deficiency. Since speech is a learned skill, all learning will thus be a difficult process and will parallel the degree of mental deficiency. These might include hearing impairment, partial or complete paralysis of the palate or muscles of the throat, a serious incoordination of tongue movement caused by damage to the nervous system, and environmental and stimulatory causes of extreme emotional shock.

It is from here that the speech pathologist will come into play. In the past it was thought that retarded children suffered some brain injury which directly interfered with speech development . . . this theory is still valid . . . though not proven.

From this point on linguistic development lies in the hands of the teacher, the pathologist, and specially designed remedial speech problems which can lead to necessary language acquisition.

speech is more than mere words

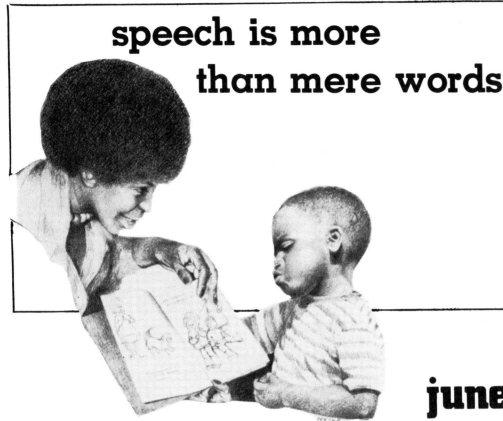

june mather

Human speech sets people apart from other living creatures. However, this ability is only one way of communicating with others. Gesture and intonation, body language, and sounds often speak louder and more clearly, especially to children. The tone of voice, the expression on a face, and the touch of another person's hand tell a small child more than can be conveyed in mere words. As a result, little children are likely to copy sounds and gestures early in their development.

This was brought home to me some years ago when I was singing a nursery rhyme—I believe it was "Jack and Jill"—with a group of preschool children. Dennis, who was nearly four years old, had never attempted to say one single word to my knowledge, and hardly ever made any sounds either, and I was beginning to despair of his ever being able to do so. Jeremy, who was sitting across from Dennis, knew the words of the song well; but he was bored and restless and, instead of joining in, he made a sound known as the Bronx cheer or raspberry! This sound was echoed without hesitation by my silent little friend Dennis. His enormous grin of delight at his achievement made me realize that noises like this are far more interesting to the child who has not yet learned to speak.

After all, the world is full of curious and wonderful sounds—footsteps, opening doors, telephones, wind, rattles, birdsong, breathing, garbage cans, cars, water running, food frying, people talking—they are all new and exciting to the child. He has not learned, as he will when he grows older, to block out many of the surrounding noises and concentrate on one sound, particularly the sound of the human voice.

Human speech, at this point in a child's life, is simply a series of sounds (happy sounds to make him smile, scolding sounds to make him cry) too complicated for him even to try to imitate. On the other hand, he can cough, laugh, sneeze, belch, cry, gurgle, and coo. He will enjoy copying these sounds when you make them—even Bronx cheers! It becomes a game he plays with you as he repeats them over and over again.

Listening to you is a good habit for him to get into, for you can gradually introduce new and more meaningful sounds for him to imitate—sounds that can be connected to objects (animal noises, the ticking of a watch or clock, the ringing of a telephone, and so forth).

Next, you can encourage him to use conversational sounds and sounds that accompany gestures. These are the kinds of noises that people use all the time without perhaps even realizing it. The "ouch!" when you hurt yourself, the "oops!" when you make a mistake, the "uh huh" of agreement (usually combined with a nodding head), the "tut tut" meaning "fancy that!" or "oh dear!" or "I can hardly believe what you are telling me," the "uh uh" and a wagging finger which means "no" or "stop," and of course the "mmm mmm" that keeps conversation going.

Various sounds and gestures are used in different cultures, but most of them are universally understood. Certainly children who do not talk yet find them more meaningful and easier to copy than words. By using sounds and appropriate gestures, they are able to carry on a conversation without actually talking. Because some children are able to speak only after many years, it should be remembered that the goal of speech is to make people able to communicate with one another. If your child is able to do this more easily with gestures and sounds, it is better to help him communicate more effectively this way. It is better to help him do what he *can* do more effectively than to set goals so high he cannot possibly reach them.

This is not to say that a child who seems to be unable to talk should only be taught to use sounds and gestures. At all times the words he is trying to say should be repeated by you as he indicates his needs. Carry on a conversation with him and, if anything, use more words yourself. Constantly be alert for what he is trying to convey and, in simple terms, put it into words for him.

This means getting down to his level and seeing the world through his eyes. It is not something you expect to have to do *all* the time, but try to spend some time each day conversing one way or another with your child. It is better to give him your full attention for small amounts of time than to *be* with him all the time and yet never really communicate with him.

Even though it is hard to realize, children who do not know words nevertheless understand a great deal of what *we* are saying. They are able to do so because they interpret our gestures, our body language, and the tone of our voice long before they understand the words that accompany them.

Timothy—only just beginning to walk—has a favorite song. It is "If You're Happy and You Know It, Clap Your Hands." He cannot say any words yet, but he laughs with the greatest glee when I come to the line "If you're mad and you know it, stamp your feet," and I put on my angriest face while I sing the words. It is the same angry face he sees when I am scolding him for pouring sand over another child's head in the sandbox. Yet he laughs at my make-believe anger,

and he respects it when it is real. Even without understanding words, he is well aware of this subtle difference and shade of meaning.

For a child like Timothy, who cannot talk yet and may not be able to for some years to come, his problem is *not* in understanding the world around him—it is in having other people understand *him*. We are so used to the idea of human speech that many of us do not appreciate the intelligence of a child who cannot talk. Yet, as Timothy showed me, even without the use of words, he was capable of a high degree of understanding. How unfortunate it is that the capability of an individual is so often measured by his ability to use words.

If Timothy, as a toddler, can tell the difference between truth and make-believe, surely we should not worry about his inability to say words yet. Let us build on the abilities he already possesses. He can tell reality from pretense—can he see the difference between up and down, in and out, over and under, stop and go, "throw it on the floor" and "pick it up," "pull it out of the closet" and "put it away," "pull your socks on" and "take your socks off"?

These are the ideas to use in daily contact with Timothy and children like him. Though we will be talking all the time, appropriate gestures should be added to point up what we are saying. In time, Timothy will copy our gestures and begin to associate them with our words. As he hears them repeated over and over he may, in time, attempt to say them himself.

As he begins to recognize the difference between things, he will start to notice similarities— not similarity of words; that comes much later in life—for example, the reflection of a familiar face in a mirror, the similarity between a picture and the object it represents.

Cindy stroked her hair and pointed to her feet when she was shown pictures of a brush and comb and a pair of red shoes. She could not say the words, but she certainly recognized the objects in the pictures.

At about the same time in her life Cindy began to show an interest in matching things—that her hands matched her doll's hands, that both she and her mother wore hats, that one red shoe matched her other red shoe, and so on.

If your child enjoys looking at pictures and matching things, encourage him to point with his finger. If there is more than one object on a page, or if there are two shoes in front of him, have him point to each one separately. This will teach him to appreciate the difference between one object and another, as well as the difference between *one* thing and a whole lot of things. This, of course, is a beginning step to counting and understanding numbers.

Pointing to different parts of her body as we named them was something else that Cindy loved to do. She was able to do this long before she made any attempt to say the words herself. Children like her will be intrigued by the fact that they have *two* feet, hands, and ears and yet only *one* mouth and nose. You can point out many things in everyday conversation that will help your child to understand the idea of number. "Take *one* cookie," "here are two apples—you may have one," "give Daddy one cake," "show me your shoe—you have two shoes, one . . . two."

When your child copies a sound you have made (like Dennis and the Bronx cheer) you have another opportunity to introduce numbers. Suppose he imitates a cough, for instance. Cough again deliberately, and if he copies it again you have a game going together. See what he will do when you cough twice in succession. You can do the same thing knocking on a door; can he copy the number of times that you knock? Banging on a drum is great fun; see what happens when you bang the drum many times. What you are doing at this stage is pointing out the difference between one sound and two sounds, one thing and a number of things.

Singing is probably the way a little baby begins to *enjoy* words—listening to them as beautiful sounds. There is something soothing and yet stimulating in hearing songs repeated over and over. Many children find it easier to sing words than to say them. Others have a whole repertoire of songs before understanding any of the actual words. Many children who do not or cannot sing love to join in with actions such as hiding their hands behind them and pointing one at a time for "Where Is Thumbkin?" or pretending to wash their faces and brush their teeth for "This Is the Way We Wash our Face."

Songs—and the best are the old ones familiar to everyone—are the way a child is introduced to his literary heritage. Nursery rhymes, folk songs, and familiar hymns need to be woven into the fabric of his being at an early age because this is one way of passing the cultural background from one generation to the next. Television, radio, and records can help here; but so often in these media the new and innovative is emphasized at the expense of the old and familiar. The result, for the slower-than-average child, is that instead of learning to join in with songs everyone knows, which would help him integrate more with society, he learns only the latest hit tunes, which, by the time he has learned them, will have become out-of-date and forgotten. Slower-than-average children take longer to learn songs. Because of this it is better to teach them the type of song that will be suitable for them later on, when they are grown up. This means including old favorites such as "I've Been Working on the Railroad" or "Row, Row, Row Your Boat" or "Daisy, Daisy" along with nursery rhymes.

Sometimes it is quite hard to remember all the old songs that you were brought up with. This is where grandmothers and grandfathers come into the picture, for they probably remember singing to you when you were a baby and can teach the same songs to their grandchildren.

While your child is listening to people singing and talking, he will discover one day that things and people have names. People to begin with— *you* to begin with. In nearly every language "ma-ma" is one of the first words a youngster says, and in nearly every language this word means mother. Perhaps this is because "mm-mm" is one of the first sounds of contentment a baby makes.

It is rather difficult for parents to accept the fact that, when their child begins to use words or sounds that represent words, he may not really understand what he is saying at all. Our son's first word was "car"—at least that is what I fondly imagined, and I even recorded the date in my baby book. Looking back, I realize he probably had no idea what he was saying on the first occasion. It simply happened that he made a "ca" sound while watching his father come up to the house in the car. We had waited so long for this first word! I grabbed him, hugged him, and raced out to tell my husband the good news. For the next few weeks, I remember, Alan called everything "car."

It is easy to confuse children this way. I should have kept my enthusiasm and pleasure to myself and encouraged him to play with his new sound, to make a game of it with me. Something like this:

Alan: ca ca
Me: ca ca

Alan: ca ca
Me: ca ca ca ca
Alan: ca ca ca
Me: car (going to the car and pointing to it)
Alan: car
Me: da da car
Alan: da da
Me: Daddy's car
And so on.

Being able to say something which somebody else understands is an exciting event for both the speaker and the listener, particularly if the speaker is doing it for the first time. The first time for Dennis happened one day when he began to do a peculiar little dance all by himself in the corner of the room. He kept repeating an unintelligible babble, and it was only when we saw he had put the candlestick on the floor that we recognized the tune as "Jack Be Nimble, Jack Be Quick." Then, as we watched him, he jumped right over the candlestick, leaving no doubt in our minds *he* knew exactly what he was saying.

Meanings and words do not always fit together quite so well. Whenever Roddy washes his hands he says, "Hot, cold, hot, cold, hot, cold"!

Conversations with children like Alan, Dennis, and Roddy are on two levels. Because they are beginning to experiment with consonant sounds and words, we must encourage them to try more of these sounds. But, at the same time, we must continue to stimulate them with the ideas, concepts, and discriminations which were discussed earlier in the chapter. What has to be remembered with slower-than-average children is that understanding is a separate skill which has little to do with the formation of recognizable words.

The ability to produce words depends on the operation of the many different parts of the mouth, throat, tongue, lips, lungs, etc. that make up the vocal mechanism. Learning to use the vocal mechanism is a long and complicated process. It takes a great deal of practice. The average baby spends an enormous amount of time vocalizing in the form of cooing, shrieking, crying, screaming, gurgling, chuckling, etc.

As a newborn baby, he uses these sounds to communicate his moods and feelings—crying because he needs something, laughing with joy and delight. But there comes a stage later on when he makes sounds and noises for the pure pleasure of hearing his own voice. This stage also comes to the slower-than-average child, but it comes later in life, when the child is no longer a baby, and it lasts for a much longer time.

It can be a very irritating time for parents who misinterpret these vocalizations and do not understand the child's need to try out the sounds he can make. Liza discovered one day how to shriek. To her it was a wonderful sound, and it had a magnificent effect on all those around her. Everyone stopped what he was doing to look at her, and that made her do it more than ever.

It was only natural that Liza's family would assume that she "only does it to annoy, because she knows it teases," to paraphrase the Duchess in Alice's Adventures in Wonderland. They tried scolding her, but this did not stop her—and anyway they did not want to discourage her from making sounds. So they decided to pretend they did not hear her shrieks, and instead they began to make other sounds and noises such as barking and mooing to play along with her. In time, she began to enjoy copying these new sounds.

With the slower-than-average child the important thing is to encourage vocalization. This gives him the practice he needs in order eventually to begin to use words. The way you can do this depends on your imagination, but whenever you are alone with him, sing or make noises or play with sounds together. Make it an enjoyable and amusing experience for both of you.

Unfortunately, slower-than-average children can be put off when too much is demanded from them. Amy, at four years of age, was just beginning to use a few words, and her father and mother were delighted. Her grandmother was a teacher of the old school, who believed she could help Amy by sitting down and working intensively with her. This she did on several occasions. Shortly after this Amy's mother noticed that she was beginning to stutter mildly—and the stutter only happened to Amy when she was taken to visit her grandmother!

Therese was a plump little girl who really enjoyed food. She was in the habit, at mealtimes, of pointing to whatever she wanted because she could not talk. Eventually she began to say a few words. Her parents decided to try to speed up her talking. When she pointed to something she wanted at the dinner table, they insisted she make an attempt to say the word before they passed the food to her. For a few days all seemed to be going well, and Therese began to repeat one or two words. But then she did something that she had not done for several past months. She began to wet herself. Her mother could not understand it, but her father wondered whether they were putting too much pressure on her to talk. They decided not to be quite so insistent with her, and sure enough, in a few days, she was as well toilet-trained as she had been before.

There is a very thin line between having a child do as well as he possibly can and pushing him beyond his capacity. One of the best ways to be sure that you are not putting too much pressure on your child is to be on the watch for signs such as Amy's stutter or Therese's wetting. These signs may be outward indications of inward frustration.

Once children begin saying words, the important thing to do is to talk to them. Conversation is the way children learn how to use words. It is one thing to learn the names of people, objects, numbers, colors, sizes, and actions; but only in conversation do these words begin to have real meaning.

When you carry on a conversation with a child you should try to give him opportunities to use those words he knows best. Do not be discouraged if your child keeps saying the same word again and again. Eloise had a favorite word— *kittycat*—and every day she found all kinds of

3. LINGUISTIC DEVELOPMENT

reasons for saying the word over and over until her family complained that she never said anything else. Favorite words can be used by adults to enlarge a child's vocabulary.

Eloise's love of cats can be used to teach her how to use more words. The way to do this is to build up conversations around her particular interest. When Eloise begins looking for her cat, her parents should say such things as "Where do you suppose Kitty is?" "Is he behind the sofa?" "Who is that under the bed?" "What is Kitty doing?" "Isn't he soft and cuddly?" and so on. Out of these kinds of (rather one-sided) conversational questions Eloise may begin to put *kitty* together with another word such as "kitty bed" or "kitty soft" or "kitty where?" and thus begin to converse. The idea of "yes" and "no" can be introduced here: "Kitty on the bed?" "No, Kitty's not on the bed." "Yes, Kitty is in the closet."

Conversations with beginning talkers consist mainly of questions which give the child a chance to use his favorite word as the answer. Adult: "What's under the bed?" Eloise (triumphantly): "Kittycat!"

At this stage correct pronunciation is less important than the attempt to say words. Children can be put off if their efforts are misunderstood or ridiculed. Whenever possible simply accept what the child says, and, if you can, correct it by repeating the word properly.

Billy, for some reason or another, used a Y sound at the beginning of his words—"yookies and yuice" for "cookies and juice." Obviously he was able to make the *c* sound, but "yookies" seemed to come more easily to him. We tried to correct the habit by pointing out things beginning with the *c* sound such as cat, camel, kangaroo, catch, car, kick. I shall never forget his amazement and then his burst of delighted laughter when he came across an animal in an alphabet book called a yak.

Books make it possible to show the whole world to your child while he is sitting on your lap. Unlike television or everyday experience, books can be looked at over and over again whenever you feel like it. Every page in a book may be different, but it never changes from one day to the next. For a child, there is something very reassuring about the rediscovery of a familiar book, something stimulating about anticipating the story, about revisiting a world that stays the same forever.

Books for little children should be chosen with care. Pictures should be clear and precise. The more realistic they are, the easier it is for a child to relate them to his everyday experience, even though he will be constantly coming across things that he has never actually seen in real life. Wild animals, farm animals, birds, and insects for city children; fire engines, smokestacks, and skyscrapers for country youngsters. All these strange and unfamiliar things become part of a child's life and experience through books.

The text of a book is as important as the pictures. Except for simple counting and alphabet books and books of pictures, choose books with texts that appeal to you. *You* are the one who has to do the actual reading, and it is your interest that will stimulate your child.

Try to find books with clear pictures, interesting texts, and not too many words on each page. Little children find it hard to sit still and listen for too long, and they usually enjoy the activity of turning the pages over one by one.

As you read the same book over and over again, your child will begin to memorize the simple text. Soon he will be able to say some of the words along with you, and eventually he will be able to look at the book all by himself and your words will echo in his mind as he does so.

While you are reading you can encourage him to talk by asking him questions about the pictures and having him point to things he knows. Discussions about the pictures can introduce counting, colors, sizes, and shapes. Conversation about the story—what is happening and what is going to happen—encourages the child to join in the reading experience. It is *not* reading, but it does set up good habits for reading later on (sitting still, concentrating on one page at a time, taking an interest in the unfolding story, listening to your voice, and learning to tell the difference between the printed word and the pictures).

It is hard for adults to realize that, just as a baby becoming aware of human speech is unable in the early stages to understand the words being spoken, so an older child, seeing printed words in a book, may not know what they are. For him written words and letters are simply squiggles. It will be many, many years before he is able to distinguish and recognize words and begin to read them for himself.

Meantime the important thing for him to learn is that the written word is different from a picture (or even from an object), even though it stands for the same thing. The word *shoe* means the same thing as the shoe in the picture; the word *milk* tells what is contained inside the carton; *John* is his name; etc. This is not reading, but it is laying the groundwork for future reading by showing the child that our world is full of things which stand for something else.

The same idea, of course, applies to numbers: 1, 2, 3, 4, 5, etc. are symbols which stand for something else. It is less important for a child to recognize these symbols than to understand what they stand for. So a child beginning to use words can be taught to count how many blocks, how many fingers, how many shoes, how many people by the actual experience of pointing to a series of objects one by one, and saying "One, two, three . . ." along with you. Eventually he will recognize the symbols; but, like recognition of letters and words, this comes later on in his life.

The beginning talker learns words not by seeing them written down, as adults do, but by hearing them spoken. So writing words on bits of paper and sticking them on familiar objects does not help children talk. Children learn to say words only when they hear words spoken.

You may find that your child makes certain sounds much more than others. And he makes these same sounds more frequently than any others. This was the case with Catherine, who went through a stage of making a lot of guttural gu-gu sounds. Because she was slow at talking (she was six at the time) her mother decided to fit words into these gu-gu sounds that she seemed to find easy to make. "Good girl" was pretty close, so whenever Catherine did anything to merit it, her mother would say "Good girl," which of course Catherine promptly repeated. So if your child seems slow to talk, see if you can pick out the sounds he *can* make and build up words on these favorite sounds.

In all things it is much better to help your child improve what he is able to do than constantly try to get him to do something he cannot quite manage. By building on his abilities—expanding, enlarging and encouraging them, whether they consist of gestures, sounds, words, or phrases—you can show him how to reach the goal of speech, which is to make it easier for him to reach out and communicate with other people.

Vocabulary Development of Educable Retarded Children

ARTHUR M. TAYLOR
MARTHA L. THURLOW
JAMES E. TURNURE

ARTHUR M. TAYLOR *is Supervisor of Programs for the Mentally Retarded, Special Education Department, St. Paul Public Schools, St. Paul, Minnesota; and* MARTHA L. THURLOW *is Research Fellow, and* JAMES E. TURNURE *is Professor of Educational Psychology, Department of Psychoeducational Studies, and RD&D Center in Education of Handicapped Children, University of Minnesota, Minneapolis. This research was supported in part by a grant to the University of Minnesota Research, Development and Demonstration Center in Education of Handicapped Children (OEG-0-332189-4533-032) from the US Office of Education.*

B ASIC research involving the procedure of verbal elaboration has shown that the learning of paired items is greatly facilitated when the items are presented within a verbal context and that the procedure is particularly effective for young children (Turnure, Thurlow, & Larsen, 1971) and retarded children (Jensen & Rohwer, 1963; Turnure, 1971; Turnure, Larsen, & Thurlow, 1973). In fact, Rohwer (1973) has concluded that elaboration is the main process necessary for efficient associative learning.

Although elaboration, the embedding of information within verbal contexts, appears to be a naturally occurring process and one that is necessarily involved in most instruction, an analysis of the use of elaboration in instructional materials reveals it is not used as consistently or as efficiently as possible. For example, elaboration appears in vocabulary instruction, where a single sentence commonly is used to present the meaning of a single vocabulary word. The use of single sentences for elaborations, however,

does not recognize recent research findings that suggest extended elaborations (e.g., paragraphs) have even more impressive effects than simple sentences (Turnure, 1971). The idea of presenting the meaning of a vocabulary word in isolation is also inconsistent with recent research that indicates elaboration facilitates learning mainly because it provides stronger relations between two or more words or concepts learned together in a single context (Bender & Taylor, 1973; Rohwer, 1971; Turnure & Thurlow, 1973).

Despite the potential educational applicability of elaboration, only a few studies have demonstrated that extended elaboration can successfully be used as a vehicle for effective classroom learning. Ross (1971) has developed math concepts via elaboration based instruction, and Bender and Taylor (1973) have used elaboration as a basis for developing social studies instruction for retarded children. Other instructional materials using elaborational techniques have been prepared by individuals interested in vocabulary development (Ammon & Ammon, 1971; Draper & Moeller, 1971). Ammon and Ammon (1971) demonstrated that elaborations involving story themes could be used effectively to develop vocabulary, and Draper and Moeller (1971) successfully used thematic elaborations (i.e., myths and fables) to develop and interrelate new vocabulary words for children in the fourth through sixth grades. Unfortunately, the benefits of using the thematic instruction were not compared to the benefits of nonthematic instruction. Furthermore, neither investigation examined the effectiveness of elaboration in vocabulary instruction for retarded children. While vocabulary instruction has long been a major focus in the education of children, such instruction is particularly critical with retarded children since these children seem to progress more slowly in vocabulary development than expected (Beier, Starkweather, & Lambert, 1969),

Purpose

The purpose of this study was to examine the effectiveness of nonrelational, relational, and mixed approaches to vocabulary instruction for educable mentally retarded children. The nonrelational condition was developed to represent traditional approaches to vocabulary instruction. In this condition, nonrelational elaborations were used during the initial presentation of words and during a final sum-

mary. The relational condition was developed to reflect the implication of recent research that the success of elaborations is primarily due to relations, at least in paired associate learning (Thurlow & Turnure, 1972; Turnure & Thurlow, 1973). In this condition, relational elaborations were used in the initial presentation of words and in a thematic summary. The mixed condition represented a blending of the other two conditions. Nonrelational elaborations were used during the initial presentation of words, but major relations between words were presented in a thematic summary.

This investigation allowed for the comparison of the two types of elaborations and the two types of summaries. The two types of elaborations were referred to as relational and nonrelational. Relational elaborations were contexts that developed specific relationships between two or more vocabulary words, and nonrelational elaborations were contexts that expanded the meaning of a single vocabulary word without relating it to the meaning of any other vocabulary word. The two types of summaries were designated as thematic and nonthematic. Thematic summaries were single integrative stories that emphasized a thematic relationship among the vocabulary words in a lesson, and nonthematic summaries were a series of single nonrelational elaborations (one for each vocabulary word in a lesson).

In addition to studying the effects of these factors on vocabulary growth, the study also assessed the spontaneous use of elaboration and related strategies by children receiving the various combinations of elaborations and summaries.

Method

Subjects

Nine self contained classes for primary age educable mentally retarded children ages 8 to 11 participated in the study. The 107 children were pretested on two instruments, the Peabody Picture Vocabulary Test (PPVT) (Dunn, 1961), and the Minnesota Picture Vocabulary Test (MPVT) (Taylor, Thurlow, & Turnure, 1974), which is a test for experimental words that was modeled after the PPVT.

The mean PPVT pretest scores were used to assign the classes to the instructional conditions. The nine classes were grouped in blocks of three, such that the first block contained the three classes with the highest mean PPVT

Vocabulary Development of Educable Retarded Children, Arthur M. Taylor, Martha L. Thurlow, James E. Turnure, *Exceptional Children*, Vol. 43 No. 7, April 1977. ©1977 The Council for Exceptional Children.

scores, and so on. The three classes within each block were then randomly assigned to the three instructional conditions. This assignment procedure not only resulted in similar mean PPVT pretest scores for the three instructional conditions but also similar MPVT pretest scores. The mean chronological ages and IQ scores were not significantly different; the overall mean chronological age was 10.0 years (SD = 0.7) and the overall mean IQ was 74.4 (SD = 5.6).

Materials

Three versions of each vocabulary lesson were written to correspond to the three experimental conditions. The lessons for the relational condition involved the use of a relational elaboration in the initial presentation of the vocabulary word and the use of a thematic summary at the end of the lesson. In the nonrelational condition, nonrelational elaborations were used during the initial presentations and also during the nonthematic summary. The mixed condition included nonrelational elaborations followed by a thematic summary.

Of the 15 vocabulary lessons written, 4 each were for the money, time, and written word units, and 3 were for the airplanes unit. Five vocabulary words were taught in each lesson. Lessons were presented on cassette tape recordings while the students followed in textbooks consisting of pictures. The content of the tapes and pictures varied among the three conditions in accordance with the experimental manipulations.

All vocabulary lessons were written in the same format, with the content of the elaborations and summaries being the only source of variation between conditions. (More specific descriptions of the make up of lessons can be found in Taylor, Thurlow, & Turnure, 1974.)

Tests

In this study, the following testing instruments were used to measure either vocabulary development or the use of instructional strategies: PPVT, MPVT, weekly tests, and utilization tests.

The PPVT was used to measure general vocabulary development (i.e., vocabulary not taught in the experimental lessons). For this study, the test was adapted for group administration by using score sheets, and all subjects were tested on the same subset of items. These 44 items were administered as both a pretest and a posttest.

The MPVT was a group administered test containing 27 items, a representative sample of the 75 vocabulary words taught. Changes in MPVT scores from pretest to posttest were used to measure vocabulary growth related to the specific words presented in the instruction.

Weekly tests were group administered tests given at the end of each week to assess the effectiveness of that week's instruction. Each weekly test had two parts—picture recognition and grouping. The picture recognition test required the children to identify pictures of words taught during the week's instruction. The grouping test evaluated the children's ability to remember the words taught in each lesson by asking them to pick from an array made up of two to four pictures of intraunit and/or extraunit intrusions the pictures showing words learned on the same day as a given stimulus picture.

The utilization test was administered individually as a structured interview in which the subject was given a 60 × 40 cm picture of a city scene (Taylor, Thurlow, & Turnure, 1974) that included representations of all 20 words taught in the city unit. The first part of the interview was designed primarily to determine how many of the 20 vocabulary words the subjects would use. The second part of the interview was used to investigate the types of contextual responses the subjects used to describe the picture. Each subject's overall response was judged as to whether or not it was thematic. In addition, all elaborational responses containing vocabulary words were classified as to the type of elaboration represented (relational or nonrelational).

Procedure

Each class was pretested on the PPVT and the MPVT, and then instruction was started. Lessons from each unit that lasted from 30 to 50 minutes were presented the first 4 days of the week. The weekly tests (picture recognition and grouping) were given at the end of each unit by a trained tester.

Instruction was presented over a period of 4 weeks, and all lessons were presented in the same manner. As the children listened to the tape, they referred to their pictures. At the same time, the teacher followed the tape script and monitored student responses.

After all units were completed, each class was posttested on the PPVT, the MPVT, and the utilization test. The utilization test was administered to 54 of the 107 subjects in the study about one month after all other testing. These subjects were the 6 subjects from each class for whom the most complete data were available.

Results

Vocabulary Development

Data related to vocabulary development are presented in Table 1. Changes in PPVT scores were used to assess the hypothesis that all conditions would show general vocabulary development as a result of instruction. The data indicated, however, that only the relational condition showed the expected significant gain from pretest to posttest (t(28) = 1.80, p <.05, one-tailed test). (See Taylor, Thurlow, & Turnure, 1974, for the rationale and derivation of the general and specific hypotheses presented in this section.)

MPVT scores, shown in Table 1, were used to assess specific vocabulary growth. Repeated measures t tests revealed that the gains were significant in all conditions (ps <.001), thus supporting the hypothesis that all conditions would result in specific vocabulary growth.

The data from the weekly picture recognition tests provided information related to the relatively short term effects of the instruction on vocabulary development. Tests on these data confirmed the findings from the MPVT. (See Taylor, Thurlow, & Turnure, 1974, for a discussion of these results.)

Usage of vocabulary was assessed by the first part of the utilization test. One measure of usage taken from this part of the test was the mean number of different vocabulary words used by subjects to describe the picture (maximum = 20). The prediction that subjects in the relational and mixed conditions would use significantly more vocabulary words arose from the assumption that an emphasis on relations would make vocabulary words more available for long term retention. A one-tailed t test of the mean numbers of different words (4.83, 5.55, and 6.06 in the nonrelational, relational, and mixed conditions, respectively) confirmed the hypothesis (t(52) = 1.80, p <.05).

A second measure of vocabulary usage was the total number of vocabulary nouns (including repetitions) used in relation to the total

TABLE 1
Means and Standard Deviations of PPVT [a] and MPVT [b] Pretest and Posttest Scores

Test Condition	Pretest X	Pretest SD	Posttest X	Posttest SD	Gain
PPVT					
Nonrelational	32.19	4.51	32.23	4.84	0.04
Relational	31.75	4.76	33.07	3.97	1.32
Mixed	31.79	5.21	32.68	4.28	0.89
MPVT					
Nonrelational	16.71	2.43	22.57	2.42	5.86
Relational	16.96	2.21	22.39	3.07	5.43
Mixed	16.87	2.00	22.60	2.37	5.73

[a] PPVT = Peabody Picture Vocabulary Test
[b] MPVT = Minnesota Picture Vocabulary Test

number of all nouns used by subjects in their descriptions. It was hypothesized that subjects in the relational condition would use relatively more vocabulary nouns than nonvocabulary nouns in their descriptions. This hypothesis was supported by planned comparisons (F(1,51) = 3.79, p <.05, one-tailed test). The percentages of the total nouns that were vocabulary words were 36.6% in the nonrelational condition, 38.3% in the mixed condition, and 49.6% in the relational condition.

Use of Instructional Strategies

The use of grouping strategies following instruction was partially assessed by means of the weekly grouping test. The mean percentages of pictures correctly grouped on each of the four tests are presented in Table 2. In

3. LINGUISTIC DEVELOPMENT

TABLE 2

Mean Percentages of Pictures Grouped Correctly on Four Weekly Grouping Tests

	Instructional condition		
Weekly test	Relational	Mixed	Nonrelational
City	70.9	69.0	55.9
Written word	92.7	89.2	90.0
Money	76.2	81.2	74.4
Airplanes	80.1	80.1	75.9
Mean percentage	80.0	79.6	74.1

separate t tests conducted to determine if subjects in the conditions receiving thematic summaries (relational and mixed conditions) were better able to group pictures of the vocabulary words according to the lesson within which they were presented than were subjects in the nonrelational condition, 3 of 4 tests revealed significant differences: city—$t(89) = 3.56$, $p < .01$; money—$t(89) = 1.90$, $p < .05$; and airplanes—$t(94) = 1.68$, $p < .05$. The relational and mixed conditions were not found to be significantly different from each other on any of the weekly grouping tests.

The main instrument for assessing strategy usage resulting from the instruction was the second part of the utilization test. The mean number of relational elaborations used to describe the picture was 0.94 ($SD = 1.20$) in the relational condition, 1.22 ($SD = 2.04$) in the mixed condition, and 1.11 ($SD = 1.49$) in the nonrelational condition. As suggested by these means, the number of relational elaborations did not differ with the conditions, and thus, the data failed to support the hypothesis that subjects in the relational and mixed conditions would use significantly more relations than the subjects in the nonrelational condition.

The mean numbers of nonrelational elaborations used in the relational, mixed, and nonrelational conditions were 1.22 ($SD = 1.16$), 3.44 ($SD = 3.43$), and 1.89 ($SD = 1.67$), respectively. Orthogonal t tests were used to test the hypothesis that subjects receiving nonrelational elaborations (mixed and nonrelational conditions) would use significantly more nonrelational elaborations than subjects in the relational condition; this hypothesis was supported ($t(52) = 2.08$, $p < .05$). The remaining orthogonal t test confirmed that this difference was due to the large number of nonrelational elaborations used by subjects in the mixed condition rather than the nonrelational condition ($t(34) = 1.68$, $p < .05$, one-tailed test).

The use of an integration strategy was measured by scoring each subject's complete response to the picture as to whether or not it represented a single integrated (i.e., thematic) story. The proportions of subjects giving an integrated story in the relational, mixed, and nonrelational conditions were .28, .39, and .11, respectively. As hypothesized, a significantly greater proportion of subjects in the two conditions receiving thematic summa-

ries (relational and mixed conditions) told an integrated story about the picture than in the nonrelational condition ($z = 1.74$, $p < .05$, one-tailed test).

Discussion

This study represents an important link between laboratory research on learning strategies and the development of instruction. Although laboratory studies of elaboration have done much to help refine knowledge of this important learning process, investigators have only vaguely intimated ways in which elaboration can actually be applied to classroom materials. This study made a direct attempt to investigate the types of elaborations and the ways in which elaborations can be used more effectively in education. A major purpose of the study was to delineate the effects of elaboration on the development of vocabulary. The finding that subjects in all instructional conditions showed considerable increases in the experimental vocabulary replicates the findings of Ammon and Ammon (1971) and extends their findings to the population of educable mentally retarded children.

The grouping and utilization tests provided measures of whether subjects from the relational and mixed conditions used their experience with different types of summaries and elaborations. The hypothesis that subjects in conditions containing thematic summaries would perform better when asked to group the vocabulary was supported on 3 of 4 weekly grouping tests. The results from the utilization test supported the hypothesis that significantly more of the subjects who had been exposed to integrative stories in the summaries would use such themes in their own responses. Utilization data also indicated that relational elaborations seldom occurred in this test format, with no significant differences across conditions. Nonrelational elaborations (contexts that expanded upon the meaning of a single vocabulary word without relating that word to a second vocabulary word), however, were used significantly more often as descriptive statements by subjects who had received instruction based heavily on nonrelational elaborations.

The findings from this study have their most important implications as they relate to the three instructional conditions, conditions which have direct applicability to the classroom. The subjects in the nonrelational condition, a condition that presented vocabulary instruction in a manner similar to the approach often taken in the classroom, performed essentially as well as subjects in the other conditions on measures of specific vocabulary development but less well on indices of strategy usage and generalized vocabulary development. Subjects in the mixed condition, who received a combination of nonrelational elaborations and thematic summaries, performed better than subjects in the other conditions on the following two measures: number of vocabulary words, and

number of nonrelational elaborations used. Relational condition subjects showed higher performances on other measures (PPVT gains, proportion of vocabulary nouns to other nouns). Both the relational and mixed conditions surpassed the nonrelational condition on organization measures (weekly grouping tests). On the basis of these differential findings, it appears that perhaps the approach selected for vocabulary instruction in the classroom should vary depending upon plans for subsequent usage (e.g., creative expression versus introduction of new subject matter areas) and even on the characteristics of the children being taught. Further study should be undertaken to explore these possibilities.

Recommendations

Several specific recommendations regarding the nature of elaboration based vocabulary instruction can be made as a result of this study. First, the combination of pictorially presented elaborations and audio tape descriptions seems to make an excellent instructional package for the population of educable mentally retarded children. However, the instruction appears to be greatly enhanced when the pictures are simple, easy to read, and present only a single context or relation. Second, it seems that 5 new vocabulary words may be too many to be introduced within one elaboration based vocabulary lesson. Two or 3 new vocabulary words appear to result in the optimal length elaboration based lesson in which adequate development of definitions and relations can be made. However, if previously learned words (i.e., ones that have been defined and elaborated upon) are to be integrated, it would seem that 5 words would result in an appropriate length lesson, a lesson containing only relations designed to summarize previous learning.

With respect to the context of elaboration based vocabulary instruction, it would appear that, for retarded individuals, concrete words are far easier to develop than abstract words. Further, in presenting any one word, only one definition of the word should be presented within a single lesson. Thus, words with multiple definitions (e.g., penny—the only brown coin, the coin that buys less than all the other coins, and the coin equalling one cent) would require several lessons to teach.

Finally, the instruction should have valid testing methods and instruments to identify the current competencies of the children and to properly sequence the instruction. Tests of both expressive and receptive vocabulary, as well as tests for related skill development, should be given to adequately evaluate progress made by the students. Research on these types of assessment methods and instruments is a crucial requirement for promoting the implementation of transitional research, research that is a necessary guide to the appropriate and efficient application of findings from basic research.

Aphasia in Children

Diagnosis and Education

EDNA K. MONSEES

APHASIA in children has been receiving increased attention in recent years. This is partly due to the new techniques and instrumentation for testing hearing, which use electrodermal (EDR) or galvanic skin resistance (PGSR) responses, or electroencephalic responses (EER). These tests are showing, in many instances, a wide discrepancy between the child's sensitivity to sound and his overt responses to and utilization of sound. About ten years ago when wearable hearing aids for children first became a reality, many people hoped that early and continuous use of a hearing aid and intensive auditory training would prevent the "deaf voice quality" and would enable most children to learn speech and language much more easily than had been possible before. Notwithstanding the truly magnificent effects of hearing aids for many thousands of children, we find that our hopes have been only partially realized.

What is aphasia?

Aphasia is the inability to use and/or understand spoken language as a result of defect or damage in the central nervous system. There seems to be wide agreement in this definition.

There is fairly general agreement also that although the aphasic condition is a result of some defect in the central nervous system, evidence of such defect may not be revealed by the usual neurological examination and electroencephalogram. That is, the finding of speech and language disability, with other possible causes ruled out, is in itself evidence of central nervous system disorder.

There are two main types of aphasia —receptive or sensory aphasia and expressive or motor aphasia. In receptive (sensory) aphasia, the child lacks understanding of spoken language, has no expressive speech, and has adequate use of the speech musculature for chewing and other functions. In expressive (motor) aphasia, the child has good understanding of verbal speech, but lacks expressive speech, has adequate use of the speech musculature for chewing, etc., but has partial or complete inability to imitate speech sounds or words. Mixed receptive - expressive aphasia may be diagnosed when the characteristics of both types are present.

Characteristics of Aphasic Children

Credit for focusing attention upon the problems and needs of aphasic children in recent years is due largely to the work of Dr. Helmer Myklebust at Northwestern University and to Miss Mildred McGinnis and Dr. Frank Kleffner at Central Institute for the Deaf. Each has set forth various criteria for diagnosis of aphasia in children and suggestions for training.

In making a differential diagnosis of aphasia both believe it important to rule out mental deficiency and deafness as the cause of the child's failure to talk and/or to understand speech. Performance type psychological tests which do not depend upon the use of verbal language, either in the instructions given or in the responses, are used to detect speech failures due primarily to mental deficiency. Often when it is not possible to obtain satisfactory results on the tests, a child may be accepted for training as an aphasic before definite conclusions about the intelligence level are reached. The problem of ruling out deafness as the cause of the child's failure to speak is much more difficult, and will be discussed in some detail later.

In considering the important factors in making a differential diagnosis of aphasia, various groups emphasize different aspects of the aphasic condition.

Myklebust states that "perhaps the most fundamental problem confronted by the aphasic child is his reduced capacity for normal integration. He sees, hears, and feels; but he cannot integrate this sensory information into an experience pattern which is logical and reliable for purposes of understanding his environment . . . "[8]

CID does not believe the aphasic child to be deficient in this respect, but rather places most emphasis in diagnosis on the nature of the language disability itself. They believe that the main characteristic of the aphasic child is the weakness in memory for speech sounds and for the sequence of sounds in a word and of words in a sentence.[*]

Hardy has expressed this memory factor as follows: "What is most obvious is that they (children with this type of language disorder) cannot naturally listen, understand, store and recall symbolic structures involving a time order and a stress pattern."

It is interesting to note that Orton, writing in 1937, said of what he called "auditory aphasia" or "word deafness": "While these children show many errors of a wide variety of kinds it is clear that their difficulty is in the recalling of words previously heard, for the purpose of recognizing them when heard again or for use in speech, and that one of the outstanding obstacles to such recall is remembering all of the sounds in a word and these sounds in their proper order . . . It is the recall of sounds in proper temporal sequence which seems to be at fault . . ."

Some writers say that motor incoordination or deficiency is characteristic of aphasic children, while others feel that aphasic children have no characteristic motor difficulties.

The behavior of aphasic children has been described by some writers as distractible, disinhibited, and perseverative. Others believe that there is no characteristic behavior pattern in aphasic children, that some show these characteristics and some do not.

Aphasia and Deafness

It is generally agreed that before a diagnosis of aphasia can be made, deafness must be ruled out as an etiological factor in the child's failure to talk and to understand spoken language. In expressive or motor aphasia this usually presents no difficulty, since normal or adequate hearing often can be ascertained through standard pure tone and speech reception threshold testing, as well as by clinical observation. Some receptive aphasics also have observably normal hearing. In the case of other receptive aphasics, however, it is most difficult to ascertain the hearing acuity, particularly since receptive aphasia is in itself an auditory disorder in the broad sense of the term. The child "hears," but is unable to utilize sound and hearing in understanding the speech of others.

Some writers believe that deafness and aphasia can be differentiated on the basis of certain observable behavior of the child. For example, they say that the deaf child uses gesture and an aphasic child does not; or that the deaf child substitutes visual clues and develops understanding of speech through lipreading, while an aphasic child does not. Or they say that the deaf child is consistent in his failure to respond to environmental sounds, while the aphasic child is inconsistent. The writer has found none of these generalizations to be valid guides in differentiating the two groups. In our experience, some aphasic children gesture, as do some deaf children; some of both groups do not. Some deaf children do not develop natural lipreading skills, while some sensory aphasic children on occasion seem to understand speech. A hard of hearing child with an audiogram showing almost normal hearing for the low frequencies and a sharp drop in the middle and high frequencies can be just as baffling to his parents and other observers in his apparent inconsistent responses to sound as the aphasic child.

Hearing tests by standard audiometric techniques as well as by EDR and EER can be almost as unenlightening in differentiating deafness and aphasia. In standard audiometry, the patient is required to indicate by some overt signal whether he does or does not hear the test tone. He indicates that he is aware of the sound—and we know that awareness of sound and sensitivity to sound (or "hearing" the sound) are two quite different things. Hearing tests by EDR and EER audiometry do not require the patient to give any overt voluntary indication of his awareness of the tone. Such tests measure only the sensitivity of the organism to the tones. Recent findings by Hardy and others have shown many cases of children who give every outward appearance of deafness but show normal hearing acuity thresholds when tested by EDR and EER audiometry. There are many instances of children who give fairly consistent audiograms from one test to the next by standard audiometry showing marked hearing loss, but who show normal thresholds by EDR and EER. Hardy says that a large percentage of the children tested in the Hopkins Hearing and Speech Center, brought in for testing because of speech and language problems and suspected deafness, have this type of auditory disorder—that is, normal end-organ or cochlear function, but with what he terms auditory imperception, or central auditory disorder or retrocochlear auditory disorder. He also states that "a great weight of evidence suggests that impairment of the inner ear does not commonly exceed an average loss of 70-75 decibels . . ."

Children who fall into the category of those with abnormal utilization of sound but with normal sensitivity to sound are by no means all of one type in regard to their speech and language learning capacities. Some would consider all such children as aphasic. The writer finds it impossible on the basis of experience to accept this concept of aphasia. We have worked with many such children and find that some of them are able to learn speech and language rapidly, when fitted with a hearing aid and provided with speech instruction that emphasizes auditory training. The following case study illustrates this type of problem:

B. V., now 4½ years old, was seven months old when the parents suspected deafness because of his failure to respond to all except very loud sounds. The prenatal and birth history were negative. There was no blood type incompatability. General development was normal. He had an ear infection at 10 months, measles at two years, and asthmatic bronchitis between the ages of two and three years. When he was 15 months old, the parents began auditory training, using a small amplifier and headphones. At 22 months, he was tested and reported as having a bilateral hearing loss of about 80 db. A hearing aid was recommended, and he has been wearing one continuously since that time. About this time, the parents enrolled him in a class for children with impaired hearing and also began the Tracy Clinic correspondence course. After about one year, the parents felt that he was not benefiting from the class training and the patient began private lessons with us. At this time, he had a large receptive vocabulary and auditory discrimination had begun to develop, but his speech consisted mostly of "dah dah," with near normal voice quality and inflection. We worked on achieving better tongue and lip movement in speech, along with oral language development. After one year, when B. V. was 3½, we discontinued regular lessons because we felt that his speech and language had become almost normal for his age. We recommended continued home training and enrollment in a nursery school with normally hearing children. We now see him at intervals of about three months, and his language has continued to develop exceedingly well under this program. We referred him to Johns Hopkins Hospital for a consulting opinion on his needs. Their audiogram, made by PGSR, shows thresholds between 10 and 25 db for the six frequencies 250 through 8000. Their report reads, in part, as follows:

"This child has independent auditory patterns if sound is loud enough. Interestingly enough, in the sound proofed room, he gave gross response to voice, masking noise, whistle, and animal sounds at a 16 db level. This was not always consistent, however, However, he functions at about a 60 db level without his hearing aid. He identified a tray of objects down to this 60 db level. With his aid worn in his left ear, he identified the same tray of objects at a 30—36 db level. He repeated a P. B. (Phonetically Balanced words) list with amazing accuracy. Most of the errors he made were his own speech substitutions. This proved to be a very interesting auditory problem and there is little doubt but that this is a brain stem problem which lies retrocochlear. . . . Certainly, this child should use moderate gain amplification. . . . It seems that this child should be able to get along in a regular classroom with adequate supportive help. . . . Impression: An intelligent child with a retrocochlear auditory problem which probably lies in the brain stem. It seems to involve an unstable loudness factor. There may be a slight conductive component." They reported also that "his language and speech are a real tool for him." They recommended continuation of the present program and speech therapy in a year or so if it is indicated.

We find that some children with central auditory disorders, such as the example just given, learn rapidly when fitted with a hearing aid and taught by methods commonly used with the deaf and hard of hearing, and with auditory training. Other children do not learn by such methods; these children exhibit the weakness of memory for speech sounds and for the sequence of sounds in words, which CID emphasizes as the crux of the problem of aphasia. In our opinion, diagnosis of aphasia cannot be properly given until after a period of diagnostic teaching which clearly reveals such memory weakness for speech sounds and sequence.

Teaching Methods

A considerable variety of suggestions have been put forth for the teaching of speech and language skills to aphasic children. Myklebust states that children with receptive aphasia usually need training only with inner and receptive language. He believes that children with receptive aphasia will begin using language after they achieve a certain level of receptive language, so that training in expressive language is not required. For children who do not start expressive language naturally, however, he recommends training in expressive language. He does not recommend correction of the child's articulation until his "language usage has met practical communication needs in daily life."[6]

Myklebust's method consists of four stages of training: (1) teaching of inner language as shown by the child's ability to play imaginatively with toys; (2) teaching the child to recognize the names of the toys; (3) teaching the child to recall the names of the toys (giving the right word in response to the question "What is that?"), and (4) at a much later stage, when the child can use speech adequately, teaching correct articulation. The method presents the whole word and words in phrases and sentences, and the child learns these words and phrases through simple repetition of them.

The writer has not seen this method demonstrated at Northwestern, nor had the opportunity to observe the children trained there. However, the method as it is described is the same as that we use in teaching speech and language to preschool deaf and hard of hearing children. In our experience we have found a fairly high percentage of children who fail to learn by this method. The children who do not learn are those who cannot remember a word from one day to the next or even from one hour to the next. They exhibit the poor memory

for the sounds and sequence of sounds discussed above. In the writer's opinion, children who have no memory problem and who learn by the method described, might rather be regarded as having speech problems due to auditory impairment or other factors.

Just as it is true that a diagnostic label may not fully describe a child or his symptoms, so should it be pointed out that children who learn by the whole word—simple repetition method and those who do not learn by this method are not two highly distinct types except at the extremes. There are gradations of ability and disability. That is, a child may not be totally devoid of the ability to learn speech and language by the whole word-simple repetition method of teaching, but he may learn so slowly and articulate so poorly that we would have to say that his problem is more like aphasia than like a speech problem due primarily to auditory impairment, central or peripheral. It is with the children who do exhibit marked deficiency in the ability to remember speech sounds or sequence that the McGinnis-CID method is achieving such successful results.

The CID method which is used for both receptive and expressive aphasia, may be described as follows: the child is taught first to articulate a number of speech sounds, then to produce several sounds in a set sequence and to read and write these sounds in sequence *before* the sequence is identified as a word and associated with the appropriate picture illustrating the word. By means of a highly disciplined and structured system of drills, the child learns first to say, for example, the sound of the letters "b" "oa" and "t." He learns to say them in sequence but separated into three distinct sounds—"b"—oa—t." He learns to read these three sounds in sequence, then to write them, and finally the sequence is associated with a picture of a boat. In order to effect the memory required to recall the sound of each letter, a multi-sensory approach is used: the kineseology of precise articulatory position, the kinesthetic and visual experiences of writing the sound and seeing it in writing. Different colors are used in writing consonants and vowels in the word in order further to emphasize separation and sequence. Thus the weak auditory memory is reinforced by kinesthetic and visual stimuli. The next steps in the process involve learning to read and write the words from memory and to differentiate by auditory stimulation alone among the sounds and letters learned. As soon as an adequate number of words is learned, the building of sentences begins; first the child memorizes the sentences by rote, then learns to

use them in other than drill situations.

Children taught by this method learn to talk, to read, and to write as parts of one integrated process. It is reported that in the process many of them learn to make use of sound so that in time, little or no evidence of auditory disorder remains. Others with more severe auditory disorders, once they have developed means of surmounting the word memory weakness of aphasia, go on to schools or classes for deaf and hard of hearing children where they are able by this time to learn by the methods used in teaching such children.

The Use of Hearing Aids

Several years ago when Dr. Hardy and the staff at Johns Hopkins began to use the term "normal end organ," many people misinterpreted the phrase and construed it to mean "normal hearing." Unfortunately this misinterpretation still persists in some quarters. Hardy has in recent writing begun to clarify the terms, and he states clearly that "normal end organ" and "normal hearing" are not synonymous, that a child may have normal end organ functioning with severe retrocochlear auditory disorder.

Others have erroneously interpreted "auditory imperception," or "retrocochlear auditory disorder" to mean "aphasia." Hardy stresses the fact that these are two separate disorders. One patient may, of course, have a dual handicap of both auditory imperception and aphasia.

No reasonable person would suggest that a child with normal hearing should wear a hearing aid. But there is some disagreement as to the use of hearing aids with aphasic children who also have auditory imperception or perhaps even peripheral hearing loss. Some teachers would postpone the use of amplification or hearing aids for all aphasic children until the language disability has been overcome through training. Hardy feels that a mild gain hearing aid in such cases serves as an "attention centering" device and as such is helpful. The writer's experience leads unhesitatingly to acceptance of the Hopkins view in this regard. A case history of one of our aphasic pupils who also has a retrocochlear auditory problem may serve to illustrate:

R. R., now 6½ years old, was first taken to an otologist at the age of three years because he was not yet talking and because of suspected hearing loss. He was referred for and tested by PGSR and the report stated that "his hearing is in the normal range from 250 through 8000 cycles." The impression was "delayed speech for various reasons" — mostly emotional and complicated by a multilingual situation. Another series of tests was made several months later at another medical center, and this report says, "It is the considered opinion of each of the consultants here that the lack of speech is basically due to his inability to hear, or at least to comprehend what he hears." By the age of 4½, R. had acquired only a few words. He communicated by means of gestures accompanied by jargon. He was examined at still another center at that time, and the diagnosis was "general delayed speech complicated by bilingual models." We had our first contact with him at this time also. We tested his hearing by standard audiometric techniques and obtained fairly clear-cut thresholds of about 60 db. We recommended a hearing aid, which he has been using continuously since that time. Since the family was living outside the country at this time, we instructed the parents in methods of teaching speech and language and suggested enrollment in the Tracy Clinic course. The family returned to Washington to live one year later, when the patient was 5½ years old. He had learned no more than 10 words during the intervening year, and his communication still consisted of elaborate gestures accompanied by meaningless jargon. Our repeated audiograms using standard techniques show some discrepancies, but generally indicate a loss of between 45 and 65 db. We started private lessons at the rate of three a week, and the family gave home training of one-hour daily lessons. We were using the whole word-simple repetition method previously. described, which we had used successfully with hard of hearing children. In a three-month period, R. learned only about twelve words and these were articulated very poorly. We then changed to the method of teaching by phonetic elements and drills leading up to a word. In six weeks of training by this method, R. had learned to recognize by hearing alone, by lipreading alone, and by reading, and could write, four vowel sounds and three consonants. He had also learned six words, which he could read, write, name orally, and match to the correct picture. His progress since then has remained steady and reasonably rapid.

Subsequent testing by EDR audiometry confirms the earlier tests showing normal thresholds. This is no longer interpreted as normal hearing, however, but as a retrocochlear or central auditory disorder. R. continues to wear his hearing aid, and it is of unquestionable benefit to him. Without the aid, he responds only occasionally to speech or to sounds in his environment. During several lessons we tried without the hearing aid, he persistently said "What?" and gestured to indicate he did not hear,

or cupped his hand to his ear. With the aid on, he responds when spoken to, notices other sounds, and attends to his lessons without apparent hearing difficulty. A recent report from Hopkins regarding this child says, in part: "His hearing aid has apparently been of considerable benefit in centering his attention on speech stimuli. . . . The test picture this time was most interesting. In the sound-field of the test room, he responded clearly to a wide variety of stimuli at 10-15 db re normal. These were stable, repeatable responses. By PGSR audiometry, the peripheral function is well in normal range. . . . There is evidently a loudness factor involved, of about 40 db, which suggests an involvement in the central, transmissive pathways. . . . Without doubt, the basic factor is an aphasoid disorder. . . . Whether the present loudness deficit is a true organic involvement or an inhibitory, behavioral thing, is speculative. The fact is that he responds better with the increased loudness of the hearing aid."

On the other hand, we confess to having attempted on two occasions to put hearing aids on children who absolutely rejected them. We concluded that the normal thresholds on the EDR tests in these cases meant truly normal hearing, not merely "normal end organ."

It is our policy to try hearing aids on an experimental basis at first, for all children who do not respond overtly to sound in a normal manner. We believe that a child with normal hearing will not tolerate a hearing aid—unless, perhaps, he has a grossly abnormal personality and drastic measures have been used in the effort to force him to wear an aid. We do not attempt to force any child to wear a hearing aid. Children with central auditory disorders as well as children with peripheral hearing impairment, in our experience, are usually delighted with their hearing aids and apparently get a great deal of help from them.

Planning the Educational Program

Just as there remains much to be discovered and learned about the nature and causes of aphasia in children, there also perhaps remains much to be learned about effective methods of teaching aphasic children. Children in general and the aphasic condition itself are not static. Close cooperation between personnel engaged in diagnosis and teaching is certainly desirable. And within the educational program, flexibility should be provided so that children with similar problems and abilities can be grouped together for teaching, and so that easy transfer from one group to another can be made as the child's needs

change. An ideal school program would provide for transfer, sometimes on a trial basis with supportive teaching and perhaps subsequent complete transfer of children from classes for aphasic children to classes for normal children on the one hand, or classes for deaf or hard of hearing children on the other. This transfer would take place when the training had given the aphasic child mastery over the tools for learning and remembering words and language forms so that he could now learn by the methods used in teaching normal children or deaf or hard of hearing children, as the case might be. There should also be ease of transfer the other way—from classes for normal hearing or hearing handicapped to classes for aphasics. The teaching in all classes, it is hoped, would be both diagnostic and creative, and designed to meet the needs of the individual child.

Summary

To summarize: there is clinically observable a group of children having a language disability characterized by failure to develop speech and/or lack of understanding of spoken language, where the disability cannot be accounted for by intellectual deficiency. In some cases, adequate hearing is evident or readily ascertainable. In other cases, accurate measurement of hearing acuity may be difficult to obtain by standard audiometric techniques, and often shows marked inconsistencies from one test to another or discrepancy between observable hearing and the test results. Tests by EDR and EER audiometry often show normal end-organ functioning or retrocochlear impairment which cannot be expressed in terms of decibels and which is characterized by normal sensitivity to sound but abnormal utilization of or response to sound.

Children in this category—with no speech and/or no understanding of speech, and auditory imperception of central nervous system origin—fall into one or two main groups in terms of their response to training:

In one group are those who through the use of hearing aids and training are able to develop good auditory discrimination fairly rapidly, and who learn to talk and to understand speech by teaching methods that present whole words and achieve memory of these words by simple repetition.

In another group are those children

who cannot remember whole words taught by techniques of simple repetition. These children require special speech memory building techniques which build upon speech sounds, not words, and use a multi-sensory approach of kinesthetic, tactile, visual and auditory stimuli to bolster the weak auditory sensory channel and weak memory. It is for this latter group that we would reserve the use of the diagnosis of aphasia.

Between these two extremes are to be found many gradations of ability and disability in speech and language learning. An adequate educational program would provide groupings of children—normal, hearing handicapped, and aphasic, according to their educational needs and abilities, and would provide the type of training suitable for the group. Such a program would also provide for transfer from one group to another as the needs of the individual child change.

1. Berry, Mildred F.; Eisenson, Jon. *Speech Disorders.* N.Y. Appleton-Century-Crofts, Inc. "Congenital Aphasia," Chap. 17, pp. 420-439.

2. Hardy, William G. "Problems of Audition, Perception and Understanding." *The Volta Review.* Vol. 58, Sept. 1956, pp. 289-300.

3. Karlin, Isaach W. "Aphasias in Children." *A.M.A. Journal of Diseases of Children.* Vol. 87, 1954, pp. 752-767.

4. McGinnis, M. A.; Kleffner, F. R.; Goldstein, R. "Teaching Aphasic Children." *The Volta Review,* Vol. 58. June, 1956, pp. 239-244.

5. McGinnis, Mildred A., "The Association Method for Diagnosis and Treatment of Congenital Aphasia." Unpublished master's dissertation, Washington University, St. Louis, 1939.

6. Myklebust, Helmer. "Training Aphasic Children." *The Volta Review,* Vol. 57, April, 1955, pp. 149-157.

7. Myklebust, Helmer. *Auditory Disorders in Children,* N.Y. Grune & Stratton. 1954.

8. Myklebust, Helmer. "Aphasia in Children—Language Development and Language Pathology" and "Aphasia in Children—Diagnosis and Training," in Travis, Lee. *Handbook of Speech Pathology.* N.Y. Appleton-Century-Crofts, 1957, pp. 503-530.

9. Myklebust, Helmer R. "Language Training and a Comparison Between Children with Aphasia and Those with Deafness," *American Annals of the Deaf,* Vol. 101, No. 2, March 1956.

10. Orton, Samuel R. *Reading, Writing and Speech Problems in Children.* N.Y., W. W. Norton Co. 1937.

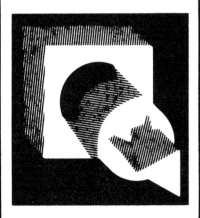

Murdering Our Mother Tongue

Condensed from "Strictly Speaking"
Edwin Newman

Edwin Newman is an NBC News correspondent and commentator.

Language is in a decline. The evidence is all around us. Most conversation these days is as pleasing to the ear as a Flash-Frozen Wonder Dinner is to the palate— "You've got to be kidding," "How does that grab you?" "Just for openers," "No way," "Is he for real?" "Like I mean," "Would you believe?" "Out of sight."

John Lindsay, former mayor of New York City, once said that his youngest child would go to a boys' school because "he needs peer stuff," and Kevin White, mayor of Boston, talks about "young juveniles." An official of the Office of Economic Opportunity was quoted as saying, "That's the loggerhead no one has yet gotten past." Dr. Oscar Sussman of the New Jersey State Health Department wondered aloud during a television interview, "Can we stop something, preventive-medicinewise, from happening?" And the New York *Times* speaks of Jim Palmer of Baltimore and Vida Blue of Oakland engaging in a "flaunted pitching classic."

Unquestionably, a world without mistakes would be less fun. I cherish the memory of the Long Island Railroad union leader who felt he was chasing "Willie the Wisp" during contract negotiations, also of a colleague in the Navy in World War II who wanted to know what a "lert" was, inasmuch as we were about to go on one. But a mistake is one thing, impreciseness another. Watergate, in the course of revealing so much else about American life, also revealed a poverty of expression, an addiction to a language that was al-most denatured. In addition to "at that point in time," John Ehrlichman spoke of "that time era," and John Mitchell of "that time frame." A discussion never took place before or after a particular date. It was always "prior to" or "subsequent to."

In March 1974, the White House press secretary, Ron Ziegler, explained a request for a four-day extension of a subpoena from the Watergate prosecutor for certain files. The extension was needed, Ziegler said, so that James St. Clair, President Nixon's attorney, could "evaluate and make a judgment in terms of a response." One wonders why he didn't say that the man wanted more time to think about it.

Language used to obfuscate or conceal or dress with false dignity is not confined to politics. We love to pump air into the language and make it soft and gaseous. Newsmen borrow the style from those they consider authoritative, such as the Air Force general who spoke one day about the nuclear deterrent—it deterred so well, the general said, that the Russians were "not in a position to attack us with any confidence factor." He did not say the Russians lacked confidence. They lacked a "confidence factor."

The war in Indochina produced a host of terms that "media folks," as Mayor Richard Daley of Chicago once called us, accepted at our peril —"protective reaction strike," "interdiction," "surgical bombing," "contingency capability," and "new-life hamlet" (which in sterner days was a refugee camp). Weathermen once spoke of thunderstorms. Thun-

---

Among all the English-speaking countries, we are the one that the others fear will drown in an ocean of verbosity. In our country, we don't have rain. We have "precipitation activity." In many countries, babies talk. We have "age groups that verbalize."

Whenever we see four or five gathered together on a television panel, we hear people who have nothing much to say, and say it in words of six syllables. We are known abroad, but don't seem to know it at home, for having the gift that Winston Churchill attributed to the first Labor prime minister of Great Britain: "He has the gift of compressing the largest amount of words into the smallest amount of thought."

If you think our politicians are verbose—and they are among the most gaseous windbags in the Western world—they are surpassed by sociologists and often by teachers and critics of the arts. For sheer gastric distention of the mind, nothing can equal a tribute or a manifesto written by the friend of an artist who is having his first one-man show.

The only bit of advice I leave you with is a sentence from Winston Churchill: "The short words are best, and the old words when short are best of all."

—Alistair Cooke, in a commencement address at the Maryland Institute, College of Art, in Baltimore

   "Murdering Our Mother Tongue," Edwin Newman, *Reader's Digest*, Vol. 105 No. 632, December 1974. ©1974 Edwin Newman.

derstorms were pumped up to "thunderstorm activity," then to "major thunderstorm activity." In the same way, headwinds no longer delay commercial airlines. "Head-wind components" do.

This desire for weightiness also creeps into the language of business. Triple and quadruple phrases come into being—"high retention characteristics," "process knowledge rate development," "antidilutive common-stock equivalents." In its report on 1972, the Allegheny Power System told its shareholders: "In the last analysis, the former, or front-end, process seems more desirable because the latter, or back-end, process is likely to create its own environmental approaches."

Benjamin Franklin was asked what kind of government the Constitutional Convention was giving the country. He replied, "A republic —if you can keep it." We were also given a language, and there is a competition in throwing it away.

I have in mind "Y'know." The prevalence of Y'know is one of the most far-reaching and depressing developments of our time, disfiguring conversation wherever you go. I take part in meetings where persons of high rank and station, with salaries to match, say almost nothing else. Some people collapse into Y'know after giving up trying to say what they mean; others scatter it broadside. For a while, I thought it clever to ask people who were spattering me with Y'knows why, if I knew, were they telling me? After having lunch alone with some regularity, I dropped the question.

To choose a lower order of speech conveys, I suppose, a certain scorn for organized, grammatical and precise expression. Object to it and you are likely to be told that you are a pedant, a crank, an elitist, and behind the times. "Right on," "up-tight" and "chicken out," to take only a few examples, are looked upon as vivid phrases that enrich and renew the language. They do enrich it, but they are exhausted, very rapidly, by overuse. When that happens, they wrinkle into clichés before our eyes.

We have a foreign influence in the United States, too, as may be seen from the free use of the word gourmet, which the dictionary defines as a connoisseur in eating and drinking. A noun, in other words. But in the United States it is used more frequently as an adjective. Foods that used to be known as delicacies are now known as gourmet foods, and you get them at a gourmet store.

Language sets the tone of our society. Since we must speak and read, and spend much of our lives doing so, it seems sensible to get some pleasure and inspiration from these activities. The wisecrack is a wonderful thing, and the colorful phrase, and the flight of fancy. So is the accurate description of a place or an event, and so is the careful formulation of an idea. They brighten the world. Direct and precise language—if people could be persuaded to try it—would make conversations more interesting, which is no small thing; would help to substitute facts for bluster, also no small thing; and would promote the practice of organized thought and even of occasional silence, which would be an immeasurable blessing.

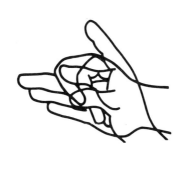

Home Language Training Program for Dysacusic and Aphasic Children

EDWARD G. SCAGLIOTTA

The Midland School in New Jersey has inaugurated a general guide to be used as the foundation for a home training program which will help dysacusic and aphasic children and their parents. The program not only helps the child attain a language foundation which prepares him for school, but it also helps the parents understand their child and the problems he experiences as he emerges from his silent world. The outline covers auditory training, voice, speech, and language development. It is replete with concrete suggestions in all these areas.

THE primary function of the home training program is to provide the child with an opportunity for continued application of learned speech, language, and related experiences in the home environment. It is a foundation supplement upon which the framework of communication is laid.

In addition, it conveys to the parents the course of action undertaken in the school program and provides concrete experiences and activities to initiate and maintain their active participation. Through this pragmatic approach, the home training program serves to mold and blend harmoniously the emotions that bind the child and parents, and as the child begins to emerge from his silent world the home becomes a better place in which to live.

The following outline is merely a general guide to elicit the child's response. Every child will not respond to all areas. What is applicable, utilize, what is not applicable, improvise.

A. Training for Auditory Figure-Ground Discrimination

1. Provide experience for identifying gross sounds (drum, clicker, bell, horn, etc., and especially incidental gross sounds such as a bursting paper bag or radiator hiss).

2. Provide experience for finer discrimination (rustling of paper, marbles in can or box, ticking of alarm clock, etc.).

3. Develop awareness to voice and speech (1/4" rubber hose attached to funnel—insert end into ear and speak directly into funnel part of apparatus).

    a) Maintain music as background while eliciting sounds or words as the auditory stimuli.

First attempt each of these activities in full view of the child; later have him turn his back and identify each sound.

B. Auditory Perception

1. Training for pitch, intensity and tempo.

    a. *Pitch*—high or low sounds.

        1) Pantomime — child holds hand over head for high pitch; holds hand near the floor for low sounds.

        2) On a sheet of paper the child draws a horizontal line at the top for high pitch and a similar line at the bottom for low pitch.

    b. *Intensity*—loud or soft sounds.

        1) Pantomime — child cups hands around mouth for loud sounds; holds index finger vertically across lips for soft sounds.

        2) On a sheet of paper the child draws long vertical lines for loud sounds and short vertical lines for soft sounds.

    c. *Tempo*—fast or slow.

        1) Pantomime — child makes imaginary circles in the air with his arm, rotating slowly for slow tempo, rotating rapidly for fast tempo.

        2) On a sheet of paper the child rapidly draws short diagonal lines for slow tempo.

        3) Child imitates the fast or slow rhythm on his own instrument (tambourine or drum).

C. Voice and Speech

1. Provide experience in imitating various animal and environmental sounds.

cow	— moo, moo
lamb	— baa, baa
pig	— oink, oink
hammer	— bang, bang
bell	— ding, ding
horn	— honk, honk

    a. Child may pick up an appropriate toy in conjunction with the sound.

2. Imitation of the consonant elements of the alphabet.

    a. To facilitate the child's ability to produce, comprehend and recall each element, identify each speech sound with some animal, human, cartoon character, or environmental sound.

    b. Consonant elements and activities.

1) Tactile sense — If specific tactile stimulus is not indicated, it is advantageous for the child to place the palm of his hand on the cheek of the speaker.

m —Mosquito sound (continuous "mmm" sound). Have the child hold index finger against one nostril and hum "mmm" as a mosquito.

s —Silly Snake sound ("ssss"). Have the child fill his cheeks with air and slowly expel as a hissing snake. (Draw a silly looking snake shaped in an "S" form.)

l —Singing Lady sound ("lah-lah-lah"). Have the child lift his tongue up and behind the upper front teeth and sing "lah-lah-lah."

p —Motor Boat sound ("puh-puh-puh"). Give the child a narrow strip of paper, which is to be held vertically under the nostrils. Make the paper move by saying "puh-puh-puh"— the motor boat sound.

j —Jumping Jim sound— ("ju-ju-ju"). Jumping Jim is a frog who calls to his frog friends. With lips pushed together and tongue pressed against the teeth, he calls "ju-ju-ju."

r —Ready Rocket sound ("errr"). Ready Rocket is poised on the launching pad, awaiting blast off time. 4-3-2-1-0 Blast Off! Child responds by providing rocket sound "errrr."

b —Babbling Baby sound ("buh-buh-buh"). Babbling Baby has not yet learned to say words. His only response is "buh, buh, buh."

n —Neighing Nellie sound ("neigh, neigh"). Nellie neighs "thank-you" whenever someone gives her sugar. (Give the child a small piece of candy to elicit "neigh-neigh.")

sh—Shaking Shirley sound ("shhh"). Shaking Shirley will only stop shaking when someone holds his index finger vertically across his lips and says "shhh."

d —Woody Woodpecker sound — ("di-di-di"). Have child hold tongue tightly against palate and make the sound of Woody Woodpecker pecking in a tree for insects.

ch—Train sound ("cha-chi-choo, cha-chi-choo"). Play train—have child alternately extend arms; first slowly, then more rapidly as the train picks up speed.

f —Funny Fish sound ("ffff"). Have child bite lower lip and blow "a bubble" as Funny Fish often does—"fffff."

v —Kazoo sound ("vvvv"). Place a sheet of tissue paper over a comb and have child "sing" the "v-v-v" sound. (Make certain the child does not say "vee", just "vvv.")

t —Talking Tess sound ("ti-ti-ti"). Have the child imitate Tess who talks incessantly saying "ti-ti; ti-ti; ti; ti-ti; ti; ti-ti; ti." (Concentrate on voice inflection.)

k —(Hard 'c') Cold Crow sound ("cuh-cuh-cuh"). Show the child how to firmly hold his tongue tip below the front teeth. Cold Crow is so cold his tongue becomes stuck tightly under his bottom teeth and can only say softly "cuh-cuh-cuh."
Soft 'c' has the same sound as 's.'

g —(Hard) Goofy Goat sound ("guh-guh-guh"). Goofy Goat has a sore throat and cannot bleat. The only sound he can make is "guh-guh-guh" way back in his throat. Soft 'g' has the same sound as 'j.'

h —Panting Boy ("hhhh"). Have the child pretend he has just completed a long fast foot race and is very tired. Show him how to breathe in deeply and pant.

w —Wind Sound—("oooo"). Have the child moisten his index finger. Using the "unvoiced o sound." have the child feel the cooling effect of the wind on his finger.

th—(voiced) Racing Car sound ("thhhh"). With the tongue protruded slightly between the teeth, have the child hold his finger on his tongue tip and feel the roar of the Racing Car engine.

th—(unvoiced) Radiator sound ("thhhh"). Have the child place his tongue just slightly between his teeth and then blow to feel the steam escaping from the radiator. (If steam radiators are available have the child feel the steam escaping from the safety valve, then allow him to feel his own escaping breath.)

z —Buzzing Bee sound ("zzzz"). Place between the child's teeth a narrow strip of paper. Have the child then pretend he is a bee and must say "zzzzzz" as he flies about looking for flowers.

y —Cowboy Yell ("yi-yi-yi"). Pretend to be cowboys. Straddle a chair and gallop away shouting "yi-yi-yi." (Wearing a cowboy hat may better set the stage.)

ng—Martian sound ("ing-ong-ung"). Have the child pretend he has just landed his space ship on Mars. As he climbs down from his space ship he meets a Martian creature who greets him with "ing-ong-ung."

3. Auditory Recall

a. Making use of animal, instrument or environmental sounds already learned, have the child listen with his back turned and attempt to identify the sound. (Child may respond by selecting appropriate object or picture.)

b. Prepare cards with markings

3. LINGUISTIC DEVELOPMENT

used in section B, part 1 of this outline (pitch and intensity). Place the cards in front of the child and continue as stated above.

c. Recall through repetition.
   1) Nonsense syllables. "ing-ong-ung," "cha-chi-choo," etc.

   2) A series of number digits "five, six, seven," etc.

   3) A phrase or short sentence. "I want a cookie." "On the table," etc.

D. Speech Motor Skills

1. Encourage smiling, laughing, sneezing, coughing, swallowing, crying, chewing, and yawning. Having the child observe self in mirror may prove advantageous.

2. Elicit spontaneous babbling making use of the phonetical elements listed under section C of this outline.

3. Physical Exercises

   a. Rotate head to the right, back, left and front.

   b. Drop the head forward as far as possible, then raise and tilt back as far as possible.

   c. Shake head from right to left.

4. Breathing Exercises

   a. Inhale and exhale through the nose with mouth closed.

   b. Inhale through the nose and exhale through the mouth; direct the breath on a strip of paper held vertically under the nose. Attempt to have the child maintain a steady flow of air.

   c. Have the child blow down paper animals, a ping pong ball across the floor, or blow out candles.

5. Voice Production Exercises

   a. Have the child imitate extended consonants already learned (lalalalala — jujujujujuju — etc.).

   b. Combine and vary with other vowel sounds (la le lo, ba, be, bo, lo la le, bu ba bo—etc.)

   c. Sing meaningless nonsense syllables or number digits.

6. Articulation

   a. Chewing—This exercise utilizes the same muscles used for speech. First eliminate the

voice, then later add voice. (The child's diet should always include coarse foods such as raw carrots, celery, apple, etc.)

b. Jaw exercises—
   1) Raise and lower the jaw.

   2) Move the jaw from right to left; slowly at first, then more rapidly.

c. Lip exercises—
   1) Show the child how to pout.

   2) Form an "O" with the lips; relax, then repeat.

   3) Pick up objects with the lips alone; drop the object and repeat.

d. Tongue Exercises—
   1) Protrude and retract the tongue; try to touch your nose!

   2) Move the tongue up and down and from side to side.

   3) Roll the tongue and protrude.

   4) Protrude the tongue and move from side to side.

   5) Protrude the tongue and bite gently — (similar to pronouncing the "th" sound).

E. Language Development

1. Introduce all words in conjunction with an object, picture, event, or situation. Orally give the name and attempt to elicit comprehension. Follow by introducing the work on a printed card. Matching the printed card to the object, picture, event, or situation is often advantageous. Save all the word cards for memory and recall exercises.

2. Instruct the child in the use of various environmental objects: hammer, fork, brush, comb, broom, and so forth.

3. Matching — either purchase the many matching activities sold at the local department store or construct your own.

   a. Matching sequence:
      1. Object to object.
      2. Object to picture.
      3. Picture to picture.
      4. Picture to word.
      5. Word to word.
      6. Word alone.

4. Provide the child with a chalkboard on which he can experiment.

5. Tactile and Kinesthetic fortification.

   a. Place several familiar, dissimilar objects in an opaque bag (2 or 3 at first.). Through touch alone have the child select the object you name, or have the child select the object after looking at a printed name card.

   b. Using medium grit sandpaper cut out letters of the alphabet both in upper (8″ size) and lower (4″ size) case, and mount on hardboard. Hand guiding may be required initially. Upon acquisition of a specific letter form, have the child attempt to transfer this activity to another media (formation of letters in the air, on chalkboard, on paper, in clay, etc.).

   c. Comparisons: Consistency (sand, flour, marble), texture (sandpaper, fur, satin, etc.), and degree (hot or cold) should be utilized to provide many tactile experiences for the child. A specific learning situation may be established or accomplished incidentally as the situation arises.

6. Quantitative Language Conceptualization.

   a. Develop a series of language activities based on environmental happenings similar to the example below.

Question	Response
What is it doing outside?	It is raining.
From where does the rain come?	From the clouds.
Where are the clouds?	Up in the sky.
What color are the clouds?	White (or gray).
What do you wear when it rains?	Response to this question will vary.

   b. If the child requests his wants and desires in one word form, attempt to provide him with desired question, i.e.:
      1) Child asks, "milk?"
      2) Parent provides the proper interrogative form, "May I have some milk?" Have the child attempt the full question. Accept gratefully his attempt to respond.

c. For the child who has some speech and language, be *ever* prepared to question him about his environment. Utilize this approach on an incidental and informal basis during the course of the day, i.e.:

1) What color are your carrots?
2) Is the stove hot or cold?
3) What is father doing?
4) How many cookies do you want?

7. Concrete and Abstract Commands.

a. Concrete commands: jump, hop, skip, walk, march, dance, put, look, show, run, etc. Utilize these commands in conjunction and correlated with a play or rhythm activity. Cards printed with these commands may be necessary to elicit response.

b. Abstract commands: in, on, under, over, where, who, on top of, how, why, into, etc. Put the ball *on* the table; *into* the box, *under* the table, etc.

8. Expansion of Child's Environment.

a. Trips are extremely meaningful—farms, zoos, museums, firehouses, pet shops, libraries, etc., provide excellent source material for both receptive and expressive language development.

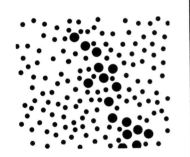

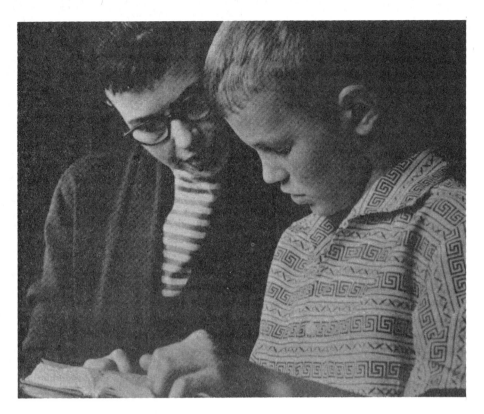

A Tangibly Reinforced
Speech Reception
Threshold Procedure for
Use With Small Children

Frederick N. Martin   Sherry Coombes

Evaluating the hearing thresholds of very young children is one of the most difficult tasks assigned to the audiologist. Traditionally pure-tone stimuli have been used in testing young children. Relatively few efforts have been directed toward testing for speech reception threshold (SRT). SRT testing, however, may be desirable for the following reasons: (1) speech materials have higher face validity for the evaluation of communicative skills than do nonspeech items (Bunch, 1934; Hardy and Pauls, 1950); (2) often there is greater success in obtaining responses to speech than to pure tones (Giolas, 1969; Hodgson, 1972); (3) closer attention is generally given to verbal stimuli than to nonverbal materials (Ewing and Ewing, 1944; Hardy and Bordley, 1951); (4) SRT scores aid in the confirmation of pure-tone thresholds (Carhart, 1946; Ventry, Chaiklin, and Dixon, 1971); and (5) speech is a more concrete test stimulus since it is usual in the acoustic environment where pure tones are not.

Although SRT testing of children is desirable, the literature discloses a lack of consistency in obtaining SRTs on subjects below the age of four years (Keaster, 1947; Siegenthaler, Pearson, and Lezak, 1954; Meyerson, 1956;

Griffing, Simonton, and Hedgecock, 1967). The most widely used procedure appears to be the Meyerson (1956) technique of having the child point to pictures of the spondaic stimulus words, but this method is frequently unsatisfactory with prekindergarten subjects.

Training the young child to respond to controlled sound stimuli often takes the form of operant conditioning. Operant behavior must be defined in terms of emitted responses, those which are willful or voluntary. Operant conditioning in audiometry differs from its classical use in learning in that the subject is not allowed complete control of initial responses to a stimulus. In audiometry the subject must be supplied with some form of verbal or visual instruction, including physical guidance, to obtain a desired response. Operant conditioning in audiometry therefore transcends its original Skinnerian definition.

In operant conditioning terms a reinforcer is any event which increases the probability of a response. Reinforcers may be tangible, that is, an object which has appraised value such as an edible item or a token. In audiometry most reinforcers are intangible, such as a nod or smile from the examiner. A structured method for difficult-to-test patients was realized by Lloyd, Spradlin, and Reid (1968) in a procedure called TROCA (Tangible Reinforcement Operant Conditioning Audiometry). The procedure consisted of (1) determining the reinforcer (either an edible or nonedible item); (2) initial training; (3) sound field screening; and (4) bilateral screening and threshold determination. Using profoundly retarded subjects, tangible reinforcers showed improved results over visual (intangible) reinforcers in obtaining responses to auditory stimuli.

Immediately prior to the present study a new device was developed by one of us (FNM) which attempts to alleviate some of the various problems encountered in determining SRTs of very young children. The present research was designed to investigate the efficacy of this device as used with a type of operant conditioning audiometry.

PROCEDURE

Response Device

The test device was a multicolored clown, approximately 48 inches in height, constructed of pressboard, and mounted on the wall of the test room. The clown consisted of 19 separate, manually depressible parts with a microswitch located behind each part. The microswitches were connected to a control box situated in the examiner's room. Twelve buttons, each labeled with a different clown part, were located on the control box. The discrepancy between the number of parts on the clown and those labeled on the control device was due to paired items such as legs, feet, or ears which were individually, yet identically wired. When a part was touched, an electrical circuit was completed and registered in the control box which acted as a decoder. Correct identification of a clown part was identified by a blue light labeled "correct" on the control device. A red light labeled "error" signaled the depression of a part other than the one programmed. Only one stimulus button could be depressed at any given time. Depression of a reset button, accompanied by a green "ready" light cleared the circuits for reprogramming. A feeder tube was situated behind the clown's right arm so that small chocolate candies could be emptied into a cup held in the clown's right hand. A switch on the control box allowed for automatic and instant release of one candy into the cup each time the correct switch was depressed and the circuit completed. An option for a partial reinforcement schedule was possible with the switch set to "manual." With the manual setting, depression of a release button on the control box was necessary to activate the feeder tube. The clown was

3. LINGUISTIC DEVELOPMENT

wired so that a light flashed above the cup to signal to the child that a reward had been presented.

Subjects

Forty normal-hearing monolingual children between the ages of 17–56 months served as subjects for our study. All of the children were from middle or upper-middle class environments. Parents were interviewed prior to testing to ascertain that there was no history of ear disease and that age of onset of speech and motor activities was normal. For purposes of analysis the subjects were grouped by age into four categories. Each age-group consisted of five males and five females. The youngest age-group ranged from 17–20 months, the second age-group ranged from 27–33 months. Age-group number three ranged from 39–45 months, and the oldest group ranged from 51–56 months.

Method

Initially all subjects were led into the test room where the examiner pointed to and named each separate part of the clown. Before the examiner left the room the subject was informed that he would often receive candy from the clown if he did as the voice instructed.

Stimulus items were played on a cassette recorder (Wollensak 4760) with an output to the audiometer. Level and linearity calibration were accomplished each day with the usual electronic equipment.

Twelve words were used as stimuli in our test: hair, hat, ball (held in the clown's hand), hand, eye, nose, ear, foot, arm, leg, tummy, and mouth. Because all our children were residents of Texas we departed from the traditional speaker with general American dialect and chose to use a speaker with a central Texas dialect (SC). All stimulus words were recorded 10 dB below the carrier phrase "Put your hand on the _____." A 10-sec pause was left between the stimulus word and the initiation of the next carrier phrase. Several scramblings of the 12 words were recorded. All testing was performed in a two-room, double-walled acoustic suite, with ambient noise levels in both rooms below 45 dBC. The experimenters sat in a separate room from the subject, although a window allowed visual supervision. The tests were administered with a speech audiometer (Grason-Stadler 1701) with a sound field system calibrated so that 0 dB HTL was equal to 13 dB SPL at a distance of three feet from the loud-speaker.

The experimental procedure included two related phases: a conditioning period and threshold determination. Initial training consisted of presentation of the stimulus words at 40 dB HTL, until the child demonstrated five correct responses in five consecutive presentations. It was felt from the interview with the parents that all the stimulus words were within each child's vocabulary. A correct response consisted of manual depression of the clown part which was named in the preceding stimulus sentence.

During the conditioning period the reinforcement switch on the control box remained set on "automatic" so that reinforcers were delivered on a continuous reinforcement schedule. Reward was automatically withheld if the subject responded (1) in the absence of a stimulus, (2) incorrectly to a stimulus, or (3) by depressing more than one clown part in response to a stimulus.

Modeling by the parents was often necessary before the younger children would attempt the task. Parents were instructed in advance that they should initially aid their children if it was necessary. Prompting, by taking the child's hand and touching it to the clown part named, also proved a valuable aid in establishing responses in some cases.

The test procedure was constructed from the same paradigm as the conditioning procedure with the exceptions of variations in the intensities of the stimuli and introduction of a variable-ratio schedule of reinforcement. Before the intensity was lowered it was determined that the subject was under control for the new contingency of less than 100% reinforcement. Then, employing a descending intensity method, the first stimulus item was presented at 25 dB HTL, followed by intensity decrements of 15 dB until the first incorrect response was obtained. From that point the intensity was increased 5 dB with each incorrect response and decreased 10 dB with each correct response. This procedure was followed until the subject indicated a level at which he responded to at least three of six stimulus words. Threshold was then defined as the level at which the subject responded correctly to at least 50% of the words presented to him. This method of ascertaining threshold also served to assure the examiner that the threshold score was indeed a hearing threshold and not the point in the test where the subject ceased to be under stimulus control due to fatigue, reinforcement saturation, or other factors. Correct responses at a 5-dB increment over the intensity of an incorrect response indicated that conditioning was still intact at the lower intensities. A variable-ratio schedule on an average of every third correct response was sufficient for most of the children.

RESULTS

Ninety percent of the two-and-one-half-year-old subjects were successfully evaluated while the remaining male child in this age-group did not meet the conditioning criteria and, therefore, did not yield an SRT. Thresholds were evaluated on all 20 of the three- and four-year-old children, however our procedure was totally unsuccessful with the one-and-one-half-year-old children, as no thresholds were determined for either sex.

DISCUSSION

We recognize that there are aspects of this study that violate some of the rules of operant conditioning, specifically with regard to the reinforcer we used. We would not argue with those who would claim that edible items are frequently inappropriate reinforcers, or even that tangibles only tend to be more reinforcing than intangibles. In fact, the subject himself should determine his own reward. The lack of conditioning for our youngest group might be explained on the basis of our operant model rather than immaturity or distractibility. The next version of our test device takes some of these problems into consideration. Our original plan was to see whether the basic concept of tangibly reinforced operant speech audiometry was workable with our device. We found that it was, and suggest it as an addition to the battery of tests for small children and not as a replacement for other, more traditional measures such as TROCA, COR, or different versions of play audiometry.

We are aware that the children who were successfully tested in this study could probably have been evaluated by more traditional means, without the requirement of a highly specialized device. Since our procedure worked well with normal young children we are encouraged to proceed with our initial goal in evaluating the hearing of mentally retarded and other difficult-to-test children. We are presently comparing our methodology with other procedures for these children.

Helping your child
speak correctly

John E. Bryant

*John E. Bryant is Director of Speech and Hearing Services at
the Mid-Island Speech and Hearing Center, Commack, New York.
. . . Illustrations by Anna Marie Magagna.*

"My five-year-old son has been talking for only a little more than a year. It's not easy to understand him. Recently, his kindergarten teacher told me his speech was very slow in developing and that I should be concerned. In every other respect he does things as well as the other children. He is learning his numbers and letters and how to write his own name. Should I really be concerned? Won't he just grow out of his speech problem?"

These questions were asked by Mrs. Peters. We shall try to answer them and also broaden the discussion to cover the entire topic of developing good speech patterns in children. This is an area too little known to the general public and one that many parents should be aware of in order to help their own children speak correctly.

It is possible for a child to have normal intelligence and still be slow in developing his speech patterns. Any number of things can impede his speech development. An overprotective mother, one who anticipates his every need, can make it unnecessary for her child to talk. He may find it far easier simply to point and gesture.

Some children have poor speech because early childhood illnesses limited their activities. The fewer experiences a child has with other children and adults, and the smaller his world is, the smaller his vocabulary.

These are merely a few of the causes of delayed speech development. Before we examine some others, it may be helpful to look first at the way a child learns to talk. This should help us understand what can cause a child's speech to be delayed.

NORMAL DEVELOPMENT OF SPEECH

Have you ever tried to answer the question: when did your child learn to talk? It is almost impossible to answer because the onset of speech in most children follows the mastery of a series of skills that begins the moment the child is born. The birth cry and subsequent crying help the baby to develop the fundamental skill of taking in air quickly and letting it out slowly while making a voiced sound. These early cries usually are cries of discomfort caused by hunger, pain, and wet diapers. They all tend to sound alike. But near the end of three months, the baby begins to make slight variations in his crying as his needs differ. This enables most mothers to tell their child's hungry cry from his wet one.

Before the child is six months old he may begin to make sounds when he is comfortable. These sounds, or babbling, provide the child with lip, tongue, and jaw exercise which helps prepare him for speech. The sounds may include *da da da da* and *ma ma ma ma*. It should be pointed out, to the disappointment of many parents, that these sounds are not real words and that the child is not calling his father or mother.

Before he is nine months old, the child starts to add inflection to his increased babbling. It is not unusual to hear an eight- or nine-month-old child imitate the demanding, questioning, and consoling inflections that adults use as they talk to each other. At this age the child may also begin using a higher pitch, much to his parents' chagrin, and may begin yelling to get attention.

Somewhere between ten and 18 months, the average child may say his first real words. But before he says them, you may notice that he attempts to imitate more often, especially if you interrupt his vocal play by saying the sound he is saying. This can stimulate him to imitate you and to continue making the sounds. He may even imitate some words that you introduce into his vocal play. He gestures a lot as he says his first words; and often he may use one word to mean many things. For example, *kah* may refer to cat, cup, and cookie.

The child continues to enjoy vocal play when he is alone; he also continues to echo much of what is said to him. He may begin to use a lot of unintelligible words and sounds when conversing with his toys or parents. These are unintelligible because he has not yet developed the vocabulary needed to express himself. As he manipulates new toys or objects, we generally supply him with their names. He begins to associate words with objects, and will use a word over and over until it is his. This is the way he builds his vocabulary.

At about the age of two, the child begins using speech to communicate. He says new words, but his articulation is faulty. He begins to build sentences, but his grammar is poor. He usually speaks too loudly, and he may not have very much conversational rhythm, but he will be *talking!*

CAN PARENTS HELP?

Not only can parents help, but they should help. In many cases parents can prevent speech problems by spending more time with the child and patiently correcting his errors. Certainly, parents can encourage normal development of speech, and, in cases where their children have defective speech, assist in the corrective program.

encouraging normal speech

As parents we spend a good deal of our time teaching our children. We teach them to use the toilet, to dress and feed themselves, to brush their teeth, and to put their toys away. But we seldom deliberately teach our children to talk. Isn't it strange that something as important as language and speech is left to chance? Most parents prefer to allow their children to learn to talk at their own speed. It is wise not to rush the child into learning skills he is not mature enough to handle, but simply letting him learn to talk at his own speed is as much a mistake as setting unrealistic goals. It ignores the fact that speech is learned and that it can and should be taught.

Parents who try to teach their children to talk generally do so by adding new words to the child's vocabulary, helping him with his pronunciation, and teaching him to correct himself when he makes a mistake.

vocabulary development

There are several ways to build larger vocabularies. A most common method is pointing out and naming objects in picture books. The best books use realistic, brightly colored pictures and have, preferably, only one picture to a page.

Another easy method is to make a game of naming objects. It can be played in the home, in the yard, anywhere — the more places the better. When the child touches or feels the object being named, it helps him build up associations. If he hears the *clock* ticking, or throws the *ball*, or feels Mommy's *hair*, he will find it easier to remember the words.

There are many opportunities to teach new words every day. For example, when the child hesitates over a word, his parents should supply the word along with a simple definition of it that he can understand.

teaching speech sounds

Speech sounds usually develop in sequence. Some are more difficult than others. Many young children have difficulty with the (s) sound, substituting (th) for (s) as in "Thilly Thally" for "Silly Sally," while relatively few children will have trouble with the (p) sound. This is because the ability to produce the (s) sound develops later than does that of the (p) sound. When testing a child's articulation skills, speech therapists use a developmental guide similar to the one printed below. This guide shows the usual order of development of sounds. A child is considered to have a speech problem if he is unable to say the sounds at the age listed.

Age	Sounds
3½	(m), (b), (p), (h), (w)
4½	(k), (g), (t), (d), (n), (ng), (y)
5½	(f), (v)
6½	(sh), (zh), (l), (th voiced)
7½	(s), (z), (r), (th voiceless), (ch), (j)

This brief summary is included here merely to point out that we could be unrealistic if we expected a child to be able to say the (s) sound before he was three or four. This doesn't mean, however, that he cannot be helped to master all — or most — of the sounds before he reaches seven and a half.

Teaching a child to say his sounds is a rewarding job, but it can be frustrating for both parent and child if it is done unwisely, without being responsive to what this particular child can do. Above all, it is important to do the teaching in a friendly way, a little at a time. If you become upset and emotional, the child will feel there is something wrong with him, when, in effect, you are trying to help him to develop normally.

It is advisable to follow two steps when teaching your child to say speech sounds. First, it is helpful if you teach him the characteristics of each sound. Children enjoy playing a game of bringing life to inanimate things, and so, for example, the (s) sound might be called the snake sound, while the (p) sound is called the motor boat sound. (Your child must, of course, know something about snakes and motor boats if the game is to have meaning.) He will become familiar with the associations rather quickly because it is easy to remember that snakes say *s s s s s* when they are angry and motor boats go *puht, puht, puht,* as they ride over the water. Once he knows them, always refer to the sounds in your games by the associations you have given them. For your convenience a list of sounds and suggestions appears below.

m — humming top	v — airplane
b — bouncing ball	sh — be quiet
p — motor boat	zh — sports car
h — panting puppy	l — ling-a-ling (telephone ring)
w — windmill	th (voiced) — airplane
k — crow	s — snake
g — frog	z — buzzing bee
t — ticking clock	r — old car
d — woodpecker	th (voiceless) — angry goose
n — mosquito	ch — choo choo train
ng — ding dong bell	j — pogo stick
y — yipping dog	wh — blow out the candle
f — angry kitten	

Using these associations for the sounds, invent games (or participate in the ones described below) to help your child learn how the sound really sounds, how it looks when someone says it, how he can say it, and also that a sound is part of a word.

Teach one sound at a time. It only confuses your child if you attempt to teach him two or more sounds simultaneously. Spend a week or two on one sound before going on to the next. Games should be played for sounds your child can already say correctly. The awareness of how these sounds are made that develops out of the games will aid him in learning the more difficult sounds.

game suggestions

The few games that are included here should serve to stimulate your own imagination. You are sure to think of variations and new ones once you begin the practice.

(P) The Motor Boat Sound: Using small balls of paper or cotton, or Ping-Pong balls, challenge your child to a game to see who can blow the balls the farthest across the table by saying the (P) sound. The winner gets a reward. This game can also be played with the (b), (h), (k), (t), (f), (sh), (th), and (ch) sounds.

2. The Store: Start the game by saying, "I own a grocery store and I sell something that has the snake sound in its name. Can you guess what it is?" Some of the possible responses may include ice cream, soda, cigars, sandwiches, etc. When the child guesses the object you have chosen, he is the store owner. The type of store can change with each game. The sounds can be varied as well.

3. Select a short children's poem or nursery rhyme. Count the number of times the sound you are working on is repeated in the piece. Several games can then be played that will help the child to hear and to identify the sounds. One such game might be to have the child clap his hands each time he hears you say a word that contains his sound. Or you may ask him to repeat the word which has the sound when he hears it.

Another game that children enjoy is called the "sound tree." Draw a picture of an apple tree. Cut out a number of apples (equal to the number of sounds you will present in the story), and place them on the apple tree. As you read the selection, the

3. LINGUISTIC DEVELOPMENT

child is allowed to pick an apple each time he hears his sound. Variations of this game include pasting ornaments on Christmas trees or pine cones on pine trees. A similar game can be played by drawing a staircase. Using a cut-out of a girl or a boy, the child moves the cut-out one step up each time he hears his sound. If he reaches the top of the stairs, he wins.

Another game every child will be sure to enjoy is the "candy dish" game. Place a number of candies (again equal to the number of sounds you will present) on the table. As you read the selection the child is to place one of the candies in a dish each time he hears his sound. Repeat the game several times until he is able to get all of the candies in the dish, at which time an appropriate reward may be given. He'll gladly accept the candy.

teaching self correction

Once your child is able to identify and say some of the speech sounds, you can begin to help him to correct his own errors in pronunciation. The sounds you want him to correct should be confined to those sounds that are expected of a child his age (see the table on page 4). Even though you have worked on sounds that children develop later, it would be unfair to expect him to correct at the age of four those sounds that usually develop at seven.

Using rhymes or word play, you can teach your child that words are made up of a series of sounds connected in sequence. Most children are unable to hear isolated sounds in a word. Instead, they hear the word as a whole — as a single sound. You will have to help your child understand that words have a beginning, a middle, and an end. Children have to be taught to say the entire word correctly. They love rhyming games, and such games will help them to know that sounds are different, yet related.

A simple game of rhyming can be played by selecting a word and then attempting to find as many words as possible that rhyme with it. For example, if the sample word is *cat*, the child can be guided to respond with *bat*, *fat*, *hat*, *mat*, *pat*, *rat*, *sat*, and *vat*. If the sample word is *rake*, then *bake*, *cake*, *lake*, *make*, *sake*, *take*, and *wake* would be appropriate responses. Keeping score will make the game more interesting by adding a touch of competition.

Another rhyming game that many children enjoy is easily made and simply played. Cut out several pictures of common objects, such as hat, car, boat, and top, for example. A department store catalog is an excellent source of colorful pictures. Paste the pictures on a large sheet of paper or cardboard. With the paper on the floor, stand back a few feet and toss a penny or a button onto the paper. If the child can think of a word that rhymes with the picture on which his penny has landed, he gets one point. Ten points wins the game.

Colorful pictures are commonly used in teaching, and two other rhyming games using pictures are suggested here.
1. The Sentence Game: This fun game is played by showing the child a picture and then saying a rhymed couplet — leaving out the final (and rhyming) word for the child to fill in. For example, hold a picture of a clown upside down and say "This funny clown is upside *down*." A picture of a pig can be used with, "Here is a pig that is very *big*."
2. The Matching Game: This is an easy-to-make game, but it may be a bit more difficult for the child to play. Paste pictures of objects that rhyme in two columns.

EXAMPLE:

cat	dish
rake	hat
fish	clock
sock	cake

Name the first picture in column one. The child is to draw a line from the picture you have named to the picture in column two that rhymes.

These are only a few of the many rhyming games that can be

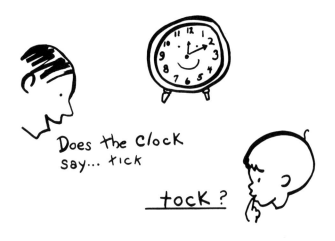

Does the clock say... tick tock?

invented. Have fun with them, and as your child learns to tell one sound from another, he will begin to use the correct sounds in his own speech.

CAUSES OF SPEECH PROBLEMS

It is not within the scope of this pamphlet to examine the many types of speech disorders and their causes, but it may be helpful if we look briefly at some of the major reasons why speech development may not proceed normally.

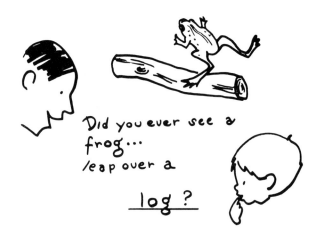

Did you ever see a frog... leap over a log?

organic (physical) problems

There are several physical problems that can cause speech to be delayed or distorted. For example, the child who is born deaf or hard of hearing, or who acquires a substantial hearing loss before speech has developed, will usually experience a great deal of difficulty in learning to talk. We learn to talk by listening to the speech of others. If we were deprived of the ability to hear, we would have no models after which to pattern our speech.

Clefts of the lip and palate can often cause a speech disorder. When the palate is absent or not functioning adequately, too much air will escape through the nose when speaking, thereby causing indistinct speech.

Other physical problems which can cause speech disorders are malocclusion (improper bite), brain injury, cerebral palsy, and deformities of the mouth, throat, or larynx (voice box).

functional problems

Functional problems include many types of speech defects that, having no organic cause, can be attributed to any one of the following causes: (1) Ill health during the first two years of

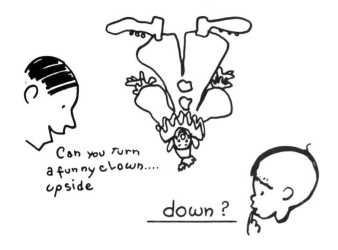

In fact, speech disorders are the most common handicaps known to man, numbering more than all other physical handicaps combined. It was estimated at the middle of the 20th century that a minimum of 2,000,000 children, which is 5 per cent of the school-age population, had serious speech defects. Another 5 per cent, it was estimated, had speech problems of a minor nature. These figures do not include those preschool children and adults who also have speech defects. The total number must be staggering and serves to point out the need for increased parental understanding to prevent the onset of many communication problems and to provide treatment of problems that do exist, the earlier the better.

do children outgrow speech disorders?

This very common question is often asked by parents who are not certain about how their children are developing. Some would like to believe that their children are really not experiencing difficulty in learning to speak; they would rather believe that their children are just slower than others in learning speech skills, as they very well may be. Others feel that their children could

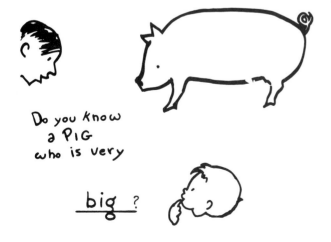

speak well if they wanted to, but are just "lazy." And then there are those who want a true picture of what their child is experiencing so that they will know if they should relax and let things take their course, or whether they have reason to be concerned — and need to do something to help him.

In order to **answer the** question posed, two things must be considered. The first is whether or not the child has a true speech disorder. It is to be expected that young children are not going to speak as well as older children because they are still learning. It has been said that it is far more difficult to learn-to speak than it is to learn to play the violin. We wouldn't expect a child who is learning the scales to be able to give a solo concert. Doesn't it seem fair, therefore, to allow the same privilege to a child who is learning to speak? Most young children make errors in their speech. It is to be expected. Before they can put sounds into words and communicate with another person, they must first learn how to pronounce the sounds. They must hear a lot of conversation, have many meaningful experiences, develop a substantial vocabulary, and have a willing listener before they will ever be able to speak in an intelligible manner.

On the other hand, many parents are overeager for their children to speak well. Some of these parents think their children are having difficulty, when in many cases the speech problem exists only in their own ears. Their children generally do not have speech problems when they grow up. This doesn't mean that they outgrew them. The truth is that they were developing normally; their parents suffered from unrealistic expectations.

The second consideration is the child who is really developing slowly. Many speech therapists feel there is no such thing as a "lazy" talker. If a young child is slow in developing speech there generally is a reason, and it should be discovered and corrected early. Instead of seeking professional advice, many parents follow the advice of a friend or relative who says, "Don't worry about it." Unfortunately, if their children do have true speech problems, the chances are they will not outgrow them. Then they will find themselves attempting to overcome the problem at a later date when it is far more difficult to correct. The longer the speech disorder remains uncorrected, the more difficult it becomes to eradicate. For some older children a speech difficulty is not a problem. That is the way they speak. Period. Others may find it too painful to admit they are having difficulty and to ask for help. When a youngster reaches this stage it generally requires more than a few simple speech exercises to correct the problem.

It is often difficult to know whether or not our children are really experiencing difficulty in learning to speak or if we are at fault in judging their speaking skills according to unrealistic standards. The wisest thing to do if we are unsure is to seek out the advice of someone who is knowledgeable about the way young children develop, such as a teacher, a psychologist, or, if one is available, a speech therapist.

other considerations

It has been found that there sometimes is a connection between children with speech problems and children who experience difficulty in learning to read. If the child's inability to speak correctly hampers his reading, in reality it affects his entire education, based as it is on ability to read.

Sometimes there is also a connection between children who speak poorly and those who reveal disturbed behavior. Any child with a defect faces rough treatment from other youngsters. Being the butt of many jokes can be especially tormenting. In response, the child may lash out at his peers or withdraw from everyone to protect himself. Both tactics are damaging emotionally to the child.

It would seem, then, that children who do not outgrow speech disorders on their own, and whose problems go uncorrected, also face the possibility of doing poorly in school and of developing defensive behavior patterns that set them apart from other children their own age.

WHO CAN "TREAT" SPEECH DISORDERS?

The specialists who can help a child with speech problems include speech therapists, hearing therapists, teachers of the speech and hearing handicapped, teachers of the deaf, and audiologists (per-

3. LINGUISTIC DEVELOPMENT

sons who test hearing).

Many speech therapists work in the public schools. These professional people must meet the requirements set up by their State Education Departments before they can be employed in the schools. This generally means that they are graduates of accredited colleges or universities and have completed a course of study in the area of speech pathology.

In addition to meeting the requirements of the State Education Departments and the various professional organizations, speech therapists adhere to a self-imposed code of ethics which helps to protect the public.

In spite of the newness of the profession, most universities provide good courses and adequate clinical practice to prepare their students to provide speech and hearing services to the many who need such specialized help.

what a speech therapist does

It is important to note that all speech disorders differ, and that even those that seem to be the same — e.g., children who lisp — vary to such a degree that it is not practical to describe the treatment in detail. However, the following is a broad description of what a speech therapist does. The therapist will undoubtedly start by collecting information (generally called the "case history"), which may range from a description of the child's birth to whether or not the child has any playmates his own age. Then, the therapist will test the child. Depending on the complaint presented by the parents and information gathered in the case history, the evaluation may include:

1) *An Articulation Test.* This is to assess the type of speech errors that are being made. A record will be kept of the sounds that are defective, how they are being mispronounced, and the number of errors made.

2) *A Hearing Test.* Hearing is generally tested to determine if a hearing problem is the cause of the speech disorder.

3) *An Auditory Discrimination Test.* This test is given to determine if the child is hearing the sounds correctly. For example, if he is unable to recognize the specific characteristics of a given sound, he will not have a good model to imitate.

4) *A Language Development Test.* This is administered to help determine the amount of vocabulary the child has acquired because vocabulary is generally a good indication of intelligence. This test is especially helpful in situations where mental retardation is suspected.

The therapist will usually examine the child's mouth to determine if there are any physical reasons for the poor speech. He will look for things such as tongue-tie. This means that the movement of the tongue tip is restricted by the presence of a small piece of tissue under the tongue. Tongue-tie is not a common occurrence, but it is looked for as part of the evaluation. The therapist will also look at the shape of the roof of the mouth and at the positioning of the child's teeth. Very often a misshapen mouth or a poor bite can be the cause of a speech problem. The soft palate, which is the soft tissue that hangs down in the back of the mouth, commonly mistaken for the tonsils, is also examined. Sometimes the soft palate may be short or not working properly, which can result in nasal and distorted speech.

This is not, by any means, the extent of the testing that goes into all speech evaluations, but it should give you an idea of the methods used to determine the presence and cause of a speech disorder.

When the evaluation is complete, the therapist will attempt to determine the cause of the speech disorder. Since most speech problems are the result of some psychological or physical defect, every effort is made first to identify the cause and then to treat it.

When the diagnosis is complete, the therapist will discuss the total situation with the parents and will make recommendations as to the best approach to correct the speech problem.

Speech therapy is an educational process. In some cases it is a matter of replacing an old habit with a new one. A process of reteaching. In other cases it is strictly an initial teaching process that requires drill and repetition. Many times the parents will be called on to practice with the child at home to reinforce what is being done in therapy.

With young children the therapy will usually be presented in the form of play. The therapist may use speech games with the child to hold his attention while subtle changes are being made in his speech.

For the most part, speech therapy is a pleasant experience, including the playing of games and the successful achievement of goals, and having a relationship with another person that is based on acceptance rather than rejection.

how long does therapy last?

It is impossible to predict how long it will take to correct a speech problem. Even though two children may have similar lisps (Thilly Thally for Silly Sally), there are too many other variables — such as intelligence, need to change, parental pressure to change, and emotional need to use an infantile speech pattern — ever to predict when the problem will be corrected and therapy terminated. Not only is it impossible to estimate the length of time it will take, but also it is unfair to the parents, the child, and the therapist to have to work against the calendar. But simple substitutions of one sound for another are usually considered short term, while speech disorders that result from physical problems such as cleft palate or hearing loss are usually considered to be long term.

It is understandable for you to want to know approximately when to expect improvement, but it must be kept in mind that speech therapy is an educational process that requires time to develop the necessary skills that are the foundation for acceptable speech. Be fair to your child and to yourself. You certainly can expect improvement in a reasonable amount of time, but do not expect overnight miracles to take place.

PARENT-CHILD RELATIONSHIPS

Progress often depends on the parents' attitude toward the child's problem. There are at least three possibilities:

1. Parents may reject their children and their speech disorder.
2. Parents may compensate for their reactions to their children and their speech disorders.
3. Or parents may fully accept their children and their speech disorders.

the rejecting parent

Experience has shown that many children who have speech and language problems come from homes which have disturbed family relationships. These in turn cause the child to feel emotionally insecure. Moreover, some parents of speech-handicapped children tend to provide less encouragement for their children to talk, but at the same time are critical of their speaking abilities.

Unfortunately, the parents who reject their child's speech problem, who need help in learning to love and accept their child, are the parents least seen by the therapist. They rarely attend P.T.A. meetings or visit school during open school time. If the child is receiving speech therapy at a center, these parents tend not to keep appointments regularly and generally fail to follow through on recommendations made by the therapist. As a result, the chances for improving the child's speech are poor.

the compensating parent

Many other parents overcompensate for conscious or unconscious feelings toward their speech-handicapped child. Overcompensation is often the result of feelings of resentment or guilt. Parents who may feel socially stigmatized for having produced a defective child tend to coddle the child.

Some people may feel that the mother who does everything for her child is being a wonderful mother, but overprotection may make the child submissive in his responses and unable to develop self-reliance.

Take, for example, the case of a child whose parents and older sister dominated his life by dressing, bathing, and feeding him, by walking him to and from school and constantly watching his play to prevent him from getting hurt. It becomes understandable why he would have infantile speech.

the accepting parent
In accepting their child's speech problem, parents are really accepting their child. They have gained the ability to provide for the special needs of their child's speech handicap while continuing to live a normal life, tending to family, home, and civic and social obligations.

Children who are accepted by their parents generally profit more from speech therapy than do children who are made to feel uneasy by parental rejection. If you expect a child to learn to speak, you must first provide him with a model he can identify himself with, a speaking person who loves him.

The most obvious thing about a successful parent and handicapped child relationship is that the child is treated as a child, not as a handicapped child.

OUR RESPONSIBILITIES
We must understand that we have a responsibility to our children, not to ourselves, and that if speech therapy is to be at all successful, we must allow our children the emotional freedom to profit from the program.

We must maintain a consistent and accepting attitude and not become discouraged or overzealous by slow or rapid progress.

We must also understand that some children may have lifelong afflictions and that it is our responsibility to help prepare them for a life that is as normal as possible.

If good parent-child relationships can be achieved early, the results will be a better emotional adjustment for both parent and child and more likelihood of a successful speech therapy.

where you can find a speech therapist
If your child is experiencing difficulty in learning to speak, or if he seems to have a speech problem, you should consult with a qualified speech specialist. If your local school has a speech correctionist on its faculty, you may arrange to meet with him and have him evaluate your child's speech. If the school does not offer speech correction services, the administration may be able to direct you to a qualified person. The local Departments of Health and of Social Welfare may also be of assistance.

Many colleges, universities, and hospitals have speech and hearing centers that provide consultation as well as therapy services to the community. In recent years a number of private speech and hearing centers employing qualified speech therapists have been set up. These centers, as well as the speech therapists who maintain a private practice, may be able to offer advice to you.

are all private speech therapists qualified?
Most states have not instituted a procedure of licensure which would permit only licensed or certified speech therapists to engage in private practice. As a result, occasionally an unqualified person will advertise himself as a speech correctionist, speech therapist, or speech pathologist, and engage in private practice. To assure yourself that you are consulting with a qualified person, it is wise to inquire as to his background and qualifications. Make sure your therapist has met the basic requirements set up by either the State Education Department, the State Health Department, the State Speech and Hearing Association, or the American Speech and Hearing Association, 9030 Old Georgetown Road, Washington, D.C. 20014. It is not possible to list the state requirements for they may differ from state to state. The requirements set by the American Speech and Hearing Association, however, are nationwide and hold that a person must have at least a Master's degree before engaging in private practice.

IN SUMMARY
Speech is a complex learned skill that takes years to develop. Its development can be delayed or adversely influenced by so many things, from infantile illness to the imitation of a poor speech pattern, it seems a miracle that no more than 5 to 10 per cent of school-age children suffer from speech disorders.

Research has shown that children who are deprived of early stimulation, who have been exposed to a limited number of experiences will demonstrate more speech disorders than will children who are considered advantaged. However, even the advantaged child is susceptible to poor speech. He may have enjoyed more exposure to his environment, but childhood illness, an overprotective parent, an organic disorder, or an emotional problem can contribute to or cause delayed speech.

Any child can have a speech problem. If your child's speech is not understandable, if he has developed a speech pattern that attracts too much attention to itself, or if his inability to communicate easily is causing him to feel uncomfortable in speaking situations, it is important to do something to help him.

Seek out a qualified speech therapist, have him evaluate your child's speech, and then try to follow up on his recommendations. You may discover what is causing the difficulty, what you can do to prevent his speech from becoming worse, and what should be done to correct the problem.

Word Retrieval
of Aphasic Adults

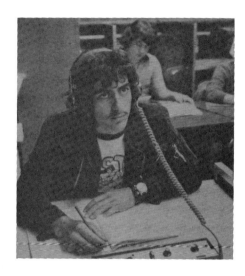

Robert C. Marshall

Word retrieval difficulties are a cardinal symptom of aphasic involvement. Substantial evidence has been reported that suggests aphasics' word retrieval efforts result from reduced available vocabulary (Schuell and Jenkins, 1961; Schuell, Jenkins, and Jiminez-Pabon, 1964; Schuell, 1974). There is further reason to believe that the inability of an aphasic to evoke a desired word is due to an underlying loss in the efficiency of the retrieval process itself. Luria (1972) explains the problem as a breakdown in the "rule of force" whereby strong and weak stimuli evoke similar responses such that no selective organization of the relevant associational processes is possible. Regarding the effects of this breakdown on language use, he suggests that speech is a highly selective multidimensional matrix whereby each word evokes a complex of semantic, phonetic, and morphological associations. For the aphasic, all associations of a given matrix are evoked with an equal probability so that the choice of the proper association becomes difficult or is blocked out entirely. Schuell and Jenkins (1961) have also emphasized the importance of the associational processes to aphasic word retrieval. They suggested that given stimuli activate portions of associational clusters and that the integrity of these clusters serves to mediate the various error types produced by the aphasic in the retrieval process. They found an inverse relationship between the number of semantic associational errors and total errors for aphasics on a naming task and that this error type predominated for mildly impaired subjects. For this reason they suggested that associational errors comprise the "best" errors for an aphasic.

For the most part, studies of aphasics' word retrieval problems have employed confrontation naming tasks (Vandette, 1964; Bisiach, 1966; Goodglass et al., 1966; Benton, Smith, and Lang, 1972). The primary concern in most investigations has usually been whether or not the aphasic successfully named the item rather than the behavior exhibited in the word retrieval process. An exception to this format was a study by Barton (1971) who presented subjects with a naming task but ascertained whether they could supply the first letter, number of syllables, and length of the words they could not retrieve. Results indicated that aphasics could provide certain information about words they could not retrieve at a better than chance level. Aphasia clinicians have also recognized

"Word Retrieval of Aphasic Adults," Robert C. Marshall, *Journal of Speech and Hearing Research*, Vol. 41 No. 4, November 1976. ©1976 Journal of Speech and Hearing Research.

that patients are able to demonstrate by gesture, association, circumlocution, or description their awareness of particular elements they cannot retrieve. Berman and Peele (1967) pointed out that some of the behaviors emitted by the aphasic in searching for a given word may be helpful in triggering production of the word. They found certain aphasic and apractic patients could increase their communicative efficiency when made aware of the utility of these behaviors.

The research reviewed to this point suggests that a descriptive study of the types of retrieval behaviors employed by aphasics may be worthwhile for two reasons. First of all, specification of the various behaviors exhibited by aphasics as they attempt to retrieve a particular word might yield some insight to the organization of language processes within the central nervous system. Secondly, certain retrieval behaviors might prove to be more useful, not only for particular aphasic patients, but for the aphasic population as a whole and thereby provide clinicians with information to design more effective therapeutic strategies. This investigation was designed to determine the types of word retrieval behaviors used by aphasic adults and to ascertain the effectiveness of these behaviors in the production of desired words in conversation.

DATA COLLECTION

For this study a word retrieval behavior was operationally defined as "a situation whereby the aphasic, unprompted by the clinician, illustrates that he is unable to retrieve a word and initiates some effort to do so without assistance from the clinician." Instances of retrieval behavior were recorded from the conversations of 18 adult aphasics for periods of time ranging from one week to three months. These data were collected within the individual treatment sessions of patients seen at the Portland Veterans Administration Hospital. All patients had reached a point in their therapeutic course where they could generate some functional conversation. Clinician-patient discussions focused on activities and problems relevant to the patient's home, work, health, family, recreation, and finances. For the most part discussions were nondirective following an approach to treatment of aphasia earlier described by Wepman (1972). Although patients were occasionally asked to respond or responded on their own to a specific therapeutic stimulus, retrieval behaviors generated for these responses were not recorded. Retrieval behaviors were either recorded directly by the clinician or taken from recordings made during the therapy sessions. Ultimately, each behavior was transcribed in context (as nearly as possible) onto an individual card. The individual transcriptions were then classified in terms of the types of behaviors observed as the patient attempted to produce the desired word and whether or not the behavior was followed by production of the intended word.

RESULTS

Identification of Word Retrieval Behaviors

There were 740 instances of word retrieval behavior recorded for the 18 aphasics who participated in the study. From these data five behaviors (specific examples are provided in the Appendix) were identified. All recorded behaviors were classified into one of the five behavior categories.

Delay. The patient takes or requests additional time to produce the word. Although some delay is certainly inherent in all retrieval efforts, in this case subjects tended to use a filled pause, unfilled pause, or some stalling tactic to let the listener know they did not want to be interrupted and needed more time to produce the word. This behavior seems analogous to what Brown and Mc-

3. LINGUISTIC DEVELOPMENT

Neil (1966) and others (Barton, 1971) have termed the "tip of the tongue" phenomena.

Semantic Association. The aphasic produces one or more words that are semantically related to the desired word. These included opposites (table-chair), in-class associations (Ford-Plymouth), part-whole relationships (branch-tree), and serially related items (one, two, three).

Phonetic Association. The patient produces a word or words which are phonetically similar to the desired word. It should be pointed out that this behavior does not resemble the groping off-target phonemic production described by Johns and Darley (1970) as apraxia of speech but seems more closely related to what has been termed a "slip of the tongue" or spoonerism.

Description. Subjects attempted to produce the desired word by describing what they were talking about. Although associational behaviors were often observed within the context of subject's descriptions, the examples in the Appendix clearly indicate the necessity on the part of the patient to tell something about the intended word.

Generalization. Here subjects produced general words or what have been described (Geschwind, 1967) as empty words in place of the desired word. In many instances this behavior seemed to represent a manipulative effort on the part of the aphasic to get the clinician to supply the needed word.

Use of Word Retrieval Behaviors

Figure 1 illustrates the number of times the various retrieval behaviors were used by the subjects and the frequency each behavior was followed by the production of the desired word. Semantic association and description were the

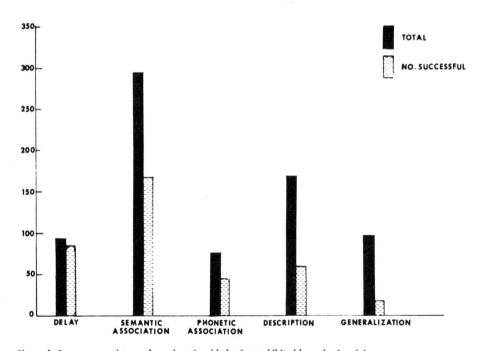

Figure 1. Frequency and type of word retrieval behaviors exhibited by aphasic adults.

most frequently observed behaviors. Phonetic associations, delays, and generalizations were observed with near equal frequency. Although subjects were far more likely to exhibit a semantic than a phonetic association, the likelihood of these behaviors being followed by the desired word was approximately equal. Semantic associations were followed by the intended word 56.7% of the time; phonetic associations were followed by the intended word 56.6% of the time. Description, the second most frequently recorded behavior, was followed by the intended word only 34.9% of the time. Delay, while used sparingly by most subjects, proved to be the most effective retrieval behavior (90.6% success). This is in contrast to generalization which prompted the needed word with 17% success.

Retrieval Behavior for Individual Subjects

Table 1 gives the proportions of retrieval behaviors for individual subjects with a minimum of 50 recorded behaviors and the percentage of times the behavior was followed by the intended word. To provide some idea about the relationship between use of a behavior and severity of aphasia, subjects are ranked (Table 1) in order of severity of communicative impairment on the basis of overall percentile scores on the Porch Index of Communicative Ability (Porch, 1967). Delaying behavior was shown to a noticeable degree only for higher level subjects. As mentioned previously, this approach for those aphasics using it was highly successful. Semantic associations were exhibited

TABLE 1. Proportions of all word retrieval behaviors (P) and success percentages (%) of various behaviors for individual subjects providing 50 or more behaviors.

Subject	PICA %	Delay		Semantic Association		Phonetic Association		Description		Generalization	
		P	%	P	%	P	%	P	%	P	%
1	90	0.250	92.3	0.481	72.0	0.000	0.0	0.115	66.7	0.153	37.5
2	81	0.109	88.9	0.378	67.7	0.085	71.4	0.256	14.3	0.170	0.0
3	72	0.232	89.4	0.368	56.7	0.049	28.6	0.249	52.1	0.102	41.4
4	71	0.018	100.0	0.342	47.5	0.342	55.0	0.154	27.8	0.145	0.0
5	65	0.043	100.0	0.609	42.8	0.109	40.0	0.130	0.0	0.043	0.0
6	61	0.038	100.0	0.731	63.2	0.038	0.0	0.076	0.0	0.115	0.0
7	59	0.038	100.0	0.423	27.3	0.115	100.0	0.308	50.0	0.115	0.0
8	57	0.000	0.0	0.146	16.7	0.171	28.6	0.317	0.0	0.415	0.0
9	45	0.000	0.0	0.578	0.0	0.000	0.0	0.115	0.0	0.368	0.0

by all subjects but tended to be most useful in triggering the needed word for higher level patients. Exceptions to this pattern were Subject 6, who used semantic association far more frequently and successfully than other subjects, and Subject 8, who used this approach infrequently and with limited success. Phonetic associations were employed sparingly or not at all by most subjects. The lone exception was Subject 4, who was marginally proficient in employing this behavior to evoke the desired word. Description was also employed by all subjects but was generally successful for only higher level aphasics. Again, some exceptions are evident. Subject 2 used many descriptions but was generally unsuccessful in producing the needed word with the behavior; Subject 7, on the other hand, was more successful retrieving words through description than any other approach. Generalization was noted to a substantial degree for only the two lowest subjects. This approach was totally unsuccessful except for two of the higher level subjects.

DISCUSSION

The clinician, through careful analysis of the aphasic patient's verbal habits, can often identify behaviors which enhance or prove detrimental to communicative efficiency. The results of this study suggest some comments as to the specificity and efficacy of various word retrieval behaviors used by aphasics. First of all, it is possible to arrange the identified retrieval behaviors in a hierarchial order of efficiency. In using the most effective behavior, that of delay, the aphasic seems to be saying, "I have the word" and requesting his listener to wait until he can produce it. Use of semantic and phonetic associations seems to prompt the patient to produce a related word or words and subsequently, with varying degrees of success, the word he wants. In description, the patient may be saying, "I can't come up with the word but I can tell you what I mean." It would appear that the likelihood a particular behavior will be used and subsequently lead to production of the needed word varies directly with the severity of aphasia. Delay, a successful approach, was predominantly employed by higher level subjects; generalization, an almost totally unsuccessful technique, was primarily used by lower level subjects. Association and description were exhibited by all subjects but were far more successful for the higher level subjects.

The findings of this study again highlight the importance of the associational processes to the problem of word retrieval (Schuell et al., 1964; Schuell and Jenkins, 1961; Luria, 1972; Schuell, 1974). It appears that the associations emitted by an aphasic in searching for a word are not random but reflective of how close he is to producing the word. For the most part, subjects' associational behaviors were semantic; however, phonetic associations proved useful for one subject. Associational processes may operate in other retrieval behaviors as well. For example, in delaying, the aphasic may be associating but on an internal basis. This type of activity would certainly be possible for the higher level subjects who tended to use delay. Similar implications might be drawn in that subjects tended to use description when searching for less common words (for example transformer, trifocals, accelerator, yeoman). This may be the result of trying to use a word that has few common associations. Only in generalization does it seem possible to divorce the associational processes from the phenomenon of word retrieval. Here it seems reasonable to assume, as pointed out initially by Schuell and Jenkins (1961), that an associational cluster has not been stimulated.

Many interesting facets of aphasics' verbal behavior emerged from this study. For example, many subjects did a great deal of negating in their retrieval attempts. At times a patient would deny a word before he had produced it ("I'm going to, not San Francisco, but Los Angeles") as though producing the association served an unlocking function to allow emission of the appropriate word. At times patients used gestures to accompany their word retrieval efforts. When possible, lower level aphasics would directly demonstrate by touch or pointing. Interestingly, the more difficult words to retrieve were *crutch, stroke, brace, arm* and other terms relating to the body and to illness. Finally, some subjects became annoyed when they could not produce a particular word and were reluctant to move on in their conversations until the clinician had supplied it. One subject, after failing to produce a book title, returned to the clinic after a week's absence and supplied the word.

Some caution is necessary in interpreting the results of this study inasmuch as data were collected from a limited sample of aphasics capable of generating conversational speech. Additional research is needed to provide information relative to the word retrieval behavior of less verbal aphasics. Moreover, this investigation employed a restricted definition of retrieval behavior. It would be interesting, but much more difficult, to ascertain similar information for aphasics who did not recognize or confront the problem. It is possible that patients who consciously or unconsciously ignore retrieval problems through circumlocution and substitution could then be taught to use an effective retrieval behavior. Finally, it would appear worthwhile to analyze aphasic word retrieval behaviors longitudinally to see if particular behaviors emerge at certain points in the recovery course and if they can be influenced by therapeutic intervention.

Cheris Kramer

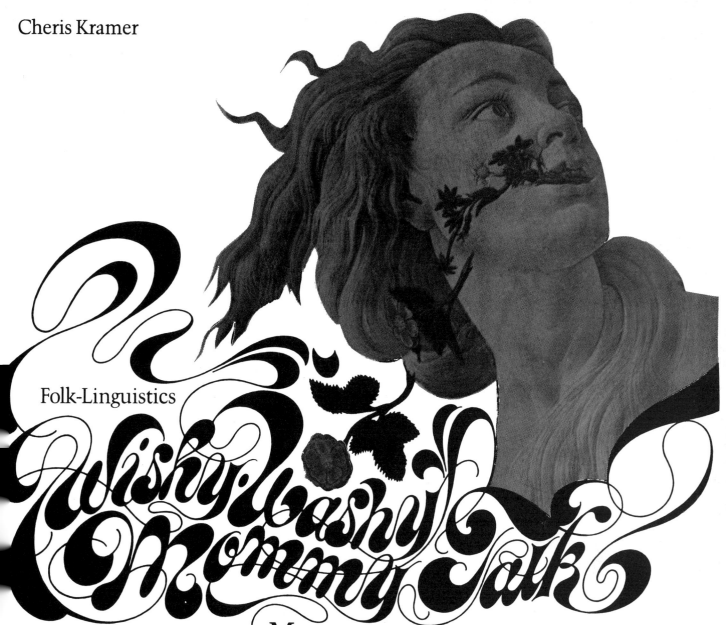

Folk-Linguistics

Wishy-Washy Mommy Talk

Men speak assertively, briefly, swear more. Women hide out in diffident sentences and flowery phrasing, but talk, talk, talk. A linguist finds those stereotypes—and they're just that—alive and well in *The New Yorker's* cartoon pages.

MEN AND WOMEN SPEAK A DIFFERENT LANGUAGE. According to popular belief, at least, the speech of women is weaker and less effective than the speech of men. Our culture has many jokes about both the quality of women's speech ("If my wife said what she thought, she'd be speechless") and its quantity ("Women need no eulogy; they speak for themselves"). Compared to male speech, the female form is supposed to be emotional, vague, euphemistic, sweetly proper, mindless, endless, high-pitched, and silly.

Such generalizations are not based on carefully controlled research. Although anthropologists have noticed sex-related differences in the languages of other cultures, there have been only a few quantitative studies of the way men and women differ in their use of English. Per-

haps this is due to the fact that many researchers view women as peculiar human beings who stand outside the laws governing mankind (i.e., males).

A noted linguist who did devote some attention to sex differences in language had some unflattering things to say about the way women talk. In his 1922 book, *Language*, Otto Jespersen wrote an entire chapter on "The Woman." (There was no parallel chapter on "The Man.") Jespersen made many claims about women's speech, among them that women frequently leave sentences unfinished, and that they are prone to jump from one idea to another when talking. These assertions rested on the author's own observations and examples drawn from literary works.

Until recently, Jespersen's chapter was one of the few published discussions of

"Folk Linguistics: Wishwasy Mommy Talk," Cheris Kramer, *Psychology Today*, Vol. 8 No. 1, June 1974. ©1974 Ziff-Davis Publishing .

129

3. LINGUISTIC DEVELOPMENT

the topic. But with the emergence of the women's liberation movement, some social scientists and linguists have begun to speculate about how language helps maintain rigid sex-role barriers. Most of these writers have derived hypotheses from their own intuitions as native speakers.

The Folklore of Female Language. In addition to the speculations of linguists, there is also a folk-linguistics of women's speech, a body of folklore about female language that permeates popular jokes and stories. These perceived differences do not necessarily correspond to real ones, but they are important as indicators of cultural attitudes and prejudices.

One way to study folk-linguistics is to examine comic art, which takes much of its material from the relationships between the sexes, including how they talk to each other. Social cartoons are especially useful, since their humor depends on the exaggeration of popular stereotypes of human behavior. In a recent study, I analyzed cartoons containing adult human speech, from three consecutive months (13 issues) of *The New Yorker*, February 17 through May 12, 1973. I chose *The New Yorker* because it is a general-circulation magazine with both male and female readers, and because many cartoonists and critics consider it to be an innovator and leader in the field of social cartooning.

In order to check my own observations and judgments against those of others, I asked 25 male and 25 female students at the University of Illinois to help me identify some of the characteristics of women's and men's speech in the cartoons. I gave each student a list of captions (but not the cartoons themselves) from four consecutive issues, March 17 through April 7. I did not identify the captions as coming from *The New Yorker*. I simply instructed the students to indicate, for each one, whether they thought the words were spoken by a male or female. At the end of the list there was room for comments about what had guided the student's choices.

For most of the 49 captions, there was a clear consensus (at least 66 percent agreement) that the speaker in the cartoon was of a particular sex. The male students were in unanimous or near-unanimous agreement on 14 captions, while females were in unanimous or near-unanimous agreement on 13.

The Silent Sex. A striking finding that emerged from my analysis was that women did not speak in as many of the cartoons as did men. According to folk-linguistics, women talk too much. But in the 156 cartoons in my sample, men speak 110 times, women only 44. In fact, the number for men goes up to 112 if we assume that a commanding voice from the clouds is that of a masculine God, and that a voice on the phone telling an elephant trainer to "Give him two bottles of aspirin and call me in the morning" belongs to a male veterinarian.

There are several possible explanations for the relative silence of women in these cartoons. Most cartoonists are men, and it may be that they depict what they know best and consider most important, i.e., men and male activities. Some students suggested that men try harder to be funny and make more comic statements. Or perhaps the cartoons reflect real life, where men like to have the last, topping word.

Women in these cartoons not only speak less, they speak in fewer places. Men speak in 38 different locations, including a courtroom, doctor's office, psychiatrist's office, police car, massage parlor, press conference, art museum, and floral shop. They are inside a home only 20 of the 110 (or 112) times they speak, excluding cocktail parties. Women, on the other hand, speak in only 16 different places, including the home, store, office and airplane. They are at home on half the occasions when they talk, again excluding cocktail parties. In four of the 13 issues I looked at, women never spoke outside the home at all.

More important, men are in control of language wherever they happen to be, but women, when they do leave home, often seem incapable of handling the language appropriate to the new location. Their speech then becomes the focus of humor. So we have a matron saying to a tight-lipped, barely patient stockbroker, "Now tell me, Mr. Hilbert, does Merrill Lynch think utilities are going to keep on being iffy?" And an enthusiastic woman at a cocktail party remarking to a man, "You have no idea how refreshing it is to meet someone raffish in West Hartford." And another woman inquiring of a book salesman, "Do you have any jolly fiction?" These cartoons are funny (subtly, in *The New Yorker* way) because in each case there is a word that does not quite belong, at least in that setting.

Politics and Pornography. The women and men who populate *The New Yorker* cartoons discuss different topics. Men

hold forth with authority on business, politics, legal matters, taxes, age, household expenses, electronic bugging, church collections, kissing, baseball, human relations, health, and—women's speech. Women discuss social life, books, food and drink, pornography, life's troubles, caring for a husband, social work, age, and life-style. Several of the students who rated the cartoon captions said they considered all statements about economics, business or jobs to be male.

We have already seen what happens when a woman steps over these boundaries and tries to discuss a topic like the stock market. In another cartoon, a woman who is listening with her husband to a TV news program and trying to keep up with current events complains, "I keep forgetting. Which is the good guy—Prince Souvanna Phouma or Prince Souphanouvong?" Forty of the 50 students rated this caption as female. A man with a similar question would probably drop the self-deprecating "I keep forgetting," and say something like, "Damn it! How are we supposed to remember which one is Souvanna Phouma and which is Souphanouvong?" This wording would put the blame for confusion on the owner of the difficult name, rather than the memory of the speaker.

In general, women in the cartoons speak less forcefully than men. For instance, they utter exclamations only five times when speaking to another adult, versus 27 times for men. Furthermore, exclamations seem to serve different functions for men and women. Males use them when they are angry or exasperated. A scowling boss yells into his intercom, "Miss Carter! Where's my input?" A husband says to his wife, "Damn it, Gertrude, Abe Beame isn't *supposed* to turn you on!" But women's exclamations are likely to convey enthusiasm, as when a woman who is admiring a picture says, "Aren't you lucky! Very few people have anything original that's nice."

Freedom to Swear. Since men do not have to be as mild as women, cartoonists let their male characters swear much more freely than their female characters. In *The New Yorker* cartoons, men use swear words (or exclamations with the word "God") 13 times. Women use them only twice, and on one of these occasions there is provocation. A woman says to her husband, who is pouring drinks at their bar, "My God, I mean is that really *all* you can say about me—I've stood the test of time?" Men curse for more trivial reasons. For example, a couple is dining in a restaurant, and the man says, "To hell with what the Sierra Club could do with the cost of a single F-111 fighter plane! Think of what *I* could do with the cost of a single F-111 fighter plane!" With the *hell*, the "masculine" topic, the emphatic *I*, and the exclamation mark, the speaker is clearly recognizable as a man.

Many of the student raters commented on the way profanity, and harsh language in general, distinguish male from female speech. They echoed an observation made by Jespersen half a century ago, when he wrote that women feel an "instinctive shrinking from coarse and gross expressions." Not all modern women agree, however. When I showed Jespersen's remark to some women living in a college dormitory, the spontaneous reaction of several of them was "Shit!"

Another comment by some of the students in the study was that men use a simpler, more direct, more assertive type of language. They are blunt and to the point, whereas women tend to "flower up" their remarks. The caption ratings reflected this view. For example, all but two of the men and two of the women assigned "I'm probably old-fashioned, but I felt much more at home with the Forsytes than I do with the Louds," to a female speaker. One female rater explained, "Women are more likely to preempt their statements with excuses for themselves, 'I may be old-fashioned, but—' . . . women are more concerned with a smooth emotional atmosphere." In contrast, men are perceived as self-assured and sometimes condescending. This came out in one of the cartoons, in which a woman complains to a man, "Can't you just say 'Scarlatti' instead of 'Scarlatti, of course'?"

Mommy Talk. Although the people of *The New Yorker* cartoons live in a world that is almost childless, there are some hints of what might be called mommy talk. For example, there is a cartoon portraying two men, one disgusted, the other puzzled, waiting in line for a public telephone. The woman using the phone gushes, "Yes, you are. You're my little snookums. Well, bye-bye for now, Sweetie Pie. Mommy's got to go . . . Hi. Was she wagging her tail?"

Finally, according to folk-linguistics, certain adjectives, like "nice" and "pretty" are typical of female speech. In the cartoons, these words sometimes serve to identify a woman as a person with traditional ideas about women's role. At other times, they are the basis for a joke, as when a woman uses them while talking about a "masculine" topic. And occasionally, a man employs them to indicate a role reversal. Unfortunately, sex-linked vocabulary differences are difficult to quantify, but in general, the cartoons do reflect the usual beliefs about feminine adjectives.

These and other findings demonstrate that stereotypical female speech is restricted and wishy-washy. The same picture emerges from other sources. For instance, the *New Seventeen Book of Etiquette and Young Living* contains a section on female speech entitled "Sweet Talk." It warns, "A pretty girl makes a good first impression with her looks, but if the sounds that come out of that pretty face are harsh, the effect is spoiled. She has to be easy on the ears as well as on the eyes."

Mary Ellmann has described the stereotyped formlessness of women's language as it appears in the works of such male writers as James Joyce, Jean-Paul Sartre, Norman Mailer, and Ernest Hemingway; the Molly Blooms of literature have just let it all flow out. The same looseness of syntax is captured in a *Saturday Review* cartoon, where a miniskirted coed says to her male professor, "If we don't know how big the whole universe is, then I don't see how we could be sure how big anything in it is either, like the whole thing might not be any bigger than maybe an orange would be if it weren't in the universe, I mean, so I don't think we ought to get too uptight about any of it because it might be really sort of small and unimportant after all, and until we find out that everything isn't just some kind of specks and things, why maybe who needs it?"

A few linguists have tried to pinpoint more precisely the devices women use to weaken their words. Robin Lakoff has suggested that women use the tag-question form for this purpose. Instead of a decisive statement, "That house looks terrible," women are apt to use an indecisive form, "That house looks terrible, doesn't it?" In this way, they ask for confirmation, and allow themselves to be persuaded otherwise. Lakoff also believes women use intonation to turn answers into questions, thus communicating subordination and uncertainty: "When will dinner be ready?" "Oh . . . around six o'clock . . . ?"

Is Folklore Fact? Both folk-linguistics and the observations of professional linguists provide useful clues to popular attitudes, and are rich sources of hypotheses about

language. These hypotheses may or may not fit empirical data about the way people actually talk. Unfortunately, there have been very few studies on sex-related differences in actual speech. Some researchers have found that women are more likely to use standard, "correct" grammar and pronunciation. Beyond that, we can make few generalizations.

Lately I have begun to explore the problem of perceived versus actual differences. My work and the work of several others at the University of Illinois indicates that while it is easy to write statements identifiable as feminine or masculine types, the sex-related cues in such statements appear relatively infrequently in the language of either sex.

In one recent study, I investigated whether men and women differ in their use of modifiers. Lakoff and others have suggested that some adjectives, like "adorable," "lovely," "divine" and "sweet," are peculiar to women; their use by a man could damage his reputation. As I noted earlier, this feature of women's speech showed up in some of *The New Yorker* cartoons. Women are also said to use certain kinds of adverbs more often than men. Jespersen wrote that women have a propensity for hyperbole which leads them to tack *-ly* onto adjectives, producing phrases like "awfully pretty" and "terribly nice." I wanted to find out if women really do use more of these forms.

I was also interested in finding out if there is an absolute difference in the number and variety of modifiers used by males and females. Opinion here is divided. Jespersen felt that men have a more extensive vocabulary, and in general take a greater interest in words. In fact, he advised people wanting to learn a foreign tongue to read "many ladies' novels, because they will there continually meet with just those everyday words and combinations which the foreigner is above all in need of, what may be termed the indispensable small-change of a language." If this is true, we might expect a greater variety of descriptive words from men. However, another linguist, Dwight Bolinger, claims that women use more adjectives than men.

Since this was an initial study, I limited my attention to *-ly* adverbs, and prenominal adjectives (words that precede and modify nouns, such as "handsome" in "handsome man"). These particular kinds of modifiers, unlike others, are unambiguous and are easy to identify.

3. LINGUISTIC DEVELOPMENT

Inanimate Objects. I had 17 men and 17 women compose written descriptions of two black-and-white photographs. Since some people have suggested that men are more interested in inanimate objects than they are in people, and the reverse is true for women, I used one photograph showing several people seated around a table, and another showing a large building adorned with pillars and statues. The subjects had 10 minutes in which to write their paragraphs.

I analyzed each paragraph by adding up the number of *-ly* adverbs and prenominal adjectives, and comparing these numbers to the total number of words used. I found none of the differences that are supposed to exist. Statistical analysis showed that women did not differ from men in either the number or variety of *-ly* adverbs or prenominal adjectives they used. Although men tended to use more words overall to describe the photographs, the differences were not statistically significant. And there did not appear to be any sex differences in the kinds of adjectives preferred.

Perhaps the differences are not in the number or variety of modifying words, but in the way they are used. A sensitive person might be able to pick up subtle cues that are not susceptible to statistical analysis. Since middle-class women are supposed to be especially conscious of stylistic variation, I enlisted the aid of 11 female students majoring in English to determine if the sex of the writers could be deduced from internal cues. I gave them 10 typed paragraphs, randomly selected from those written by the participants in the first part of the study. Five had been written by women, five by men; all described the photograph of a building. In only six of the 10 paragraphs was a majority of the English majors able to identify the writer's sex. In all, there were 59 correct guesses and 51 incorrect ones.

Interestingly, none of the English majors questioned the reasonableness of trying to assign paragraphs to male or female authors, and they were all able to give reasons for their choices. Most of these had to do with the number and type of descriptive words used. In *incorrectly* ascribing to female authors paragraphs

that were actually written by males, some of the women explained that the passages were graceful, sensitive, and contained a lot of detailed description.

Many questions remain. A greater number of sex differences may exist in spoken than in written language. Differences in written work might show up under other circumstances. For example, an important factor may be whether a woman is writing or speaking to another woman, to a man, or to a general audience. Age and socioeconomic position may affect the writer's style. Since women are individuals, researchers must be careful not to make the error of simply grouping all women together.

Vacant Chambers of the Mind. Words, phrases, and sentence patterns are not inherently strong or weak. They acquire these attributes only in a particular cultural context. If our society views female speech as inferior, it is because of the sub-

ordinate role assigned to women. Our culture is biased to interpret sex differences in favor of men.

For example, Jespersen reports an experiment in which male and female subjects had to read a paragraph as quickly as possible, then write down as much as they could remember of it. Women were able to read the passage more quickly and recall more of what they had read. But they lost anyway. Jespersen paraphrases Havelock Ellis' ingenious explanation of the results: "... with the quick reader it is as though every statement were admitted immediately and without inspection to fill the vacant chambers of the mind, while with the slow reader every statement undergoes an instinctive process of cross-examination. ..."

Thus, beliefs about sex-related language differences may be as important as the actual differences. As long as women play a subordinate role, their speech will be stereotyped as separate and unequal.

Linguistic Performance In Vulnerable And Autistic Children And Their Mothers

SHELDON M. FRANK, M.A., M.D., DORIS A. ALLEN, ED.D., LORRAYNE STEIN, AND BEVERLY MYERS

The authors studied the language patterns of schizophrenic mothers and their 4-year-old children, and compared them with the speech of normal mothers and children and normal mothers with autistic children. They found that children of schizophrenic mothers showed lags in language development and language distortions less severe than but in some ways similar to those seen in autistic children. Schizophrenic mothers were more likely to produce more deficient and/or distorted language in interactions with their children. Mothers of autistic children produced language that was equal to or above that of mothers of normal children on most parameters and adjusted their language to the chronological rather than the linguistic age of the child.

EVIDENCE OF LINGUISTIC aberration in schizophrenic patients has been compiled from the time of the earliest clinical literature on this disorder. Broadened and refined investigation of language in schizophrenia continues in the work of such psycholinguists as Chaika (1), who found that many schizophrenic patients fail to make specific semantic and syntactic distinctions.

The increasing study in recent years of the role of the family in schizophrenia has included important findings on language and communication. Wynne (2)

Revised version of a paper presented at the 128th annual meeting of the American Psychiatric Association, Anaheim, Calif., May 5–9, 1975.

Dr. Frank is Assistant Professor, Department of Psychiatry, Millhauser Laboratories, HN 408, New York University Medical Center, 550 First Ave., New York, N.Y. 10016. Dr. Allen is Clinical Instructor in Psychiatry, Albert Einstein College of Medicine, Bronx, N.Y. When this paper was written, Ms. Stein and Ms. Myers were Research Assistants, Department of Psychiatry, New York University Medical Center; Ms. Stein is currently a student in the School of General Studies, Columbia Univ., New York, N.Y., and Ms. Myers is now a graduate student, Department of Linguistics, University of Michigan, Ann Arbor, Mich.

This work was supported by research grant U2366 from the Health Research Council of the City of New York and by the New York University Medical Center.

The authors would like to thank Carolyn Goodman, Ed.D., and her staff at the Bronx Psychiatric Center Parent and Child Education Program for referring subjects for this study.

found high "communication deviance" scores in the fathers and mothers of adult schizophrenic and normal groups. These scores included variables pertaining to communicative intent, logic, semantics, and syntax.

Goldfarb (3) found that mothers of patients with childhood schizophrenia were poorer instruction-givers to their children than mothers of normal children; they were less responsive and provided sparser and more ambiguous information. His work has focused on childhood schizophrenia, which shows particularly strong and characteristic language deviations. This focus has been carried further by Shapiro (4), who found a predominance of echoing and of distorted, underdeveloped morphological and communicative parameters. The implications of Wynne and Goldfarb's work on the etiological nature of deviant parental communication in childhood schizophrenia are not supported by recent work by Howlin and associates (5, 6), whose preliminary findings showed that language of parents of autistic children is similar in communicative style to that of parents of non-psychotic aphasic children.

Recent nonclinical psycholinguistic research has also focused on family communication while examining the normal process of language acquisition. In the late 1960s one of us (S.M.F.) collaborated with Alfred and Clara Baldwin and their associates on work in this area (7–9). We found that mothers adjust their language when speaking to their preschool child to a level much less complex than the one used in speaking with other adults but slightly more complex than the language level of the child. As measured both by MLU (mean length of utterance, in words) (10) and other linguistic parameters (11), the mother's complexity level rises with the rising level of the child from age 2½ to 5 years, remaining at what we have called a "syntactic distance," which diminishes slightly with the child's age.

This is shown in figure 1, which also illustrates how much a mother simplifies her speech when addressing her child instead of another adult; her MLU falls from 12.0 words to 3.7 words. Snow (12), Clarke-Stewart (13), and Nelson (14) have also found that mothers regularly modulate their language according to the child's level of language development.

The data of Baldwin and Frank (7) and others (15–20) have led to a special focus on question-response behavior as an important aspect of normal mother-child

"Linguistic Performance in Vulnerable and Autistic Children and Their Mothers," Sheldon M. Frank, M.A.,M.D.,Doris A. Allen, E.D.D., Lorrayne Stein, Beverly Myers, *American Journal of Psychiatry*, Vol. 133, pp 909-915, August 1976, ● 1976 The American Psychiatric Association.

133

3. LINGUISTIC DEVELOPMENT

FIGURE 1
Language Complexity of Normal Mothers* and Children**

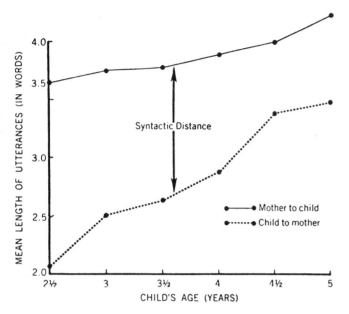

*The mean length of utterance of a mother speaking to another adult is 12.0.
**Based on data presented more fully in (7–9).

FIGURE 2
Number and Types of Utterances by Normal Mothers and Children*

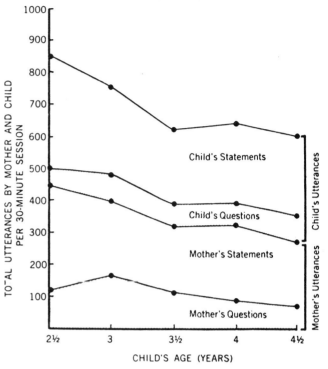

*Based on data presented more fully in (7–9).

interaction. In general, verbal interaction between mothers and their very young children (2 to 2½ years) consists of questioning, labeling, behavioral instructions, fantasy, and talk about the child's immediate desires.

As seen in figure 2, the mother dominates the interaction to the degree of contributing about 60% of the dialogue. By the time the child reaches its fourth year, the dialogue becomes more balanced, with the child contributing nearly 50%. More time is spent on communication of specific and general information and more on past and future as well as present circumstances. Fantasy diminishes as a focus. Questions are still an important means of interaction, but comprise only about one-fifth rather than one-third of the dialogue, and increasingly take on a more distanced and complex character.

When the child is 2½, most questions are of "Wh-type," comprised of "what," "who," "where," and similar questions. Within this Wh-type, the questions are predominantly ostensive, that is, they seek the label of a concrete object that is present. The interaction between a 4-year-old child and its mother contains a greater proportion of predicative questions. These deal with more complex issues such as manner, time, and cause (e.g., "how," "when," and "why") and are constructed in a more abstract manner, with the object not necessarily at hand.[1]

Our present work, a psychiatric-linguistic collabora-

tion, attempts to study with linguistic sophistication families in which a parent is schizophrenic and a child is in the early stages of language development. We wanted to assess language development in a situation in which mother-child communication may be deviant and there is the possibility of prospective study of linguistic and psychological precursors of schizophrenia. We hypothesized that many vulnerable children would show quantitative and qualitative differences from the norm in language development and that related deviant qualities would be found in the parental language. Specifically, we predicted that vulnerable children would show lags in the development of syntax, questioning behavior and responding behavior, and that their parents would fail to provide well-modulated norms in those aspects. We were also curious to see whether any deviant patterns would resemble those found in autistic children, the most linguistically deviant of "childhood schizophrenics."

We have concentrated on mothers who are schizophrenic simply because we were primarily referred subjects who were offspring of schizophrenic mothers, not fathers; certainly father-child communication deserves equally serious study.

METHOD

The data reported in this paper were collected as part of a longitudinal study of chronic schizophrenic

---

[1]These distinctions are more fully elaborated in reference (21), which discusses concepts proposed by Allen (20).

mothers and their preschool children. All of the mothers were outpatients living with and actively caring for their children. However, 7 of the 8 mothers studied had had inpatient care when their children were between 18 and 31 months of age, and all were being maintained on moderate doses of phenothiazine medication. All were native speakers of some dialect of American English and were of working class or welfare class status. Six of the 8 families had a father present in the home. The mean age of the children in this "vulnerable" group was 4 years.

A control group consisted of 8 normal mother-child pairs studied in an earlier collaboration (7, 8). This group was equivalent to the vulnerable group in socioeconomic class and age, and nearly identical in other characteristics.

A third group of 11 autistic children and their mothers was also studied. These families were of a slightly higher socioeconomic status but were otherwise comparable to the other groups. Diagnosis of autistic symptoms prior to age 2 was necessary for inclusion. The children were outpatients who could profit from a part-time therapeutic nursery and most had language abilities which placed them at the highly functioning end of the autistic spectrum.

All the mothers and their children were studied in a naturalistic playroom setting equipped with a standard set of toys including a doll house, books, puzzles, ring toss, and a toy telephone. The mothers were instructed to act with their children as they might at home. All 30-minute sessions were recorded on both audio and video tapes.

The tapes were transcribed to show all verbal interchanges between mothers and children as well as the nonlinguistic context in which each verbal exchange took place. In a preliminary analysis of the data, we looked at the following parameters for mothers and children in each of the three groups:

1. *Total number of utterances*, with proportion contributed by each member of the dyad.

2. *Mean length of utterance (MLU)*, in number of words (10).

3. *Number of transformations*. (A measure of linguistic repertoire consisting of the number of different rules used in forming sentences more complex than a simple declarative statement—e.g., a question, a negation, a sentence with a conjunction [22].)

4. *Relationship of mother's to child's language:* a) "syntactic distance" (the difference between mother's and child's values in MLU's and number of transformation, and b) correlation coefficients between mother's and child's values on these parameters (ρ and Spearman rank order).

5. *Questioning behavior:* number and types of questions employed, and time orientation (now versus not now).

6. *Responding behavior:* proportion of "good responses" (appropriate to the nature of the question) and of nonresponses to the other's questions.

RESULTS

Linguistic Production in Vulnerable Children

The vulnerable children spoke less than did the normal group (see table 1). Although the percentage contributed by the child was not significantly lower, we observed a much wider range in this group, including 3 mother-child pairs who showed patterns of nearly total silence, overwhelming mother-dominated (76%) interaction, or overwhelming child-dominated (85%) interaction. (None of these patterns was seen in the normal group.) The trend in the remaining dyads was toward a stronger-than-normal mother dominance for this age. The vulnerable children's language had shorter MLUs and significantly fewer transformations than the normal children's. Moreover, language stages, calculated according to Brown (10), were one to three levels below normal in all but 1 child. These language levels, estimated to be about one year behind normal, may even be overestimated because of the children's tendency to overemploy a small number of transformational types.

Linguistic Production in Schizophrenic Mothers

Table 2 shows that these mothers spoke only slightly less frequently to their children than did the normal group, but that their structural level was significantly simpler. Thus it appears that they simplified their language when speaking to their developing (and language-deviant) children. However, a look at the values measuring syntactic distance shows that they may have exaggerated the optimal modulation and provided too little syntactic distance between themselves and their children. A clue that their children at this age may be especially sensitive to the language model provided appears in the right-hand portion of the table. Whereas in the vulnerable group there is a significant tendency for an individual child's complexity level to correlate directly with the mother's, this is not true for the normal group at this age.

Questioning Behavior of Vulnerable Pairs

As seen in tables 3 and 4, mothers in the vulnerable group tended to ask fewer questions per half hour than normal mothers, and their children asked about half as many as those in the normal group. Both mothers and children asked relatively few questions of the complex predicative form. The right-hand column combines mothers' and children's questions in considering their time character: more than 16 times as many of the normal group's questions involved past or future time. Moreover, only 1 of the vulnerable dyads engaged in fantasy interaction, and that mother-child pair did little else.

Responding Behavior of Vulnerable Pairs

As measured by our parameters of "good responses" and "nonresponses," there seemed to be no differences on means between mothers in the vulnerable and normal groups. There were trends toward

3. LINGUISTIC DEVELOPMENT

TABLE 1
Language of Normal, Vulnerable, and Autistic Four-Year-Old Children

Measure	Normal Children (N=8)	Vulnerable Children (N=8)	Significance*	Autistic Children (N=11)	Significance*
Mean number of utterances per 30-minute session	284	210	p<.05	184	p<.10
Mean percent of total (mother and child) utterances	46.1	44.6	n.s.	32.1	p<.10
Mean MLU	2.88	2.65	n.s.	2.07	p<.01
Mean number of transformation types	15.3	10.6	p<.05	6.7	p<.01

* Compared with normal children; two-tailed t test.

TABLE 2
Language of Normal Mothers, Schizophrenic Mothers, and Mothers of Autistic Children

Measure	Normal Mothers (N=8)	Schizophrenic Mothers (N=8)	Significance*	Mothers of Autistic Children (N=11)	Significance*
Mean number of utterances per 30-minute session	329	283	n.s.	351	p<.10
Mean percent of total (mother and child) utterances	53.9	55.4	n.s.	67.9	p<.10
Mean MLU	4.11	3.43	p<.05	3.74	n.s.
Mean number of transformation types	24.3	14.6	p<.01	20.3	p<.10
Syntactic distance from child					
In MLUs**	1.23	0.78	n.s.	1.67	n.s.
In number of transformation types***	9.0	4.0	p<.05	13.6	p<.05
Correspondence of mothers' and children's MLUs					
Correlation coefficient	.33	.64	p<.10	.71	p<.05
Rank order coefficient	.07	.64	p<.10	.56	p<.10

* Compared with normal mothers; two-tailed t test.
** Mean MLU of mothers minus mean MLU of children (see table 1).
*** Mean number of transformation types used by mothers minus mean number used by children (see table 1).

fewer good responses and more nonresponses in the vulnerable children.

Parameters in the Autistic Group

As we might expect, there was a significantly lower quantity and complexity of language production in the autistic children (see table 1). Their mothers, as shown in table 2, showed a trend toward an increased amount of verbal production. The mothers' complexity level looks lower than that of the normal group, but they provided a higher than normal amount of syntactic distance. That is, despite the low absolute level of complexity, their language is pitched at a relatively higher level in relation to their children's language. We found mothers' and children's language complexity to be highly correlated.

In their questioning (table 3), mothers of autistic children showed high values of total Wh questions but normal levels of Wh-predicative questions. Their children were below normal in both of these categories. The joint value for time character shows an overwhelming predominance of present time context. There is also equal to superior responding behavior by mothers of the autistic group, with many good responses and few nonresponses. Their children are dramatically deviant from normal levels on both measures, with directions reversed from those of their mothers—namely, few good responses and an extremely high level of nonresponses.

DISCUSSION

We have seen a lag in and distortion of language production in the group of 4-year-old children of schizophrenic mothers. Quantitatively, the abnormalities were always less than those seen in autistic children, but in the same direction from normal values. Qualitatively, none of the frequently seen autistic features (reversal of pronouns, lack of a vocative term for mother, echoes, abnormal prosody) was present, except in one child later diagnosed as schizophrenic. Neither were

136

TABLE 3
Questioning and Responding Patterns of Mothers in Normal, Vulnerable, and Autistic Mother-Child Pairs

Item*	Normal Mothers (N=8)	Schizophrenic Mothers (N=8)	Significance**	Mothers of Autistic Children (N=11)	Significance**
Questions					
Number	78.5	67.8	n.s.	100.9	n.s.
Percent of total utterances	24.8	24.3	n.s.	31.0	n.s.
Number of Wh questions	30.5	27.1	n.s.	45.0	p<.10
Number of predicative Wh questions	19.1	11.1	p<.10	17.3	n.s.
Percent of "not-now" questions	8.3***	0.5***	p<.01	0.4	p<.01
Responses					
Percent of good responses	44.7	42.3	n.s.	63.3†	n.s.
Percent of nonresponses	25.0	27.6	n.s.	18.3†	n.s.

* Mean per 30-minute session.
** Compared with normal mothers; two-tailed t test.
***Joint mother-child value.
†N=7 for these variables.

TABLE 4
Questioning and Responding Patterns of Children in Normal, Vulnerable, and Autistic Mother-Child Pairs

Item*	Normal Children (N=8)	Vulnerable Children (N=8)	Significance**	Autistic Children (N=11)	Significance**
Questions					
Number	64.8	34.2	p<.10	28.3	p<.10
Percent of total utterances	22.9	17.0	n.s.	12.2	n.s.
Number of Wh questions	27.4	22.5	n.s.	20.3	n.s.
Number of predicative Wh questions	19.0	4.4	p<.05	2.3	p<.01
Percent of "not-now" questions	8.3***	0.5***	p<.01	0.4	p<.01
Responses					
Percent of good responses	52.3	41.9	n.s.	25.6	p<.01
Percent of nonresponses	24.9	35.3	n.s.	43.8	p<.10

* Mean per 30-minute session.
** Compared with normal children; two-tailed t test.
*** Joint mother-child value.

there any of the gross abnormalities seen in adult schizophrenia, such as word salad, clang associations, or the poetic linguistic devices mentioned above. Despite the quite obvious qualitative differences between the language of the vulnerable and autistic children, both manifested such features as rigidity, perseveration, stereotypy, and restriction of repertoire and context. Examples of these traits were seen in one mother-child pair who exchanged a set of three or four questions and responses about the price of a toy ("How much?"; "Thirty-eight cents."; "Is that thirty-eight cents?") for a major portion of their 30-minute session.

A major feature of the vulnerable group was the presence of these abnormal qualities in the communicative language of the mothers as well as that of their children. Whereas a normal group mother might ask elaborate ostensive questions such as "Who is that little boy riding on the truck?" and rephrase the question if not answered, the schizophrenic mother would ask a simple "What's this?" and turn to a different ob-

ject and question if not responded to. Furthermore, fully one-third of the times a schizophrenic mother asked a question she did not allow the child time to respond; she looked away, changed the subject, or asked further questions. The fact that our response categories in their present form do not yet measure this tendency, as well as a qualitatively different "feel" to responses in the vulnerable group, has led us (in other work in progress) to subdivide the global categories of good response and nonresponse into measures such as appropriateness, correctness, and no time given for response. We will test our hypothesis that vulnerable and normal groups are farther apart on some of these more specific parameters. Despite the limitations of the present global categories, however, some striking differences were seen.

Subsequent to this study, one child in the vulnerable group was independently diagnosed as schizophrenic. In retrospect, we found that her mother had had the highest percentage of nonresponses (49%), and had asked the highest percentage of Wh questions (61%);

however, she also asked the lowest percentage of Wh-predicative questions (19%)—i.e., more than four-fifths of her Wh questions were requests for a label. Her child's language level, typical for the vulnerable group, did not warrant this simplicity. In this case and others, we may add infantilization and lack of mother-child coordination to the abnormal psycholinguistic qualities seen in the vulnerable group. Our preliminary conclusion about this child and others of her group is that she is being given a deficient, distorted, and mis-matched language model by the mother, which contributes to her own developing language deficiency.

The group of mothers of autistic children showed, by contrast, a normal to superior level in all parameters studied. Typical of these were good responses, in which 5 of 7 mothers scored over 70%, and syntactic distance, in which 9 of 11 pitched their language to a level one or two words higher than their children's level of language complexity. It is interesting that the 2 mothers who were outside this range—one lower, one higher—also had the fewest good responses. By comparison, 5 of 8 mothers in the vulnerable group had fewer than 44% good responses, and 6 of 8 had less than one-word syntactic distance. The only 2 mothers who made 100% good responses were both in the autistic group. Both a didactic aim and a pitch at the chronological—rather than the linguistic—age of the child can be concluded both from these results and from observer impressions of their interactions.

In our preliminary analysis of the autistic group, we see the high mother-child complexity correlation as comprised largely of the mother's "tuning-in" to her developing child, just as we feel that much of the high mother-child correlation in the vulnerable group was a result of the child's tuning-in to the mother. That the mothers in the autistic group did not pitch their language level quite as low in relation to their children's as normal group mothers is probably due to a "floor effect." That is, an adult cannot readily simplify her language below a certain natural lower limit if she is to say anything substantial. Therefore it would seem to be a combination of the adult's floor effect and the autistic child's extremely low MLU that accounts for the greater syntactic distance in the autistic group.

Among other possible sources of variance that need to be further explored are the following: 1) the heterogeneity of both abnormal groups, especially the autistic children, who have a verbal, questioning subgroup and a very silent subgroup; 2) the socioeconomic status of the autistic group, which is higher than that of the others; 3) the early mother-child separation due to mother's illness in the vulnerable group; 4) the influence of phenothiazine medication on communication; and 5) the effect of mental illness in general, rather than schizophrenia in particular, on family communication.

Longitudinal and statistical extension of our study should clarify and may modify our preliminary conclusions and their scope. Although the communication patterns in both experimental groups are at variance with those of the normal mothers and children, there are differences between the two disturbed populations as well as similarities. Mothers of autistic children function linguistically more like normal mothers than like schizophrenic mothers on most variables, in spite of the fact that their children are very deviant. That they adjust to their children's chronological rather than linguistic age has been noted. We cannot disprove that this is inappropriate rather than beneficially didactic, but it is striking that other studies, as well as these preliminary findings, indicate that mothers of autistic children are not schizophrenic in behavior or diagnosis, and, more important, that schizophrenic mothers do not appear to produce autistic children. This suggests the need for considerable reevaluation of the nature, etiology, and sequelae of communication disturbances in families in which one or more members is psychotic if our work is to have diagnostic and clinical relevance to psychiatry.

REFERENCES

1. Chaika EO: A linguist looks at "schizophrenic" language. Brain and Language 1:257–276, 1974
2. Wynne LC: Communication disorders and the quest for relatedness in families of schizophrenics. Am J Psychoanal 30:100–114, 1970
3. Goldfarb W, Yudkovitz, E, Goldfarb N: Verbal symbols to designate objects: an experimental study of communication in mothers of schizophrenic children. J Autism Child Schizo 3:281–298, 1973
4. Shapiro T: Imitation and echoing in young schizophrenic children. J Am Acad Child Psychiatry 9:548–567, 1970
5. Howlin P, Cantwell D, Marchant R, et al: Analyzing mothers' speech to young autistic children: a methodological study. Journal of Abnormal Child Psychology 4:317–339, 1973
6. Cantwell D: Personal communication, 1975
7. Baldwin AL, Frank SM: Syntactic complexity in mother–child interactions. Presented at the biannual meeting of the Society for Research in Child Development, Santa Monica, Calif, March 30, 1969
8. Baldwin AC, Baldwin CP: Study of mother–child interaction. Am Sci 61:714–721, 1973
9. Frank SM, Seegmiller MS: Children's language environment in free play situations. Presented at the biannual meeting of the Society for Research in Child Development, Philadelphia, March 30, 1973
10. Brown R: A First Language. The Early Stages. Cambridge, Mass, Harvard University Press, 1973
11. Frank SM, Osser N: A psycholinguistic model of syntactic complexity. Lang Speech 13:38–53, 1970
12. Snow CE: Mothers' speech to children learning language. Child Dev 43:549–565, 1972
13. Clarke-Stewart KA: Interactions Between Mothers and Their Young Children: Characteristics and Consequences. Society for Research in Child Development Monograph 153. Chicago, Society for Research in Child Development, 1973
14. Nelson K: Structure and Strategy in Learning to Talk. Society for Research in Child Development Monograph 149. Chicago, Society for Research in Child Development, 1973
15. Brown R: The development of wh-questions in child speech. Journal of Verbal Learning and Behavior 7:279–290, 1968
16. Ervin-Tripp S: Discourse agreement: how children answer questions, in Cognition and the Development of Language. Edited by Hayes JR. New York, John Wiley & Sons, 1970. pp 79–107
17. Blank M: Teaching Learning in the Preschool: A Dialogue Approach. Columbus, Ohio, Charles E. Merrill, 1973
18. Klima ES, Bellugi U: Syntactic regularities in the speech of

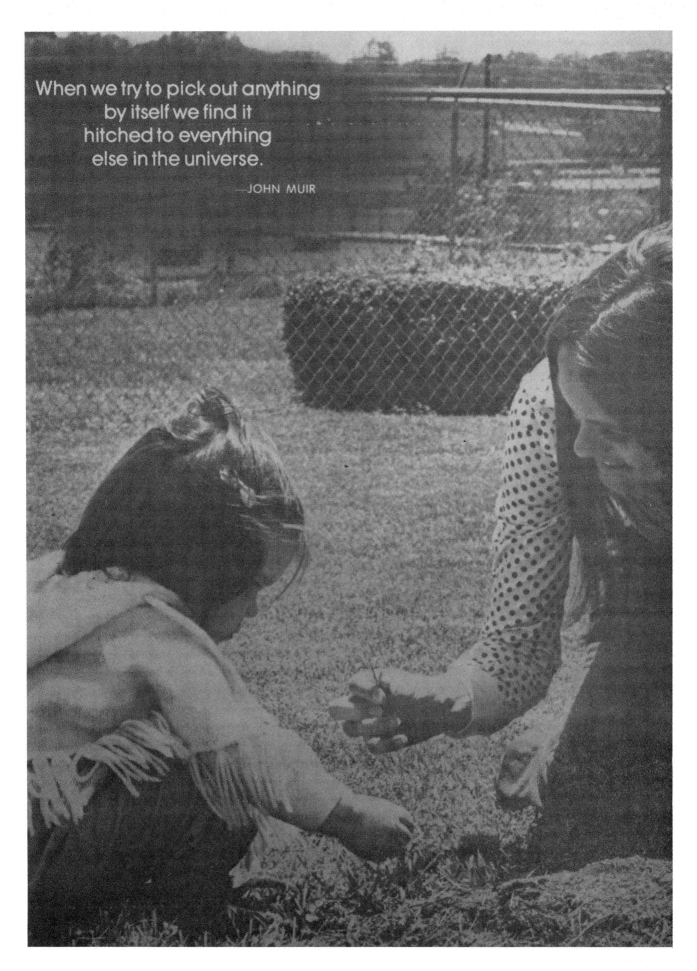

When we try to pick out anything
by itself we find it
hitched to everything
else in the universe.

—JOHN MUIR

139

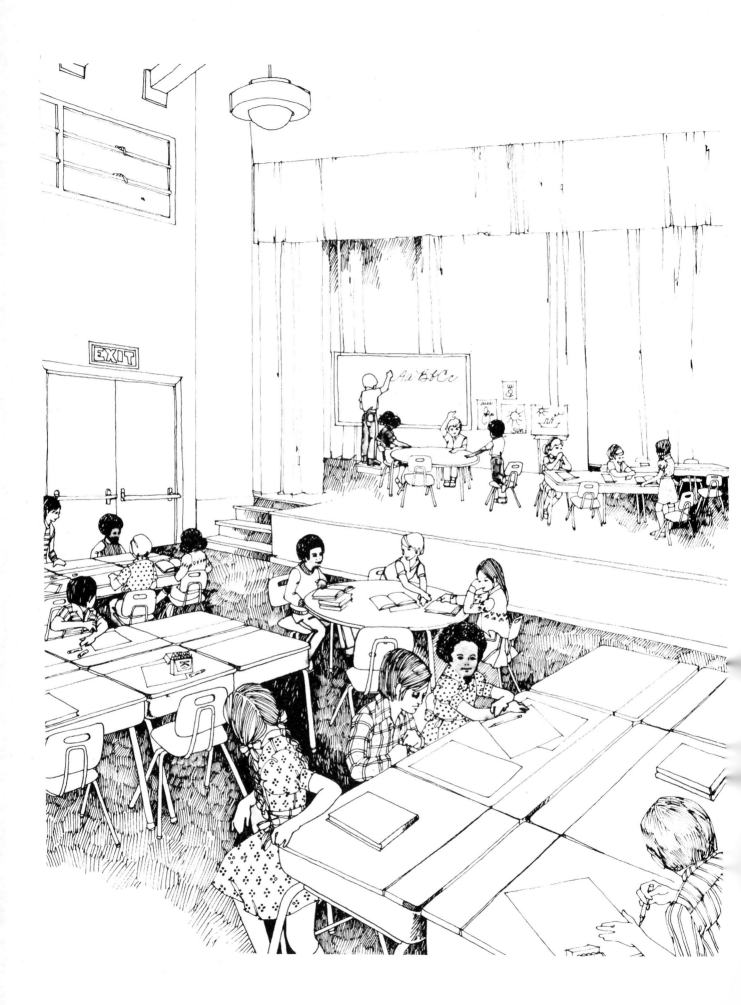

Educational Services

In the process of delivering effective and appropriate educational services to children with auditory and speech disorders, professionals must first examine the nature and needs of each child individually. Selecting educational programs based on stereotyped models of children with this disability, can only result in ineffective education. With the use of current modes of testing and assessment procedures, the trained professional may now start the child on the path to appropriate educational programming. Once the educational objectives for a child with auditory or speech defects have been identified, educational placement procedures may begin. Considering the current emphasis on mainstreaming the exceptional child into the regular classroom, the linguistically or auditorially hand-icapped child may now find himself/herself placed in an environmment with normal children. For the child whose needs are so mild that a small amount of additional remedial therapy will suffice, this placement is fine. However, for the child with moderate or severe auditory-speech impairments, full time remediation may be called for. Recent developments in preventitive and corrective programs call for a diminished need for segregation. Acoustic hearing aids, speech reading, and the development of enlightened speech programs have entered the picture today, increasing the chance for progress. New public awareness, federal legislation, and an overall concern for quality educational services for all handicapped children will only benefit these children in years to come.

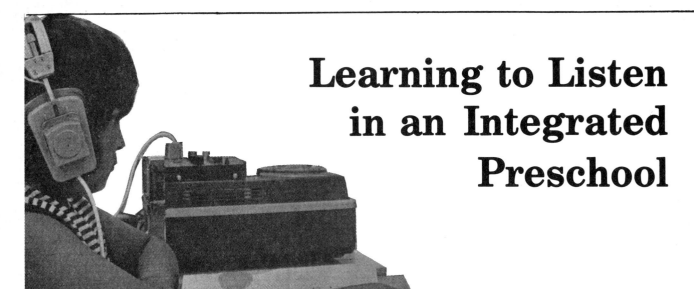

Learning to Listen in an Integrated Preschool

Doreen Pollack and Marian Ernst

A young child goes through specific stages of development when he acquires certain types of learning more easily than he ever will again. This applies to verbal communication almost more than to any other skill. However, until the advent of equipment to test infant hearing and the manufacture of the modern wearable hearing aid, the opportunity to learn speech and language in the early years was denied to the youngster with a hearing loss.

why integrate?

Most hearing impaired infants today can be fitted with hearing aids which give, at the very least, the opportunity to hear voices at a conversational level. The educational pendulum therefore is swinging away from their segregation in a special learning environment. It is now felt that the preschooler with a hearing loss should go to a normal preschool where he will be encouraged to use his hearing and to listen to the natural speech and language of his peers. In an environment where everyone else talks, he, too, will be motivated to speak. Even if his own speech is extremely limited, he will be exposed to normal child-centered activities and to more challenging concepts which will aid in his own conceptual development.

He will also learn at an early age to cope with the mainstream and to pattern his social behavior after the norm. Too often, we overprotect a child with a handicap, make excuses for unacceptable behavior, and set our expectation levels too low. Professionals, no less than lay people, are guilty of setting limits on what the hearing impaired child can do, instead of giving him the benefit of the doubt — the opportunity and support to try and succeed!

It is natural for teachers to feel misgivings when they are asked, for the first time, to take into the group a child who is different. But they may experience more rewards than problems, particularly when they see the awakening of understanding and compassion in the normal-hearing child and the progress made by the limited hearing youngster.

prior considerations

Although hearing impaired children have been integrated into all types of programs with very successful results, not every preschool offers the right program for every child. Initial placement should be preceded by consideration of the child's needs and of the goals which each program sets

"Learning to Listen in an Integrated Preschool," Doreen Pollack, Marian Ernst, *The Volta Review*, 1973. ©1973 The Alexander Graham Bell Association for the Deaf, Inc.

for its enrollees. Ideally, there should be only one hearing impaired child in a preschool group, but a ratio of one to each four or five normal-hearing children is workable. The child should also be within two years of the average chronological age of the group. The hearing impaired child needs to interact verbally in activities involving normal youngsters, but if there are too many "special" preschoolers in one room, they tend to form their own nonverbal group — and very rapidly, too.

Most preschoolers with a hearing loss attend a speech and hearing clinic, and the clinician may well be the most knowledgeable person to recommend a specific program. Usually placement is not advised until the child has worn his hearing aids continuously for some length of time and has developed some communication skill, particularly in the area of cooperation and attention.

In addition to the child's developmental and interest levels, the preschool teacher will need to know how the child communicates and how adults and other children normally communicate with him. Some parent-infant programs emphasize listening and learning through the hearing aids, some stress speechreading, and others encourage sign language.

The teacher will also need to know what types of abilities the child brings into the situation. Two children with identical hearing losses, as tested by an audiometer, will probably function quite differently. One may learn quickly in spite of the loss, while another may have a loss which is secondary to other problems, such as perceptual motor disabilities.

understanding the hearing aid

Although the responsibilities of the teacher do not really change when a hearing impaired child enters her class, she may find that she has to assume a more active role in structuring the verbal environment; and she should maintain close contact with the parents and with the clinician who is working to develop the child's speech and language skills. She may enjoy visiting the clinic program and should try to attend inservice meetings.

It is the responsibility of the parent or the clinician to demonstrate to the teacher the working of a hearing aid. A modern hearing aid is easy to handle. It is worn either behind the ear or upon the chest. A small wheel on the aid controls the volume so that sound is amplified with a slight turn of the wheel just like a radio. Some aids have a separate on-off switch or a lever which is pushed to the M or microphone position.

The sound is conducted from the aid through a cord or tube attached to an earmold which must fit snugly into the child's ear. Sometimes the mold slips out a little, and a squealing or whistling sound is produced. It is easy to push it back without hurting the ear.

A hearing aid is battery powered and the parent should test the battery or batteries before the child leaves for school; it is also helpful to have a spare battery at school in case the aid stops working. Parents should be sure that the child's teacher knows how to find out if the aid is not working even if the child is too young to tell her. The teacher should hold the receiver — and the ear insert which clips onto it — close to the hearing aid and turn the on-off switch (or the volume control into which it is incorporated). She should hear a clear feedback whistling sound. A crackling sound may indicate a broken cord, and no sound usually means the battery is dead. When inserting a new battery, she should be sure that the positive sign (+) is placed by the same sign inside the battery compartment of the aid.

A hearing aid should be worn throughout the child's waking hours — but not in the swimming pool! If there is going to be water or sand play, the teacher can cover the aid with a piece of plastic to protect it.

4. EDUCATIONAL SERVICES

Two booklets which are helpful in familiarizing adults and children with the use and maintenance of hearing aids are *Tim and His Hearing Aid* by Eleanor Ronnei (The Alexander Graham Bell Association for the Deaf, 3417 Volta Place, N.W., Washington, D.C., $1.75) and *Caring for a Child's Hearing Aid* by Charlotte Dempsey (Zenith Hearing Aid Sales Corporation, 6501 West Grand Avenue, Chicago, Illinois 60635).

what can the teacher tell the other children?

Remembering that youngsters accept a child for what he is, it is not really necessary to bring up the subject of a hearing aid until someone notices it and asks questions. It may be days or weeks before this happens unless the aid is worn conspicuously in a large harness outside the clothes. The easiest way to explain the aid is the most direct way: "Some of us do not see well. Our eyes do not work the way they should so we have to wear glasses. Bobby's ears do not work the way they should so he has to wear a hearing aid. It makes everything louder so Bobby can hear better. Do you want to listen to it?"

The other children should be told not to pull the cords – which break easily – or to bump Bobby's ears. Everyone should be reminded not to shout at Bobby but to talk naturally and close to him so that they can be heard more clearly. It is not unusual for some of the other children to want a hearing aid, too!

The questions which most puzzle the first-time teacher of a child with a hearing loss (especially if the child does not respond immediately) are: "Can he really hear me? How much can he hear? Will he talk clearly? Do I have to wait until he looks at me before I speak to him?"

For too long, the word *deafness* has been understood as *total;* that is, you can either hear or not hear. In reality, there are all degrees of hearing loss, from mild to profound, and most children labeled "deaf" do possess residual hearing. When fitted with hearing aids at an early age and given the training necessary to make optimal use of his aided hearing, the "deaf" child of today does not have to grow in silence. Although a hearing aid does not give him normal hearing, he can develop auditory skills following a normal sequence, and these can be supplemented with visual clues.

the development of auditory skills

All children move through several levels of listening before reaching a conversational level. The first level involves developing *awareness* of and *attention* to sound. We are stimulated by noisemakers, music, environmental noises, and the human voice. These sounds come from different directions and from different distances. It helps the young "deaf" child if we clap our hands to our ears and say, "I hear that. Listen!"

On the second level we develop the ability to *localize* the source of each sound. It helps to turn the hearing impaired child in the right direction if he does not do so himself.

The third level involves *discrimination,* or the ability to sort out the stimuli and organize them into meaningful patterns. For example, each child can hold up the correct animal picture to match the sound he hears on a tape recording. This happens only after much stimulation.

On the fourth level we learn the appropriate *response* to sound. If we hear the door bell, we open the door. If our name is called, we turn around, and so on.*

Hopefully, by the time the hearing impaired child enters preschool he has been taught not only to listen, but also to *imitate* what he hears so that speaking (even if it often sounds like jargon) will accompany his

---

Educational Audiology for the Limited Hearing Infant, Doreen Pollack. Springfield, Ill.: Charles C Thomas, 1970.

growth in understanding language. Unless proved otherwise, he *does* have the innate ability to perceive the structure of his native language through his hearing aids, providing he receives enough input. Once he can use one-word phrases, he should be encouraged to increase his *memory span* and his ability to recall the correct *sequence* of words in a sentence. If the teacher knows what he is trying to express, she should say the sentence or phrase naturally, encourage him to imitate one word at a time, and then say the phrase again naturally. From a two-unit span, such as: *Help me* and *no more,* he will move on to a three-unit span, like: *Put it back, I want more, Where's my ball?;* and then to a four-word span: *I hear the airplane.*

Activities which develop good listening skills will benefit the whole group. Rhythm band, dance and song, nursery rhymes, finger plays, puppet shows, and counting rhymes are some of the activities for which there are attractive materials available today.* The children must also learn to follow directions, answer questions, and associate sounds with printed symbols.

Some inattention may be anticipated if the hearing impaired child is required to sit for a long period of time listening to a story, a recording, or group discussion without any visual supplements. He should be seated next to the teacher where he can see the pictures in a book or be "cued into" the subject under discussion. If the child has very little speech or language comprehension it may be necessary to arrange another activity for him, but it is not wise to make too many exceptions.

suggestions for the teacher — how to communicate

1. To get the child's attention, always call his name until he turns around; there is no need to touch him. If a teacher acts as though she does not expect him to hear, he will become conditioned to not listening.

2. Give the child time to respond. Listening is temporal and requires auditory processing within the brain. Do not rush an answer if you feel that the child should be able to get it for himself. On the other hand, if he has trouble maintaining his attention, guide him to the correct response and then repeat the word or phrase again.

3. Keep within fairly close range when providing instruction or doing any formal teaching. Many hearing impaired children have difficulty hearing clearly if the speaker is more than five feet from the hearing aid. It helps to bend down to the level of the aid. If speechreading is used, try to speak with the light on your face.

4. Use a normal conversational tone of voice. Very quiet voices are of course difficult to hear; and when voices are too loud they become distorted. Use interesting inflections and animated facial expressions; this helps all young children.

5. Use normal speech patterns. A child best learns to understand communication when it occurs in sentences as part of an activity. He may not respond, but that does not mean he did not hear what was said.

6. Encourage speech development by providing good models. Use short, clear phrases, speak at a moderate pace, and do not gesture too much. Sit beside the child when working individually, and place him next to children with good voices for group activities, such as finger plays.

7. Verbalize often and give frequent repetition. Use unfamiliar words many times in meaningful contexts. For example, "Push the wagon, push, push, push," or "That's *soft.* Feel it. It's so soft. It's soft like the bunny. It's soft like your hair."

8. Try to use the same phrases for the same activity until the child knows them. Then change the wording. For example: "Put it back. Put it

---

Auditory Perception, T. Oakland and F. Williams. Seattle: Special Child Publications, 1971.

4. EDUCATIONAL SERVICES

in the box. Put it on the shelf. Clean up time!"

9. Reinforce with the same phrases: "Good boy!" "Good try!"

10. "Clue the child in." When he joins the group, tell him: "Mary is talking about her new dog. She said he is little-bitty. His name is . . ."

how to encourage verbal interaction

Activities in which the teacher, a normal-hearing child, and the hearing impaired child all participate are usually more successful at first than those which involve a larger group of children. When the activity is proceeding well and the children are working cooperatively and using appropriate verbal expressions that the teacher has incorporated into the activity, the children should be left to continue by themselves. After a few minutes, they may abandon the activity, usually because something else attracts their attention, or perhaps because the hearing impaired child does not yet have the verbal skill to keep up with the others. Far from being discouraged, however, the teacher should look upon this as a beginning, for with repeated experiences the child's interactive abilities will improve and expand.

Activities designed to stimulate social and emotional growth can also provide concrete opportunities to develop communication skills. Having tea parties, washing dishes, planting seeds, or teaching a dog to "sit" will be more valuable when the teacher initially takes an active role in setting up the verbal patterns which then become an integral part of the activity. "Would you like a cookie? Yes, please. Would you like some tea? Pour! Pour!"

Most games appropriate for young children have very simple rules. If these rules are translated into simple verbal expressions which the hearing impaired child can learn, he can then move toward a more interactive role. If the teacher encourages all of the children to incorporate such expressions as "my turn" and "your turn" into the activity, the hearing impaired child will be assisted in his attempts to use the expressions and to interact appropriately.

Knowledge of the child's vocabulary can also be helpful. For example, if the child knows the names of colors, a game using color words offers the opportunity for his active verbal participation.

how to develop communication ability

The teacher should first provide the child with appropriate verbal patterns or speech models and then expand upon the child's own utterances. Verbal expression may be encouraged by observing the items and situations which interest the child and providing a model for his response.

1. Helping the child make verbal *observations*.
Teacher: "Jane has a funny hat. Say, 'That's funny.' "
Child: "That's funny." Or, "That's a funny hat."
Teacher: "Billy's daddy is tall. Say, 'He's tall.' "
Child: "He's tall."
Teacher: "Mary has a pretty dress. Say, 'That's pretty.' "
Child: "That's pretty."

2. Helping the child express *needs* and *wishes*.
Teacher: "You'd like a cookie? Say, 'I want a cookie.' "
Child: "I want a cookie."
Teacher: "You need some scissors. Say, 'Where's the scissors?' "
Child: "Where's scissors?"

3. Helping the child ask for *assistance*.
Teacher: "You need help with your shoe. Say, 'Help me tie my shoe.' "
Child: "Help me," or "Help me, shoe," or "Help me tie my shoe."

146

4. Helping the child express his *feelings*.

Teacher: "You are hungry. You want to eat. Say, 'I'm hungry.' "
Child: "I'm hungry." Or "I'm tired," or "I don't want to play," or "I'm sick."

5. Helping the child remark about *events*.

Teacher: "Johnny hurt his foot. Say, 'What happened to Johnny's foot?' "
Child: "What happened, Johnny's foot?"
Teacher: "Say, 'It hurts.' "
Child: "It hurts."
Teacher: "What's Johnny doing? Say, 'Johnny's crying.' "
Child: "Johnny's crying."

6. Helping the child note *daily routine*.

Teacher: "Good morning, It's time for school. Say, 'Time for school.' "
Child: "Time for school." Or "Time to play," or "Time for lunch," or "Rest time," or "Story time."

Expanding language may mean using the child's own language patterns as a vehicle to encourage him to incorporate more information in his verbal expressions. Provide additional vocabulary for him to use to expand his utterances:

Child: "car"
Teacher: "That's a car."
Child: "That car."
Teacher: "That's a blue car."
Child: "Blue car."
Teacher: "Push the car."
Child: "Push car."
Teacher: "Push the blue car."
Child: "Push blue car."

Expanding a child's concepts often means helping him associate a new word with familiar vocabulary or earlier learning. For example, if "hydrant" is a new word, the teacher might say:

It's a hydrant. What's a hydrant for? It's for water. It's a water hydrant. Who uses it? A fireman uses a water hydrant for fires. A fireman uses the water to fight fires. He gets the water from a fire hydrant.

guidelines for parental interaction

1. Help parents know their child's school.

Understanding of the school's program and good relationships with its staff members will encourage effective communication. If a problem arises or the teacher has a particular concern, the parents will know about it early and be able to help.

2. Prepare a written copy of the words to songs and finger plays so that parents can teach them at home.

These new words are usually very difficult for the young hearing impaired child to learn in a group. If they are taught to him at home, he may find it easier to participate in school.

3. Let parents observe their child in school.

Many parents are reluctant to visit the classroom, but periodic observations will help parents recognize the child's immediate needs and the ways they can help. Although hearing impaired children are often immature for their chronological age, it is often encouraging for parents to see that their child is more *like* the normal-hearing children than he is *different*. The teacher's emphasis on the child's abilities rather than disabilities will be a positive factor in his overall emotional adjustment to school.

4. Pin a note on the child's pocket or talk to his mother about the school day.

Many hearing impaired children are not ready to relate events that happen away from home. A knowledgeable parent can do a great deal to help a child verbally reconstruct his school day and can reinforce vocabulary and concepts.

5. Arrange periodic conferences between parent, teacher, and clinician to discuss the child's needs and the ways to meet them. In some schools, a teacher's best aide is a parent.

developing appropriate attitudes

Obviously, the preschool or kindergarten teacher must understand the values of developing programs which help the hearing impaired child learn normal patterns of speech and language and of behavior and acceptance as well. The teacher should be cautioned to resist the tendency to overprotect or to allow things to be too different for this child. Normal patterns of behavior must always be encouraged, and sometimes this means holding back a bit to allow the child ample opportunity to learn and develop his own resources.

Attitudes of other children

Children of preschool age accept a hearing impaired child as one like themselves. Curiosity about the hearing aid may not arise until after they have been around the child for some time. With somewhat older children, a spontaneous attitude of helpfulness may emerge among them when the hearing impaired child is not "tuned in." Attitudes toward others develop on a day-by-day basis through experience; teachers often note that having a hearing impaired child as part of the class has a positive value for all the children.

Attitudes of other parents

The majority of parents of normal children will support having the child with special needs in the nursery. Only in very rare cases do they object, and when this occurs, the staff must consider their own attitudes, too. Prejudice is sometimes caused by a lack of understanding or insufficient knowledge. A better understanding of the purposes for placing the child with his normal peer group can lead to more tolerant attitudes.

Young children will someday become adults. Whether a child has had difficulties to overcome — or whether he has known *another* person who eventually found ways to resolve *his* problems — affects the kind of world in which these children will one day live.

Teaching Aural Language

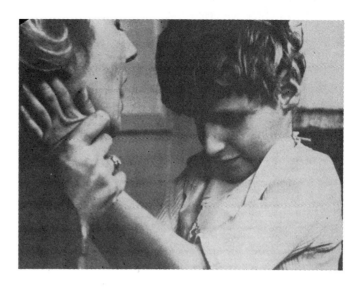

AUDREY ANN SIMMONS, Ed.D.

WHEN WE BEGIN THE EDUCATION of the hearing impaired child we are besieged by a battery of questions from parents. "Will Johnny talk?" and "When will he speak?" occur with the greatest frequency. With something akin to cathechismal acceptance, they listen to our perennial response, "Of course Johnny will talk, *after* he has acquired language."

When the parents read the literature appropriate to their needs they find the areas of speech and language treated almost as if it were speech *or* language. In fact, there are those who would have us believe that one can exist without the other.

Articles on the subject of language of the deaf tend to dismiss the spoken aspect completely and direct all the attention to the grammar of the written form which has been shown by psychologists to be of very complex nature for hearing children. On the other hand, if the article that deals with the vocal production of language (speech) appears in our journals, it usually treats only articulatory problems of speech. We may be fostering the speech-language dichotomy by studying only those aspects of language which lend themselves to the tools we have available to measure them, and by dismissing the several aspects that force us to consider the interrelation of the two, because they are elusive.

The concept that language and speech are separate entities may also be inferred when we set aside certain periods for training of speech. Fre-quently, individual speech teachers concentrate on articulation of single sounds and single words to the exclusion of other aspects. Other teachers may do auditory training in other periods when nonlinguistic noise-generating instruments (bells, whistles, records) provide the stimuli.

The linguists have been telling us for some time that language is both an auditory and vocal process which incorporates phonology, syntax, and semantics as shown in Figure 1.

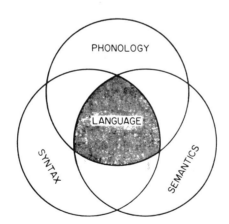

FIGURE 1   *Linguistic components of language*

Linguists agree that the *spoken language* is the language and that its most stable features are phonologic. Syntax and grammar are constantly undergoing change. Look at what is happening to the word *like*. "Winstons taste good like a cigarette should," while ungrammatical, is still language. Certainly the English language is abused, if not changed, with every issue of *Time Magazine*.

PHONOLOGY

Consider the three features which make up the phonologic portion of the interrelated aspects of language as shown in Figure 2.

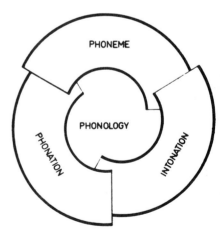

FIGURE 2   *Components of phonology*

Phonology is the sound or vocal system of the language. It includes the smallest unit in the process as well as the largest. Since children learn from the general to the specific, the smallest units are usually the last to develop in their repertory and with hearing children are not perfected until they are 7 or 8 years old.

PHONEMES

The smallest units are the phonemes of the language, which in our case is the English of our region. There are approximately 46 of these phonemes or speech elements which follow a predictable pattern. For example, children deduce at an early age that a vowel usually follows a consonant. Indeed, they have absorbed sufficient information that they observe the rule without ever knowing it exists.

They know, also, that a number of these units must be said in a given interval of time. Frequently, they misarticulate the sounds while giving appropriate timing to their utterances.

Deaf children, on the other hand, may take three to four times longer to articulate each phoneme and distort the relative durations among phonemes (Calvert). It may be that these distortions and inappropriate timings result from the speech teaching taking place away from the rest of the linguistic task. This may also be due to the overemphasis given single words or single sounds.

Sounds that look alike in print and that may be pronounced one way if taught alone or in single words are something quite different when put into meaning-bearing units for language. For example, "see Mabel" is different from "seem able" yet they contain the same phonemes. When we give the child such exercises as *p, t, k, f, th*, we may be failing to provide him with the correct data with which he can induce the consonant-vowel-consonant principle.

PHONATION

Phonation, as distinguished from phonemes, has to do with production, in particular the amount and quality. All of us are pleased that our children learn to talk, but there remains a problem that their voices are not always pleasant. Sometimes they are nasal, breathy, or harsh (Hudgins and Numbers).

It has been my experience that if a hearing impaired child has a model to follow with the emphasis on the meaning-bearing unit, the child tends to be relaxed in his imitation patterns. For the severely deaf child, the patterns may be given through multisensory modalities whereas, for the partially deaf child, it may be unisensory. When the stress is on *communication* and less on precision in the early periods of

instruction, the child has a purpose for the vocal effort. Given patterns that are meaningful to imitate, the hearing impaired child has less tension in his vocal output.

It may be that some of our activities should be examined. For example, the breath we use to extinguish a candle or to blow tissue paper may be more than the amount of breath we need to use to produce the sounds being taught that way, e.g., *p, t, k*. As a matter of fact, we could produce a large number of spoken words on that same amount of breath.

Furthermore, the timing of utterance can help to improve quality. If a child is encouraged to imitate the teacher's model of the sounds produced in the interval of time in which she spoke them, his speech should have good rhythm and not have a choppy quality.

Normal breath units, of course, are meaning units. It is very desirable that the hearing impaired child imitate normal units from the beginning. This would mean that classroom teaching would use simple phrases made up of several words rather than single words or words in carrier sentences. If the child has at least phrase units to attempt, he can't possibly build the habit of pumping out word by word.

INTONATION

This brings us to the third area of phonology, referred to by many linguists as intonation. They have shown that with hearing children, speech production proceeds by patterned wholes instead of by segments. Large patterns of intonation usually develop before the child begins *consciously* to develop the basic speech phonemes. When one listens to a young hearing child, he hears him employing genuine native intonations for statements, questions, and requests entirely without intelligible phonemes, words, or word groups. This is vocal language even though there is no observable meaning to adults, no statement by adult standards, but only the melodic and rhythmic contour-suggesting utterances (Leopold). We have found that when hearing impaired children are encouraged to talk when given meaning-units to follow, they too, pass through this phase.

Later, after the child has acquired phonemes, and some meaning-bearing units, he will fill these general configurations of sound with specific words and speech elements.

The child seems to develop linguistic control by working in from larger structural patterns to smaller ones. He understands a sentence because he

understands the "Bububu" as different from the "Bububu?" and quite different from "Bububu!" This is not because he has learned a rule that a sentence must have a subject and a verb, or that it must tell something, ask a question, or give a command. Nor is it because he understands a period, a question mark, or a comma. It is because intonation patterns are part of the grammar of his language. Intonation can be meaningful to the hearing impaired child in the same manner it is to the hearing sibling.

Prosodic patterns can tell even more about an utterance than what kind of sentence (statement, question, or exclamation). It can also denote internal meaning as well. For example, note the comma in "John, put the cat out" and its omission in "John put the cat out." These tools of intonation lead to grammar for hearing children and should help hearing impaired children also.

The meaning of a pattern can be altered entirely by the intonation used, e.g., Why did *you* come to Dallas? *Why* did you come to Dallas? Why did you come to *Dallas?* The hearing child derives emotive meaning from the intonation pattern. "The sad girl" and "the happy boy" take on meaning from their intonation before the abstractions, sadness and happiness, are truly understood. It is easier to generalize from the pattern than from the units taken singly.

As teachers, we must not forget that the very prosodic pattern of utterance changes the meaning conveyed by a speaker, for example, contrast the meaning of "Aw, you poor thing" said in sympathy and "Aw, you poor thing" said in sarcasm. Even the part of speech of a word can be changed by its stress pattern. Take the word "contrast" as used above in "contrast the meaning" and then the noun, "They are in sharp contrast." The features of phonology are always a part of the grammatical and syntactical structuring of American English. Intonation, in particular, is basic to our language.

SYNTAX

The language system is a totality, we hear it, speak it, and respond to it all of a piece and all at once. The aim of our teaching then is to approximate this totality of intake multisensorially, through mastery of the system. Here, space permits me only to direct your attention to the role of function words and urge you to seriously consider them in the early education of the children.

This talk was delivered at the Southwest Regional Meeting of the Alexander Graham Bell Association for the Deaf, held in Dallas, Tex., Oct. 6–7, 1967.

When I gave the students in our teacher education program the bibliography for their course, I marked it as follows:

- Books that must be read
- Books that should be read
- Books that might be read
- Books that could be read
- Books that may be read

The lexical words are all identical, but because of the function words, *must, should, might, could,* and *may,* I know which list will be used. Only one of those words forces the issue. A child who spends most of his time gaining meaning from single words does not have the opportunity to gain control of function words.

Certainly these are words which above all can never be taught in isolation, but only as they structure language—in syntactical patterns. They take on meaning only as they mark the lexical words which receive the primary stress. It is because function words usually get secondary stress that they are omitted from the early speech of hearing children; not only are *a, the, my, am, is, if, up, on, and* low in acoustic power, but they are also low in visibility. Deprived of these words, as the child is who has word lists to master, he may never gain control over these features. This is another reason the hearing impaired child needs meaning units to process through his multisensory vocal mechanism.

A sequence of language teaching in a classroom at Central Institute for the Deaf, where the teacher is following a linguistic program illustrates this point.

These children were able to imitate a model which was meaningful. The lesson grew from an activity all the children had experienced, the feeding of fish. The teacher gave training in auditory discrimination when she asked the children to identify the sentences they had listened to and seen earlier.

She corrected speech, particularly the faulty "sp" in *spots* and the timing of the sentence, by requiring the child to give a better imitation. She had the child process all the information through his vocal system, thereby helping him store linguistic information for later automatic use. All of these tasks, along with the teaching of concepts and providing opportunities for induction of rules, require a broadened view of language.

BIBLIOGRAPHY

CALVERT, D. R., "An Approach to the Study of Deaf Speech" in *Report of the Proceedings of the International Congress on Education of the Deaf.* Washington: U.S. Government Printing Office, 1963, pp. 242–245.

HUDGINS, C. V., and F. C. NUMBERS, *An Investigation of the Intelligibility of the Speech of the Deaf,* reviewed in *The Volta Review,* Jan., 1943, p. 42.

LEOPOLD, W., "Patterning in Children's Language," in S. Saporta (ed.), *Psycholinguistics.* New York: Holt, Rhinehart & Winston, 1961.

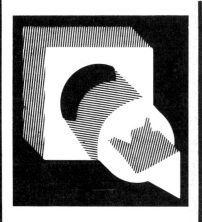

Characteristics of an Adequate Auditory/Oral Program—

A Guide for Parents and Educators

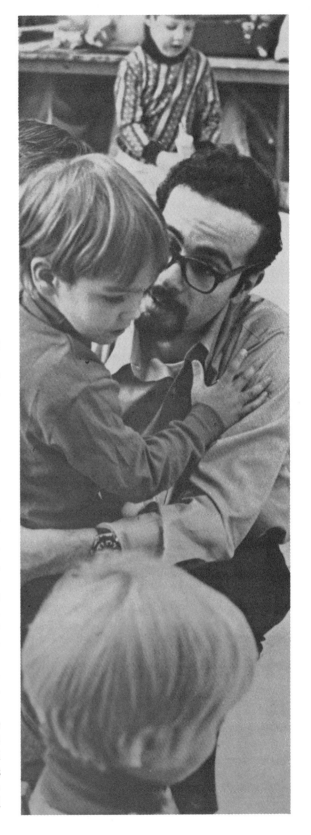

Of continuing concern to those involved in education of the hearing impaired is that of program evaluation. Dr. S. Richard Silverman, Chairman of the National Advisory Committee on Education of the Deaf, concluded the 1967 National Conference with a summation which included:

> Common sense requires that the effectiveness of any procedure, or change therein, be tested by the most objective investigations we can devise, so that substantive grounds are established for eliminating, amending, or modifying our arrangements and practices. In education this is difficult to accomplish. Many of these outcomes we seek resist satisfactory measurement, and some results must await the passage of years before an attempt at evaluation is even appropriate. Evaluation is a crucial issue demanding more concentrated attention.

As the urbanization of our nation continues at an accelerated pace, the proportion of deaf children being served in state residential schools and in large inner city centers is declining. Today approximately 60% of the educationally deaf are being programmed in day schools and classes.

Many of these programs are in small communities. They were initiated through parental pressures. They lack supervision and often operate with multi-graded classes having age ranges from 3 to 10 years. By 1965 the trend toward day schools and classes had become of sufficient magnitude to result in a federally sponsored conference to determine possible national, state, and professional measures to correct apparent weaknesses and limitations in services and administration.

As a result of this conference, which has since become known as the Lake Mohonk Conference,* some 35 priority recommendations were made. While it was acknowledged that due to financial and parental factors, small programs could not be eliminated, recommendations were made for the development of guidelines to assist in the evaluation of current programs and to assist in the establishment and operation of additional units in the future.

preparation of guidelines

No follow-up on the recommendations within the profession took

---

*Mulholland, A. M., & Fellendorf, G. W. (Investigators) *Final Report of the National Research Conference on Day Programs for Hearing Impaired Children.* Washington, D.C.: A. G. Bell Association for the Deaf, 1968.

"Characteristics of an Adequate Auditory/Oral Program—A Guide for Parents and Educators," *The Volta Review,* Vol. 77 No. 7, 1975. ©1975 The Alexander Graham Bell Association for the Deaf, Inc.

place until 1969 when the American Organization for the Education of the Hearing Impaired, the professional section of the Alexander Graham Bell Association for the Deaf, commissioned an ad hoc committee to draw up guidelines which could be utilized by parents, teachers, and administrators. The final report contained some 88 items, divided into 10 sub-areas. The guidelines were accepted by the Board of Directors of the parent organization in May, 1971.

In an effort to determine if the items represented the judgments of the hundreds of teachers, supervisors, and administrators currently assigned to programs for the hearing impaired, a project was carried out during the 1971-1973 school years to identify and rank in order of priority, characteristics of adequate auditory/oral programs.

The original 88 items were expanded to 129 in order to insure that only 1 attribute per item was being measured. A pilot study involving 25 teachers, 10 administrators, and 10 supervisors was conducted to identify any ambiguous material or faulty items. The final phase involved the distribution of the proposed rating scale to some 200 teachers, 30 administrators, and 30 supervisors, in 51 schools or classes, in 22 states and 2 Canadian provinces. Names were obtained from the current directory of the American Organization for the Education of the Hearing Impaired. All of the supervisors, 29 administrators, and 181 teachers responded. Participants were requested to rate each item on a value scale of from 0-7. Items were rank-ordered according to obtained scores.

In order to provide a simplified version of the rating scale for use by schools and parent groups, the 52 characteristics receiving the highest scores in the research project have been rank-ordered and placed into the 1975 revision of *Characteristics of Auditory/Oral Programs*. Those characteristics receiving an equal number of points are ranked together, giving a total of thirty-five levels in the rank-order. It is felt that this presents a realistic identification of adequate auditory/oral educational programs of the hearing impaired. Therefore, readers should keep in mind that these items are those deemed of prime importance and that there are other characteristics in evidence in most programs.

The relatively low rating given parent-infant services was of concern to those administering the original study. In a random check of participants, it was found that many of those responding assumed that a parent-infant program was the responsibility of another agency—and not the educational unit. In areas where parent-infant programs are not in operation, it would be assumed that the responsibility would then shift to the educational unit.

rank order of chosen characteristics

1. Faculty of classes for hearing impaired having philosophy and basic skills to insure that a majority of profoundly deaf children can be educated in an auditory/oral environment.

2. Appropriate amplification in each room.

3. Supervisors of local programs for hearing impaired having philosophy and basic skills to insure that a majority of profoundly deaf children should be educated in an oral environment.

4. Administrators of local programs for hearing impaired having a philosophy that a majority of profoundly deaf children should be educated in an oral environment.

4. EDUCATIONAL SERVICES

5. Supportive services available for teachers of normally hearing who have hearing impaired students integrated into regular classrooms.

6. Parents of hearing impaired children having a philosophy that a majority of profoundly deaf children should be educated in an oral environment.

7. Cumulative folders maintained on each child and available to faculty.

8. Decisions as to class placement, recommendations for transfers, curriculum modification, and parental participation made by supervisory and teacher personnel.

9. Periodic conferences for parents.

10. Public education activities to identify hearing impaired children prior to age 2.

---

11. Pertinent student information collected by the supervising teacher and made available to classroom teachers.

12. Sufficient space for physical activities and equipment, for children under age 6.

12. Periodic evaluation of speech and language curriculum outlines to measure attainment of short- and long-range objectives.

13. Supportive services by teachers of the deaf available through high school, whether integration is full or partial.

13. An audiologist.

14. Repair facilities for one-day service on amplification and instructional media equipment.

15. Curriculum procedures designed to stress self-responsibility and decision making on the part of hearing impaired students.

15. Yearly evaluation of students' progress toward attainment of long-range objectives developed by faculty.

15. Yearly evaluation of students' progress toward attainment of short-range objectives developed by faculty.

16. Typewriter, duplicator, and Thermo-fax equipment available for teachers.

17. Yearly staffing of all students to determine if changes in individual scheduling or placement are warranted.

17. Yearly evaluation of students' proficiency in oral communication through use of tests, tapes, and listeners.

18. On-going curriculum evaluation conducted by administrators, supervisors, and teachers in a coordinated effort.

19. Current audiological report as part of formal applications procedure.

20. Speech curriculum providing for systematic attainment of specific skills and competencies, preschool through junior high school.

20. Language arts curriculum characterized by continuity of methodology from preschool through junior high school.

20. Yearly evaluation of students' use of their residual hearing.

---

21. Parent interview as part of formal application procedure.

22. Yearly report to parents on the academic level attained by child.

23. Personnel in state department of special education having a belief that a majority of profoundly deaf children should be educated in an oral environment.

24. Supervisors and administrators who evaluate total school program yearly relative to attainment of short- and long-range objectives.

25. Selection of new personnel (administrators, supervisors, and teachers) by experienced educators of the hearing impaired.

26. Short- and long-range objectives (academic, communicative, and social) expressed in observable and measurable form.

26. Written evaluation of child's status sent to parents at least three times yearly.

27. Provision for junior and senior high students not recommended for integration to be served by teachers of the deaf.

27. Library in building with extensive listings of high-interest, low-reading-level books.

27. Faculty budget for special supplies, field trips, and materials.

28. Class size limited to six in preschool.

28. Provision for operation of classes within a district or in cooperation with other districts to provide homogeneous grouping not to exceed two grade levels per class.

28. Acoustically treated classrooms.

29. Public education program to orient the community as to the academic and vocational capabilities of the hearing impaired.

30. Yearly evaluation of total school program by faculty and presentation of recommendations to supervisors and administrators.

---

31. Class size limited to seven in primary grades.

32. Vocational rehabilitation specialist for programs with students over age 14.

33. Content of workshops and seminars determined jointly by supervisors and teachers.

34. Diagnostic services at a medical center or speech and hearing unit.

35. Psychologist or psychiatrist with experience in serving the hearing impaired.

35. School district administrators having a philosophy that a majority of profoundly deaf children should be educated in an oral environment.

35. Proximity to facilities used by normally hearing children.

35. Physical education facilities. (For certain climates this would include both indoor and outdoor.)

35. Reference materials available in library or classrooms for student use throughout day.

35. Parent counselors for work with families having hearing impaired infants, ages 0-3.

Innovation in Speech Therapy:
A Cost Effective Program

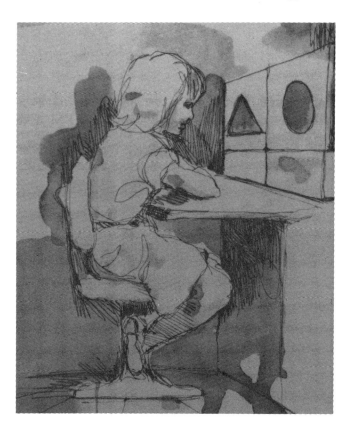

Abstract: Results of a program for treating mild to moderately speech disordered children through the use of trained paraprofessional aides are discussed. Data reveal that the use of trained aides in treating mild to moderately speech disordered children resulted in no significant difference in achievement when compared to achievement of clinician treated children. A reduction in clinician case loads of mild to moderately speech disordered children was also achieved through the program, thus leaving more time for clinicians to work with severely disordered children and to increase the incidence of work with individual children.

DAVID J. ALVORD

F UNDED under Title III of the Elementary and Secondary Education Act, the special speech therapy program described below serves 741 speech disordered children in three Iowa counties. Of this total, only about 50% of the children were receiving speech therapy prior to project implementation.

Based upon the need for additional speech services, the project developed a delivery system to improve the quality and efficiency of clinical speech services by training paraprofessional aides to work directly with mild to moderately articulatory disordered children in correctly reproducing defective sounds in isolation in a syllable, in a word, and in a sentence. This was done through the use of a token reinforcement technique. The elements that have produced educationally significant advances in speech therapy delivery systems and are worthy to serve as exem-

plary models are defined within the following set of goal statements.

1. Communication aides will provide therapy to mild or moderately articulatory disordered children that will not differ significantly in its effect from therapy provided by certified speech clinicians.
2. Students with mild to moderate articulatory disorders will benefit from speech therapy provided by project trained communication aides.
3. The use of project trained communication aides will significantly reduce the case loads of certified speech clinicians in the three county area served by the project thereby allowing more time for clinicians to work with severely speech disordered children.
4. The use of project trained communication aides will significantly reduce the number

"Innovation in Speech Therapy: A Cost Effective Program," David J. Alvord, *Exceptional Children*, Vol. 43 No. 8, May 1977. ©1977 The Council for Exceptional Children.

of speech disordered children who do not receive speech therapy.

Scope and Purpose

About 80% of the pupils served by the project are in grades K to 6 and the remaining 20% are in grades 7 to 12. Potential project participants are identified through diagnostic speech screening procedures administered by certified speech clinicians.

Certified speech clinicians were responsible for the initial 3 day training sessions and approximately 6 days of periodic instruction and supervision throughout the school year for the paraprofessional aides.

Costs

The nine communication aides were paid a total of $26,100, which is an average cost of approximately $3,000 per aide. Costs for instructional materials were $2,600 for the first year and about $1,700 per year for the second and third years. The total per pupil cost including materials and supportive personnel salaries is $80. This cost is figured on the basis of support personnel working with approximately 40% of the total case load of mild to moderately articulatory disordered children.

Cost Effectiveness

The cost effectiveness of the project can be demonstrated in terms of per pupil costs prior to and during project operation. In addition, the factor of effectiveness (pupil growth or change) prior to and during project operation must be reviewed. Preproject per pupil costs amounted to $120, while per pupil costs during project operation were $80. This is a reduction in the cost of speech therapy for mild to moderately articulatory disordered students of 33⅓%.

Further, evidence presented under goal number 1 supports the effectiveness of project services in that no significant difference was found in the treatment provided to mild or moderately articulatory disordered children when trained communication aides were used in place of certificated speech clinicians in providing therapy to children.

While per pupil costs have been reduced by approximately one-third, two other benefits have also accrued: 1) case loads of certificated clinicians have been reduced, thus freeing clinicians to work with more severely affected children; and 2) waiting lists have been sub-

stantially reduced thus more children with speech disorders can be served. Further, the project has been cost effective from the standpoint that clinician treatment of speech disordered children has changed from a group therapy centered approach to an individually centered therapy approach due to the effectiveness of the new speech therapy delivery system.

Evidence of Effectiveness

Goal 1

Communication aides will provide therapy to mild or moderately articulatory disordered children that will not differ significantly in its effect from therapy provided by certified speech clinicians.

The sample for analysis of the attainment of goal number 1 consisted of 84 mild to moderately speech disordered children. Of these, 56 were male and 28 were female. Of the 84 students, 20 composed the control group and the remaining 64 constituted the experimental group.

The design employed paralleled the pretest-posttest control group design described by Campbell and Stanley (1963). The notable exception was the absence of random assignment of subjects to groups. The instrumentation on which the data analysis was based was the McDonald Deep Screening Test of Articulation (McDonald, 1968). The following informal checks on this test were completed with respect to establishing reliability and validity:

1. Reliability was viewed in terms of an interrater scheme. Each of the three county speech clinicians made separate diagnoses of a given number of students with speech disorders. Diagnoses were then compared and a reliability coefficient of .87 was obtained.
2. A validity check was completed by having each clinician check the diagnosis standard employed on all test items with diagnoses of other clinicians on the same items across a large number of students. The agreement across all items and students resulted in a coefficient of .85.

The separate variance t statistic was used to test whether significant differences existed between improvement made by children treated by clinicians (control) and improvement made by children treated by aides (experimental). Although pretest mean scores differed slightly (control, 2.35, experimental,

4. EDUCATIONAL SERVICES

2.71), the scores were not significantly different when the t test was applied, as shown in Table 1. Thus, pretest scores of the groups can be said to be equal from a statistical standpoint. Analysis of covariance was not employed in this instance since an interaction effect did not appear to be present in that experimental and control groups maintained the same relative positions from pretest to posttest.

TABLE 1

t Value for the Difference between Pretest Scores for Speech Disordered Children in Control and Experimental Groups

Group	N	$\overline{X}$	t
Control (clinician treated)	20	2.35	.43
Experimental (aide treated)	64	2.71	

A second statistic was computed to determine whether differences in posttest scores were significant. Results indicated in Table 2 suggest that no significant difference existed between control and experimental groups. Thus, the use of aides in treating mild to moderately speech disordered children appears to be as effective as the treatment provided by certified speech clinicians.

TABLE 2

t Value for the Difference between Posttest Scores for Speech Disordered Children in Control and Experimental Groups

Group	N	$\overline{X}$	t
Control (clinician treated)	20	7.70	.93
Experimental (aide treated)	64	8.39	

Goal 2

Students with mild to moderately articulatory disorders will benefit from speech therapy provided by project trained communication aides.

To judge whether or not aides were able to produce positive gains in speech disordered children, a series of speech sounds that subjects had difficulty in producing was delineated. These sounds were then randomly sorted into two groups. One group constituted the control sounds that were not treated and the other group constituted the experimental sounds that were treated by the aides. Sixty-four students were then randomly assigned to the two groups. Pretest and posttest measures were taken on both the groups and were analyzed using the separate variance t statistic.

Two t tests were computed. The first was to assure that initial differences in means for the control and experimental groups were nonsignificant. Results of the test are reflected in Table 3. As the table suggests, no significant differences in pretest scores were found. The second t test was computed to determine whether posttest scores of the control group and experimental group differed significantly. Results are indicated in Table 4.

TABLE 3

t Test between Initial Differences in Pretest Scores for Control and Experimental Groups Treated by Aides

Group	N	$\overline{X}$	t
Control sounds (untreated)	32	3.02	.64
Experimental sounds (treated)	32	2.71	

TABLE 4

t Test between Posttest Scores for Control Group (Untreated Sounds) and Posttest Scores for Experimental Group (Aide Administered Treatment of Defective Speech Sounds)

Group	N	$\overline{X}$	t
Control (untreated sounds)	32	4.31	4.97*
Experimental (aide treated sounds)	32	8.39	

*$p < .05$

Evidence presented in Tables 3 and 4 suggests that aides can be successful in producing positive results with mild to moderately speech disordered children and that if such defective sounds are left untreated, in all probability, they will not be self correcting.

Goal 3

The use of project trained communication aides will significantly reduce the case loads of certified speech clinicians in the three county area served by the project.

This particular goal was judged attained by

resented an average case load of 33 children per clinician).

Data were collected and were compared to the prespecified criterion levels and judged accordingly. As evidenced in Table 5, the reduction in clinician case loads for the project's first and second years of operation both exceeded the prespecified project criterion level of 50%.

Goal 4

The use of project trained communication aides will significantly reduce the number of

TABLE 5

**Comparison of Clinician Caseloads Prior to and during
Project Implementation with Criterion Level**

Time frame	Clinician case load	$\overline{X}$ case load	Percent Reduction from base year	Criterion level
Base year Prior to project implementation	539	77	—	—
1st year of project operation	242	34	55% [a]	50%
2nd year of project operation	231	33	57% [a]	50%

[a] *Exceeds criterion level*

using criterion referenced measurement techniques. The project set the criterion level for success at an average of 50% reduction in the clinician case loads.

The samples consisted of: (a) all diagnosed speech disordered children receiving clinician therapy during the base year, the year prior to project implementation (this included 539 children and represented an average case load for each of the seven clinicians of 77 students); (b) 242 speech disordered children who were treated by speech clinicians during the first year of project operation (this represented a case load average of 34 children per clinician); and (c) 231 speech disordered children who were treated by clinicians during the second year of project operation (this rep-

speech disordered children who do not receive speech therapy.

The samples for purposes of this goal are depicted in Table 6. Table 6 indicates that the percentage of untreated speech disordered children decreased from 46% at the base year (prior to project implementation) to 21% during the first year of project operation and 29% during the second year of project operation. The average decrease in untreated speech disordered children over a 2 year period was 24½%. Also, it is educationally significant to note that while the percentage of children receiving therapy increased, the therapy dismissal rate also increased from 23% at the base year to 46% during the first year of project operation and 42% during the second year

4. EDUCATIONAL SERVICES

of project operation. In addition, the quality of therapy as noted earlier was not reduced.

Maintenance of Therapy Effect

To determine if positive results obtained in therapy were maintained over time, a special investigation was undertaken at the request of the project staff. The investigation was conducted by three staff members from the University of Northern Illinois' Division of Communication Disorders.

Conclusions and Implications

This project has demonstrated that in some instances paraprofessional personnel can be trained to effectively work with pupils who have mild to moderate articulatory disorders. It has also demonstrated that speech clinician caseloads can be significantly reduced through the employment of trained paraprofessionals, thus allowing more pupils in need of help to be served. Evidence provided substantiates that, in this instance, there was no

TABLE 6

Comparison of Treated to Untreated Speech Disordered Children Prior to and during Project Operation

Time frame	Treated	Percent treated	Untreated (waiting list)	Percent untreated	Total cases
Base year	384	54	328	46	712
Project year 1	585	79	156	21	741
Project year 2	621	71	250	29	871

From the total group of project treated articulatory disordered children in the three county area, a stratified random sample of children was drawn. Children from the following kinds of schools were represented (a) rural, (b) school for mentally retarded, (c) small urban school, (d) school located in a low socioeconomic area, (e) school located in a high socioeconomic area, (f) junior high school, and (g) elementary schools.

Thirty children from the variety of schools described above were selected at random; examined by independent judges for the purpose of identifying misarticulated sounds; evaluated during normal informal conversation periods for articulatory disorders; and tested using the McDonald Deep Screening Test of Articulation. Results indicated that 90% of the children who had previously received project speech therapy for articulation disorders reproduced the treated speech sounds with 90% accuracy. Although no mean length of time from therapy dismissal to retesting was calculated, the shortest time lapse between dismissal from therapy and retesting was four months.

significant difference in mild to moderately articulatory disordered pupils' ability to cor-

rectly reproduce defective sounds, whether treated by certificated speech clinicians or by trained paraprofessionals.

The trend of an ever increasing public school clientele who require special professional services, coupled with a cry for reduced educational expenditures and the local school districts' inability to afford the extra certificated personnel necessary to cope with the needs of these pupils, presents a serious problem.

The direct service approach for meeting the needs of pupils requiring speech therapy as well as other special education services may become more and more limited to severely disordered children and to initial and periodic work and more emphasis placed on indirect services provided via paraprofessionals trained and casually supervised by certificated personnel. This trend has already become quite evident in other professional fields such as medicine. It also seems likely that professionals in special education will more and more assume the role of chief diagnostician and team leaders of various levels of trained people who will work directly with pupils in the schools in carrying out treatments and programs prescribed by the certificated specialist.

Acquisition of American Sign Language by a Noncommunicating Autistic Child

Robert L. Fulwiler and Roger S. Fouts
University of Oklahoma

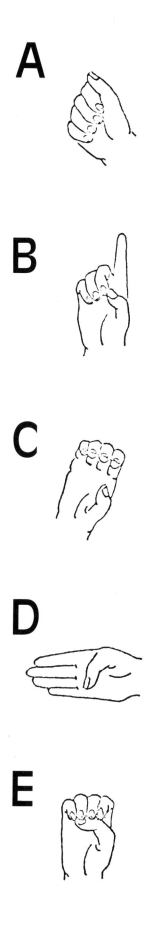

Experiments in the perception and language abilities of autistic children indicate that the children have auditory–visual association problems. These findings, combined with the findings that autistic communication is primarily gestural, led to the teaching of elements of American Sign Language to a 5-year-old nonverbal autistic boy. Results after 20 hours of training indicate that the child did acquire signs, that increasing signing led to increasing vocal speech, and that the child has rudimentary English syntax. The use of Ameslan signs spontaneously generalized to other situations and the training resulted in increased social interaction.

Hewett (1965) and Lovaas (1966) reported the establishment of verbal behavior in the repertoire of autistic children through the use of operant conditioning procedures. Though these and other studies since (e.g., Schell, Stark, & Giddan, 1967) have reported some success, many problems have become evident. First, the procedure is time-consuming and often relatively unproductive. A good example is the study by Hingtgen and Churchill (1969), who reported that the vocabularies of four children, after working with each one for 5 weeks at 6 hours per day, were 25, 60, and 16 words and one of nine "sounds." A second problem is the seeming lack of response generalization outside the therapy situation. Lovaas (1966) reported generalization, but Schell et al. (1967) reported that the increase in speech only occurred in the therapy situation. Sulzbacher and Costello (1970) and Hartung (1970) reported that the generalization of speech outside the therapy situation had to be specifically taught; it wasn't spontaneous. room. Psychiatric diagnosis was 295.8 (DSM-II) Schizophrenia, Childhood Type: Infantile Autism. The clinical psychologist's diagnosis was Infantile Autism. During initial observation the child engaged in spinning, darting, "wringing of hands," unintelligible vocalizations, and generally disorganized and unoriented behavior.

Apparatus and Materials

The training was conducted at the Timbergate Clinic, Oklahoma City. Training aids such as objects and puzzles were those available at the clinic.

4. EDUCATIONAL SERVICES

Items or stimuli to be used as reinforcers were those that were deemed effective and appropriate by the experimenters upon observation of the preferences and likes of the subject.

Procedure

The child was trained to use elements of Ameslan. The signs in Ameslan are analogous to the words in spoken English (Stokoe, Casterline, & Croneberg, 1965). Each sign consists of a particular hand configuration and movement, in addition to specific positions relative to the signer's body where the sign begins or ends. The signs to be taught were decided in vivo by the trainers as appropriate circumstances for particular signs presented themselves, or on a prearranged schedule. The method of training was the total communication method (Schlesinger & Meadow, 1972). The experimenter spoke the word while demonstrating, molding, or prompting the sign. Hence, while Ameslan signs were used, the syntactical relationships were those of signed English. The data recorded are the prompted and unprompted signs produced by the child, as well as more general behavioral observations (e.g., attentiveness, behavioral appropriateness, interpersonal interactions).

Training sessions were ½-hour periods twice a week.

RESULTS

After 20 hours of training, the child used several signs appropriately. Since the stress was on functional vocabulary rather than diversity, the signs were highly related in that they were amenable to combination among themselves. The most interesting result was that as the use of signed speech increased, the use of vocal speech increased in both amount and appropriateness. Signed words were emitted during the first hour, signed phrases were language, but also he spontaneously used the signs to give others commands such as "sit down." It is worthwhile to note that the sign language training was started after the standard behavior modification technique for language had been singularly unsuccessful. These authors also reported that they were "struck" by the way the child attended to their facial expressions. This seems to be one of the fortunate benefits of the use of sign language because much of the "emotional" component of the sign is conveyed through facial expression. Fant (1964), in discussing manual language, states, "The face is the focal point. Therefore, it carries most of the burden of enriching the meaning of signs and finger spelling." He further states, "Our voices rise and fall to add meanings to our words. The face functions for manual communication as inflections of the voice for words." As such, facial expressions are not just amusing and entertaining, they are vital to the communicative process. Hence, the child learns to attend to facial expressions and maintain "eye" contact. Miller and Miller (1973) in a study involving 19 autistic children reported that all acquired and used some signs appropriately to gain desired objects or goals. They also reported that one of the children made the transition from signed language to expressive spoken language while all children learned to respond to words which had been systematically paired with the relevant signs. Thus, it would seem that the use of a manual language would take advantage of the propensities of the autistic child while avoiding some of the problems associated with the teaching of vocal language only.

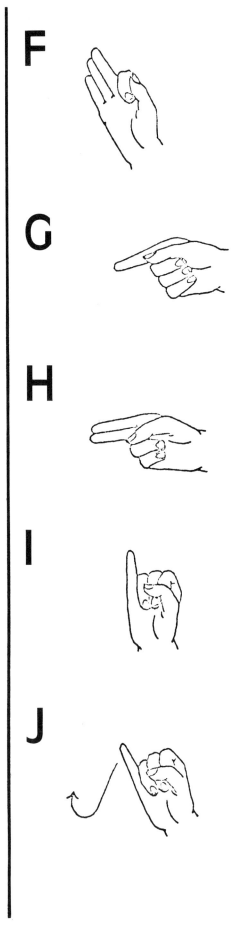

METHOD

Subject

The subject was a 5-year, 1-month-old male child who lived at home with his mother and no father. Mother reported extreme hyperactivity and bizarre behavior which included uncontrollable periods of laughter and crying, self-destructive behaviors, biting and scratching others, frequent running away, and unintelligible verbalizations.

The child had been seen by a family physician, a private neurologist, a pediatric neurologist and staff psychiatrist at a medical center, and a clinical psychologist at a private treatment center for children. Since age 3 he had attended a nursery school, a private Montessori school, and a private school for learning disordered and emotionally disturbed children. All of the schools had discontinued placement due to their inability to meet the needs of the child. The child had been denied placement in any public school class-

Table I. Signed Expressive Words

Noun	Verb	Adverb	Pronoun
dog	tickle	more	you
drink	want		me
key	gimme		
hot (coffee)	open		
listen (wristwatch)	catch		
	thank you		
	look		
Roger	hug		
food	hurry		
nut	go		
comb	up (pick up)		
shoe			
smoke			
look (kaleidoscope)			

word class frequencies, and phrase structure parallels that of the normal language acquisition process (McNeill, 1970) (see Tables I–III).

DISCUSSION

The success in the acquisition and utilization of Ameslan signs supports the hypothesis that the use of a manual language would be appropriate for developing communication in an autistic child. The increased use of vocal speech is a pleasant and common occurrence reported by others who have also used this mode of training (Miller & Miller, 1973; Webster et al., 1973). One finding which is not shown in the results is the combination of the manual and vocal forms. These were of two forms: (1) The child

Table II. Vocal Expressive Words

Noun	Verb	Adverb	Adjective	Pronoun
key	up	more	big[a]	it
drink	help[a]	down	bad[a]	me
kitty[a]	tickle	here	my	you
cake[a]	go			
car	give			
tractor[a]	sit (down)			
ball				
comb				
shoe				
hug				

[a]Not used in training.

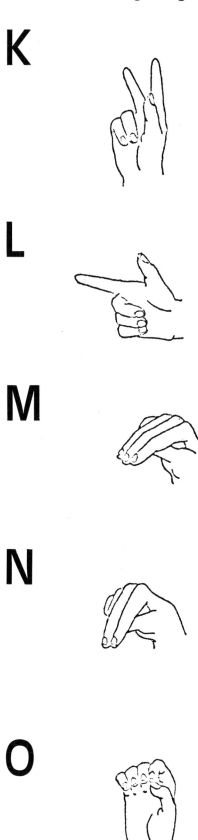

K

L

M

N

O

4. EDUCATIONAL SERVICES

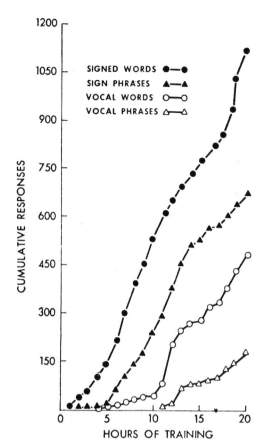

Fig. 1. Cumulative expressive signed and vocal words and phrases.

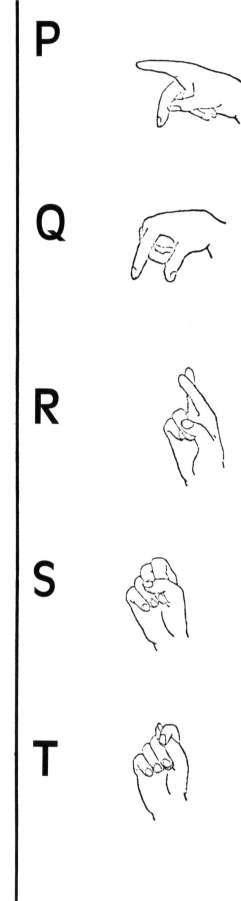

first emitted in the second hour, single vocal words were first used appropriately in the fourth hour, and vocal phrases were first emitted in the eleventh hour (Figure 1).

An analysis of both signed and vocal words reveals that the most frequent class of words used was nouns, followed by verbs, pronouns, and adverbs. The emitted sign phrases appeared in an expected order, namely, verb-object ([you] gimme key) or adverb-noun (more key). The sign "gimme" is an outstretched hand palm up, which is a natural request gesture, hence it is not an explicit "give me" verb-object phrase. The child then combined these two forms into verb-adverb-noun forms (gimme more drink or more gimme drink). The child then progressed to noun-verb-object forms (you gimme key). Hence, acquisition of individual words (signs), evidenced by the signed phrase construction which, while showing variation, did follow appropriate English syntactic order which would follow from the use of the total communication procedure.

The anecdotal reports of the use of signs outside the training situation is of great importance. The child's use of Ameslan signs (and increased vocal speech) were reported by both the child's "school" teacher and his family. This finding is in accord with Webster et al. (1973) and Miller and Miller (1973). It signifies that the autistic child is capable of using language when given the appropriate tools. It carries the implication that one of the main factors in autism may not be a cognitive malfunction, but a perceptual nonfunctioning in the crossmodal array.

The child's behavior (nonlanguage) also changed over the course of the investigation. When first seen, the child was nonattentive, highly distractible, and seemed to be lost in his own world—a common description of

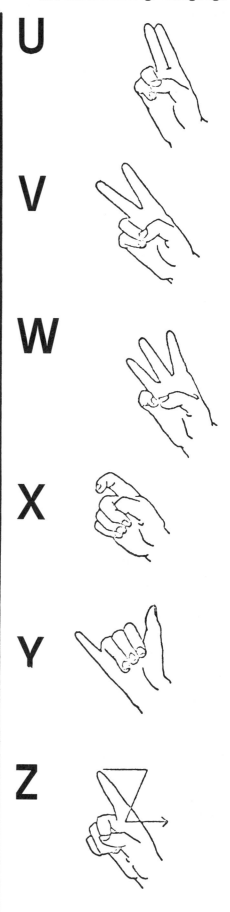

an autistic child. During the course of training, he became attentive, often sitting and working for 45 minutes at a time when extended sessions could be arranged. He would also initiate contact at the beginning of a session and would sign spontaneously to be "tickled" which involved tickling, wrestling, and general mayhem. He also, upon occasion, would mold the experimenter's hand into the tickle sign and "attack" to initiate the game. During hours 18 to 19 the child initiated a game by placing the keys in the experimenter's shirt pocket and then removing them while speaking phrases such as "find a key," "back a key," "gimme back key," "going out," and "back key going out."

At the end of a training session, other children would often enter the room where the training was conducted. During the first few sessions, the child would withdraw completely from contact, but later would actively (sometimes aggressively) seek the experimenter's attention. Toward the latter sessions, he would initiate contact with the other children, usually as an attempt to get a toy. In these attempts he would often use the "gimme" sign toward the other children. One of the children was fond of hugging everyone and the child would receive this "affection" and upon occasion would hug back. The family reported that the child anticipated and seemed to look forward to the sessions. The family also reported that the child toilet trained about midway in the investigation, and became more manageable at home. Similar occurrences were reported by his teacher. Hence, it would appear that the large amount of attention and social and physical contact, and the acquisition of effective, acceptable communication involved in manual language training had rewards beyond the mere acquisition of words.

In summary, while the scope of this investigation is admittedly limited, it demonstrates the potential usefulness of the technique and

Table III. Time Sequence of Initial Appearance of Signed Phrases

Hours	Phrases	
1–5:	gimme key more key gimme drink	
6–10:	drink that want key more gimme key more drink that gimme drink Roger key you gimme (key)	drink me gimme more comb gimme food eat (feed) me me drink gimme more drink you eat
11–15:	more that gimme more key more thank you gimme key more gimme you gimme more key	key gimme key gimme key gimme key me
16–20	my keys that shoe that gimme more you drink	gimme more that want gimme key that gimme

signed and spoke the word simultaneously, and (2) combined the forms in a phrase such as "gimme" (signed) "key" (vocal). The first form (the word being simultaneously signed and spoken) appeared in the sixth hour of training and seemed to provide a transition from sign to vocal use since hours 6 to 10 was the period when vocal speech began to increase reliably. The second form first appeared in the seventh hour of training and seemed to form a similar transition at the level of phrases. These forms of combination were also reported by Musil, Schaeffer, Kollinzas, and McDowell (1975). Another interesting result not shown in the numerical results is that the child would express preferences among the items used as reinforcers. Often when given a particular reinforcer, he would refuse it and when asked, "What do you want?" would sign for an alternate item, usually with the noun sign (drink, key, tickle) but would often use a phrase such as "gimme that" ("gimme" sign and pointing to the desired object). Thus, he was not only asking for something, but a particular something. The child seemed to have acquired some vocal expressive vocabulary as evidenced by Table II. While the number of vocal words is not large, there were some words emitted which were not part of the training program. Indeed, there was no overt attempt per se to train vocal speech. Hence, the child has acquired some language and from the emitted vocal phrase structure must also have acquired at least the rudiments of English syntax. This is also demonstrates that autistic children will, when given the means, act as do other children; which, after all, is the goal.

REFERENCES

Bryson, C. Q. Systematic identification of perceptual disabilities in autistic children. *Perceptual and Motor Skills,* 1970, *31,* 239-246.

Bryson, C. Q. Short-term memory and crossmodal information processing in autistic children. *Journal of Learning Disabilities,* 1972, *5,* 81-91.

Davis, B. J. A clinical approach to the development of communication in young schizophrenic children. *Journal of Communication Disorders,* 1970, *3,* 211-222.

Fant, L. J. *Say it with hands.* Silver Spring, Maryland: National Association of the Deaf, 1964.

Fouts, R. S. Unpublished report. Department of Psychiatry Grand Rounds, University of Oklahoma Health Sciences Center, 1973.

Gillies, S. M. Some abilities of psychotic children and subnormal controls. *Journal of Mental Deficiency Research,* 1965, *9,* 89-101.

Hartung, J. R. A review of procedures to increase verbal imitation skills and functional speech in autistic children. *Journal of Speech and Hearing Disorders,* 1970, *35,* 203-217.

Hewett, F. Teaching speech to an autistic child through operant conditioning. *American Journal of Orthopsychiatry,* 1965, *35,* 927-936.

Hingtgen, J. N., & Churchill, D. W. Identification of perceptual limitations in mute autistic children: Identification by the use of behavior modification. *Archives of General Psychiatry,* 1969, *21,* 68-71.

Hingtgen, J. N., & Coulter, S. K. Auditory control of operant behavior in mute autistic children. *Journal of Perceptual and Motor Skills,* 1967, *25,* 561-565.

Jakab, I. The patient, the mother, and the therapist: An interactional triangle in the treatment of the autistic child. *Journal of Communication Disorders,* 1972, *5,* 154-182.

Lovaas, O. I. A program from the establishment of speech in psychotic children. In J. K. Wing (Ed.), *Early childhood autism: Clinical, educational and social aspects.* London: Pergamon Press, 1966.

McNeill, D. *The acquisition of language.* New York: Harper & Row, 1970.

Miller, A., & Miller, E. E. Cognative developmental training with elevated boards and sign language. *Journal of Autism and Childhood Schizophrenia,* 1973, *3,* 65-85.

Musil, A., Schaeffer, B., Kollinzas, R., & McDowell, P. *Signed speech: A new treatment for autism.* Paper presented at Southwestern Psychological Association, 1975.

Pronovost, W., Wakstein, P., & Wakstein, P. A longitudinal study of the speech behavior of fourteen children diagnosed as atypical or autistic. *Exceptional Children,* 1966, *33,* 19-26.

Ruttenberg, B. A., & Gordon, E. G. Evaluating the communication of the autistic child. *Journal of Speech and Hearing Disorders,* 1967, *32,* 314-324.

Schell, R. E., Stark, J., & Giddan, J. J. Development of language behavior in an autistic child, *Journal of Speech and Hearing Disorders,* 1967, *32,* 51-64.

Schlesinger, H. S., & Meadow, K. P. *Sound and sign.* Berkeley: University of California Press, 1972.

Senn, M. J. E., & Solnit, A. S. *Problems in child behavior and development.* Philadelphia: Lea & Febiger, 1968.

Stokoe, W. C., Casterline, D. C., & Croneberg, C. G. *A dictionary of American sign language on linguistic principles.* Washington, D.C.: Gallaudet College Press, 1965.

Sulzbacher, S. I., & Costello, J. M. A behavioral strategy for language training of a child with autistic behaviors. *Journal of Speech and Hearing Disorders,* 1970, *35,* 255-276.

Webster, C. D., McPherson, H., Sloman, L., Evans, M. A., & Kuchar, E. Communicating with an autistic boy by gestures. *Journal of Autism and Childhood Schizophrenia,* 1973, *3,* 337-346.

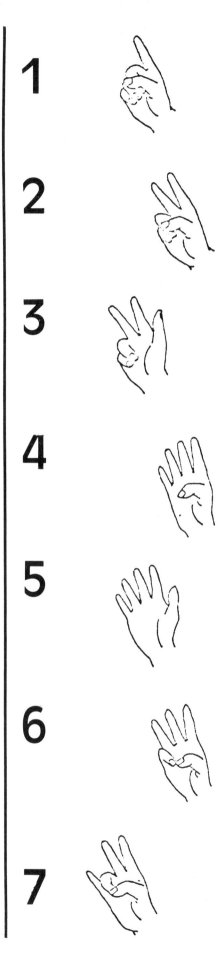

Information Processing of Visually Presented Picture and Word Stimuli by Young Hearing-Impaired and Normal-Hearing Children

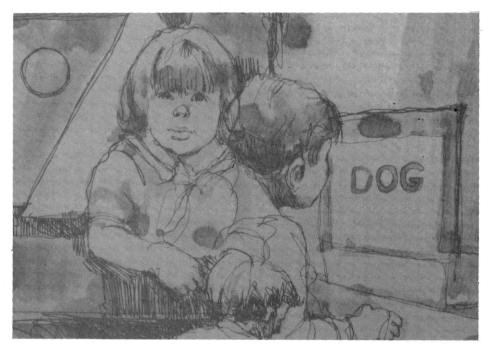

Ronald R. Kelly

C. Tomlinson-Keasey

The extensive and careful research program conducted by Paivio and his colleagues (Paivio, 1965; Paivio, 1969; Paivio and Csapo, 1969; Paivio and Madigan, 1968; Paivio, 1971) has highlighted the existence of imaginal and verbal processes which are available for the coding, storage, and retrieval of information. A multitude of studies pertaining to perception, information processing, and psychophysiological aspects have confirmed the distinction in cognitive functioning that exists for visual and verbal material (Milner, 1974; Teuber, 1974; Sperry, Gazzaniga, and Bogen, 1969; Sperry, 1974). The research to date, however, has had little impact on applied areas of psychology even though the implications of alternate modes of functioning might well be important in the overall educational process (Rohwer, 1970; Rohwer et al., 1967). One area of possible application is with persons who are handicapped in a particular processing mode. The dominance of the visual mode over the verbal, for example, may well exist in persons who are auditorily handicapped. The educational enterprise for such handicapped groups might be greatly facilitated if it were clear how these groups most easily processed information. Therefore the present study was undertaken with the primary objective of comparing information processing in a group of normal (hearing) and handicapped (hearing impaired) children.

"Information Processing of Visually Presented Pictures and Word Stimuli by Young Hearing Impaired and Normal Hearing Children," Ronald B. Kelly, Tomlinson-Keasley, *Journal of Speech and Hearing Research*, Vol. 19 No. 4, December 1976. ©1976 Journal of Speech and Hearing Research.

167

4. EDUCATIONAL SERVICES

In comparing the hearing impaired and normal hearing, one is struck by the differences in input which they are able to process. Hearing people easily process visual and auditory information simultaneously and store it in both modes (Bower, 1972; Paivio, 1972; Paivio, Rogers, and Smythe, 1968). As a result, they have dual storage modes which contain information that is easily integrated into a verbal communication system. By contrast, the hearing impaired must process most information (reading lips, signing, pictures, printed words, and so on) in a visual mode, supplemented at best by a distorted and inadequate auditory input. Such a visually oriented processing system may provide the hearing impaired only one primary storage mode. Even when someone is speaking, the hearing impaired probably transform an oral verbal message into a visual code in the form of lip movement and other observable characteristics in order to process it (Myklebust, 1964). This situation requires the hearing impaired to make at least two cognitive transformations if they are to interact with others. Not only must they transform a verbal code into a visual mode for processing but they must again transform it back into a verbal code in order to communicate. This transformation problem may well be the source of many obstacles in the information processing and communication of deaf children (Odom and Blanton, 1967).

In terms of development, being limited to a visual processing system may be extremely important. Several investigators (Piaget, 1952; Flavell, 1970; Bruner, Olver, and Greenfield, 1966; Ryan, Hegion, and Flavell, 1970) have suggested that iconic mediation appears very early, prior to verbal rehearsal, in the normal development of a hearing child. These iconic mediators would presumably develop similarly in a hearing-impaired child (Tomlinson-Keasey and Kelly, 1974). However, the normal-hearing child from two to five years of age increases the use of verbal rehearsal as he overlearns verbal-label responses to object stimuli and becomes more skillful at rapid articulation of labels (Flavell, 1970). It is supposed that the emphasis which both parents and schools place on verbal skills helps foster the complete integration of iconic and verbal input in the hearing child. For the hearing-impaired child, however, such dual coding would not be as automatic. The input for him, whether reading lips, observing signs, or reading print, would logically be coded into the visual memory, at least initially.

The above analysis suggests that normal-hearing and hearing-impaired children should exhibit differences in the relative efficiency of information processing depending on the mode in which the material is presented and the way in which it must be retrieved. In the present study subjects were presented with visual stimuli, consisting of either pictures or words, to store in their memory. In a subsequent recognition phase, subjects were given cue cards of either pictures or words to help them retrieve the stimulus information. Hence, subjects could be asked to process a pictorial sequence and be given word cues to aid recognition, or vice versa. They were then required to recall the stimulus sequence by properly arranging the cues selected. In addition, subjects were also asked to process, retrieve, and sequence using like modes (picture/picture or word/word). It was hypothesized that (1) both groups would be able to process the pictorial information more effectively than the word materials, (2) the task of recognition would be easier than recall for both groups, and (3) the normal-hearing subjects would do better on recall than the hearing impaired. Furthermore, it was predicted that (4) the hearing impaired would perform significantly better on the storage and retrieval of information that required no transformations, such as in those trials utilizing either pictures or words for both processing and retrieval, and (5) the normal-hearing children would exhibit no differences in dealing with either like or unlike modes.

METHOD

Subjects

Twenty-two subjects were used. Eleven were hearing-impaired children, ranging in age from four years to six years eight months (mean = four years 11 months). Nine subjects were considered congenitally hearing impaired, while the other two were considered as hearing impaired at nine and 16 months. The average hearing loss across 500, 1000, and 2000 Hz in the better ear ranged from 60 to 110 dB (ANSI, 1969), or from moderate to profound. Table 1 presents the hearing loss and education of each hearing-impaired sub-

TABLE 1. Descriptive information on hearing loss and education for the 11 hearing-impaired subjects.

Subjects	Age at Onset of Hearing Loss	Average Hearing Loss in Better Ear°	Number of Years in Educational Program
1	16 months	102	2
2	birth	67	2.5
3	birth	105	2.5
4	birth	102	3
5	birth	100	2.5
6	birth	83	2
7	birth	92	2.5
8	9 months	90	4
9	birth	100	2.5
10	birth	65	3
11	birth	60	5

°ANSI (1969), decibel average across 500, 1000, and 2000 Hz.

ject. All subjects had been in a formal educational program for the hearing impaired for a period of two to five years. The other 11 subjects had normal hearing and were matched by age with the hearing-impaired subjects. Only two of the normal-hearing subjects had begun elementary school.

Procedures

Nonverbal-imitative training procedures were used to assure that both groups of subjects would clearly understand what was expected of them in the experimental task. Furth (1966) and others have found in their research with the deaf that one must use nonverbal techniques in the instruction phase of the experiment to obtain valid results (Myklebust, 1964). Thus, the instructions were provided by a super-8mm film of a six-year-old boy. In the three-and-a-half minute movie the six-year-old actor watched as three stimuli were projected sequentially with a slide projector on a rear screen. After a five-second delay he was then provided with five cards (which contained either pictures or words) and he selected the three that corresponded to the stimuli he had seen. As each of the experimental subjects observed the movie, a set of cues that matched the film scene were provided for him. Thus, the subjects were able to imitate the film actor for each of the four experimental modes: (1) picture stimuli/picture cues (P/P mode); (2) picture stimuli/word cues (P/W mode); (3) word stimuli/picture cues (W/P mode); and (4) word stimuli/word cues (W/W mode). Having them imitate a film model assured that all subjects learned the experimental task in a consistent manner during the practice session.

Because it has been shown that meaningful materials are remembered better than nonmeaningful materials (Smith and Smith, 1966), the items selected for the experiment were ones that the subjects interacted with on a regular basis. For the hearing-impaired subjects, two experienced preschool teachers of the

4. EDUCATIONAL SERVICES

hearing impaired recommended the specific items that were selected. They were self, mama, mama's car, book, toy, shoes, coat, teacher, name of classmate, school, and the color blue. Because of their unique language problems, and to insure that they knew these materials, a set of personalized slides were produced for each hearing-impaired subject based on these 11 items (that is, pictures of his mother, shoes, favorite toy, and so on). Experimental items for each hearing-impaired child were personalized to insure that any processing differences between the two groups would result for reasons other than their unfamiliarity with the stimuli. In addition, for the word cues the teachers worked with the hearing-impaired subjects on lipreading and recognizing the printed name of each item for two weeks prior to the experiment. It should be mentioned that these children had been in a formal school setting for two or more years and were already familiar with the lipreading and printed forms of these items. In addition, this kind of word-to-picture association is a standard part of the preschool curriculum for the hearing impaired and seemed to pose no problem for these children. For the hearing subjects, a similar list of 11 items was used: book, shoes, coat, dog, TV, doll, cup, boy, girl, baby, and the color blue. However, since they did not have the same language limitations as the hearing-impaired children, and they were all familiar with the items, it was not necessary to personalize the stimuli for each hearing subject. Thus, the same set of experimental materials was used for the 11 hearing subjects. In addition, the parents of the hearing subjects also worked with them on the printed name of each item for two weeks prior to the experiment.

Both the hearing-impaired and the normal-hearing subjects were tested individually in the experimental booth. In addition to the practice, the experiment consisted of 12 trials. Following is a brief description of one complete trial in which the information was presented pictorially and cued with words (P/W mode). Slides of three objects were projected sequentially on the rear screen. During the three seconds that each slide was exposed, the experimenter named the objects aloud to provide an opportunity for dual coding. Hearing-impaired subjects were in a position to speechread the experimenter after they looked at each slide. Three seconds following the third stimulus slide, subjects were given five cue cards on which the words for the objects were printed. The subjects had to perform two tasks: (1) recognize the three appropriate cues from the five cards by selecting those that corresponded to the stimulus set of pictures, and (2) recall the sequence of the pictures by placing the three selected cue cards (words) in the correct order on a tray. There were 12 experimental trials–three for each of the four experimental modes (P/P, P/W, W/P, and W/W). The presentation order was the same for all subjects, although the actual sequence of trials was determined randomly.

For each trial, the subjects received one point for each correct cue card selected (recognition), and one point for each cue card placed in the appropriate order (recall of sequence). It was possible for subjects to recognize and select only one cue card and still sequence it on the tray in the correct place. In terms of chance scores, each trial of the recognition task represents a hypergeometric distribution problem (Huntsberger and Billingsley, 1973). There is a 1/10 probability that the subjects would select by chance the three correct cue cards from the five choices. Thus, for the recognition task, the expected chance score for each mode (P/P, P/W, W/P, and W/W) would be 5.4. The recall task presents a somewhat different problem for determining chance score. Assuming that a subject recognized and selected all three correct cues, then there would be a 1/6 probability that the subject would sequence them correctly by chance. To address all hypotheses, the data were analyzed in terms of a combined score, as well as separately for the dimensions of recognition and recall.

RESULTS

It was predicted that both the hearing-impaired and normal-hearing subjects would process the pictorial information most effectively, while differences would occur between them on the mode and recognition/recall dimensions. The data presented in Table 2 show that these predictions were accurate. With both recognition and recall tasks, the pictorial (P/P) processing resulted in the highest performance means for the two groups. However, differences are apparent when comparing the groups on specific mode combinations, such as P/P and W/W under recognition. In addition, the recognition task generally

TABLE 2. Means and standard deviations of both subject groups on the four experimental modes for the recognition and recall dimensions.

Subjects	Recognition				Recall			
	P/P	W/W	W/P	P/W	P/P	W/W	W/P	P/W
Hearing impaired								
Mean	7.82	7.00	6.64	6.55	5.09	3.27	3.82	3.00
SD	(1.78)	(1.48)	(1.43)	(1.29)	(3.33)	(2.45)	(2.79)	(2.45)
Normal hearing								
Mean	8.55	6.64	6.82	7.09	6.64	2.82	4.55	4.82
SD	(0.93)	(1.21)	(1.83)	(1.30)	(2.73)	(3.09)	(3.14)	(2.96)

resulted in higher means than the recall dimension. Other subtle differences are also evident.

Initially, a $2 \times 4 \times 2$ (groups $\times$ modes $\times$ recognition/recall) analysis of variance with repeated measure was conducted (Kirk, 1968). The analysis indicated no significant differences between groups ($F [1,20] = 0.68$, $p > 0.05$), but showed significance for the main effects of modes ($F [3,60] = 10.18$, $p < 0.05$) and recognition/recall ($F [1,20] = 76.39$, $p < 0.05$). However, the significant interaction between modes $\times$ recognition/recall ($F [3,60] = 3.92$, $p < 0.05$) revealed that the two groups performed differently with these main effects, which makes it difficult to interpret them. To look at the simple main effects, as well as to respond to the specific hypotheses of the present study, additional analyses were required.

For the recognition data, a 2×2 (group $\times$ P/P-W/W modes) analysis of variance with repeated measures showed a significant interaction for the performance of the groups on the picture/picture and word/word modes ($F [1,20] = 6.90$, $p < 0.05$). A subsequent analysis showed that the hearing-impaired group performed no differently with the picture/picture mode than the word/word mode ($F [1,10] = 2.87$, $p > 0.05$). By contrast, the normal-hearing subjects performed significantly better with the picture/picture mode when compared to the word/word mode ($F [1,10] = 26.89$, $p < 0.05$). Thus, in terms of the recognition dimension, the hearing-impaired subjects performed equally well on the picture/picture and word/word modes, while the normal-hearing subjects' performed better with the pictorial mode. These results suggest that the hearing-impaired subjects either had more experience with printed verbal material, or they could be processing the words as pictures.

In terms of the recall dimension, a 2×2 (groups $\times$ P/P-W/W modes) analysis of variance with repeated measures indicated that P/P was significantly easier than W/W for both groups of subjects ($F [1,20] = 20.77$, $p < 0.05$). There were no differences between groups ($F [1,10] = 0.44$, $p > 0.05$) and no interaction occurred for modes $\times$ groups ($F [1,20] = 3.73$, $p > 0.05$).

As predicted, both groups performed better with the recognition task than the recall of sequence: $F (1,10) = 42.87$, $p < 0.05$, for the hearing impaired; $F (1,10) = 33.53$, $p < 0.05$, for the normal-hearing subjects. However, contrary to one of the initial hypotheses, there was no difference between the hearing impaired group and the normal-hearing group on the dimension of recall ($F [2,20] = 0.97$, $p > 0.05$). Apparently, the recall task turned out to be equally difficult for both groups of subjects.

In addition to the separate dimensions of recognition and recall, this study was concerned with the total performance of the two groups. Hence, additional

4. EDUCATIONAL SERVICES

analyses were conducted on the subjects' combined scores for the four modes (P/P, W/P, P/W, W/W) which consisted of both recognition and recall. A 2 × 4 (groups × modes) analysis of variance with repeated measures indicated that the main effect of experimental mode was significant (F [3,60] = 10.28, $p < 0.05$). Interestingly, the hearing-impaired and normal-hearing subjects did not differ significantly on overall performance (F [1,20] = 0.68, $p > 0.05$), nor was there a significant interaction (F [3,60] = 1.70, $p > 0.05$). Scheffe's (1953) method for multiple comparisons was used to test the subjects' performances in the P/P mode versus the other three modes of W/W, P/W, and W/W. There was a significant difference in favor of the P/P mode: $F = 5.41$, $p < 0.05$. Thus, in terms of combined data, both groups of subjects performed better when information was presented and retrieved pictorially.

The final hypothesis predicted that the hearing-impaired group would perform significantly better on storage and retrieval where no transformations from one mode to another were required (see Table 3). This prediction was

TABLE 3. The overall performance of the hearing-impaired and normal-hearing subjects on like modes versus unlike modes.

Subjects	Like Modes (P/P and W/W)	Unlike Modes (W/P and P/W)
Hearing impaired		
Mean	11.59	10.00
SD	4.34	3.70
Normal hearing		
Mean	12.32	11.64
SD	4.73	4.11

based on the belief that young hearing-impaired children probably do not dual code when processing information. If this is true, then they should perform better with like modes (P/P and W/W) where dual coding is not necessary, in contrast to unlike modes (P/W and W/P) which would require it.

A directional t test comparing the hearing-impaired subjects' performances on like modes (P/P and W/W) versus unlike modes (W/P and P/W) indicated that the like modes were significantly easier (t [10] = 1.84, $p < 0.05$, one-tailed test). By contrast, and consistent with the final hypothesis, the normal-hearing subjects showed no differential performance on like versus unlike modes (t [10] = 1.15, $p > 0.05$, one-tailed test). Furthermore, it is interesting that the normal-hearing group performed slightly better on unlike modes than the hearing-impaired did on either like or unlike modes. Although this difference is not great, it does suggest that normal-hearing children are further ahead in transformation skills at this age level.

In regard to the first hypothesis, both groups of subjects did best on the overall processing (combined recognition and recall) of the P/P mode as compared to the other three modes (W/P, P/W, W/W), all of which contained the dimension of words. This was expected in view of previous research in imagery and associative learning and probably reflects a normal developmental sequence which proceeds from iconic to symbolic storage (Bruner et al., 1966; Piaget, 1952).

Analysis of the P/P and W/W modes for the recognition task also indicates that subtle differences occurred between the two groups. The hearing-impaired subjects performed equally well with these two modes, while the normal-hearing subjects did better with the pictorial mode. It should be noted that the hearing-impaired subjects had spent considerable time in a formal educational program, whereas only two of the normal-hearing subjects group attended school. The educational experience of the hearing impaired could have caused this difference in performance. An alternative explanation could be that the hearing-impaired group treated both the P/P and W/W modes as visual data and hence took advantage of their major sensory input. Perhaps their educational experiences and visual processing combined gave the hearing impaired equal facility with the P/P and W/W modes.

On the much more difficult recall phase of the experiment there were no differences between the two groups of subjects. We predicted that the normal-hearing subjects would outperform the hearing impaired on the recall of sequences. That this did not occur is probably an additional tribute to the educational experiences of the hearing impaired.

Another interesting result is the subtle difference between the groups for overall processing of like (P/P and W/W) versus unlike (W/P and P/W) modes. The fact that unlike modes were significantly more difficult than like modes for the hearing-impaired children supports the hypothesis that the children have difficulty in transforming information from one mode to another. One could argue alternatively that this difference is due largely to the one like mode (P/P) which proved to be the easiest for both groups of subjects. A look at the results of the hearing children, however, makes this hypothesis less attractive. The hearing group also performed significantly better on the P/P condition yet did not show a significant difference in the like versus unlike modes. In fact, the hearing children scored best on those experimental modes in which they could take full advantage of imagery and symbolic verbalization (P/P, W/P, and P/W). As they processed the input, they verbalized the names aloud whether it was pictorial or symbolic stimuli. Two children even sang the words to themselves, perhaps achieving a rhythmic imagery. It is obvious that these rehearsal strategies would assist dual coding for the hearing subjects.

These differences between the two groups may indicate an area of focus for the schools. Perhaps multisensory experiences for the hearing impaired would improve their ability to transform information. This could be done by strongly emphasizing the auditory dimension for young hearing-impaired children in conjunction with either a good oral technique or a comprehensive total communication approach. An alternative approach might focus on transformations within a single mode. One example might be multiple visuals of an object transformed into the word for that object, such as shown on "Sesame Street" (Children's Television Workshop). It is believed that either educational procedure could successfully encourage the transformation of information.

A final point which deserves comment is the lack of an overall significant difference between the normal-hearing and hearing-impaired children. This result is in accord with numerous other studies comparing both the intellectual and conceptual development of deaf and hearing children (Springer, 1938; Pintner and Lev, 1939; Hiskey, 1956; Brill, 1962; Mira, 1962; Furth, 1964; Furth, 1966; Furth and Youniss, 1969; Furth and Youniss, 1971). These studies all agree that the educational programs for the hearing impaired are dealing primarily with subjects of normal capabilities.

Several problems in the interpretation of the results could be remedied by further research. For example, no measure of the subjects' response times was obtained. Thus, it was not possible to ascertain whether the two groups exhibited any time differences in processing. This would have been a valuable comparison and should be explored in a subsequent study. Also, one must note that the presentation order was the same for all subjects in both groups. In spite of the order being randomly determined, there is always the possibility of some order effect existing in the data. Because of the repeated measures design, the order of presentation should probably be randomly changed for the subjects. This is a factor that will also require additional research.

In summary, this study has noted both similarities and differences in information processing for the hearing-impaired and normal-hearing groups. For some dimensions, the educational experiences provided the hearing impaired have obviously improved their processing skills. However, some of the data of the study suggest that hearing-impaired children in their preschool years may not use their cognitive abilities in the same manner as their hearing peers. Most experienced educators of the deaf would probably agree and say that is true because of their language deficit. However, we would suggest that this may be true due to a differential sensory input which results in the development of cognitive structures and means of processing information that are qualitatively different from those of the hearing. It seems possible that the hearing-impaired subjects' loss of a major sensory modality may have significantly altered the way in which information is processed and stored. Studies comparing the hearing-impaired and normal-hearing subjects of all ages should be conducted to follow the normal developmental course of information processing. The subtle differences in information processing detected in the present study might well lead to modifications in theories of information processing in hearing-impaired children and further clarify the multiple processing of normal children.

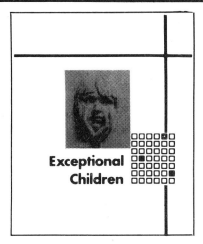

TEACHING THE NONVERBAL CHILD

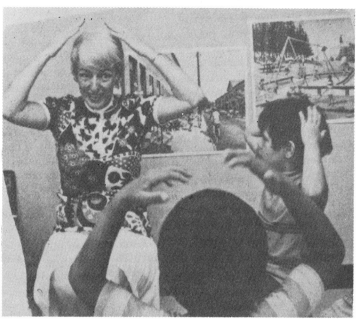

RUTH E. BENDER

THE THEME OF THIS ARTICLE IS AN oft-repeated one—what to do with the child who, by reason of a variety of handicaps, does not develop verbal language without special assistance.

He is a controversial child. No one label seems to fit him and his classmates equally. He is not deaf, although many of his symptoms simulate deafness. He may have a hearing loss, but this is not his major handicap. His problems are variously called by such names as central auditory disorder, aphasia, language disorder, minimal brain damage, autism, and mental retardation. Often he exhibits some combination of these disorders.

Most of all, he seems to live in a shadow between sound and silence.

This is almost as far as we can go in naming a common denominator for the problems involved, so we cannot really consider these children in the singular because they differ so sharply from each other. Any commonality they may have is seen more readily in what they cannot do. They cannot use sound appropriately, whether they receive it or not. They are clumsy in motor coordination to some degree, however minimal. They are often faulty in perception, visually as well as auditorally. They lack the ability to retain, with consistency, the symbolism of oral language. They lack, most of all, the ability to reproduce oral language by direct imitation of a whole word. Our concern now is not to name these children but to teach

them. But how to teach them is the question.

During the past 4 years in the Preschool Hearing Program of the Cleveland Hearing and Speech Center, we have made a special effort at exploratory teaching in this area. We lay no claim to any spectacular new discovery. Rather, our methods are a blend of previously developed and often contradictory philosophies, plus some contributions of our own. No statistical studies have been done yet on this work, but we feel that the progress of our children warrants sharing our experience with our professional colleagues.

ADMITTANCE

We begin with the child as young as is practical.

Experience has taught us that a developmental age of 18 months is a most profitable beginning. With a child who is peripherally deaf and nothing more, this may mean at 12 or 13 months of chronological age. For the children who are more involved neurologically, we have been forced to revise our standards. They seldom mature as early, and are usually not ready for our program before 2 or 2½ years of age.

This does not prohibit earlier parent counseling. Nor does it preclude periodic group situations for observation with the parents present.

Every child who applies for help through the Center enters by means of an initial evaluation. This includes referrals from his physician, interviews

with his parents, and every means available to us for evaluating his potential in speech and hearing. If the results seem to indicate that the child will profit from our program, he is accepted for teaching.

Exceptions do occur. With the best efforts of the diagnostic team at initial intake, some children remain enigmas. This does not greatly disturb the diagnosticians, as long as there is a place for these children in the educational program. There, the opportunity for long-term observation and the children's response to diagnostic teaching will help to clarify the situation.

We are wary of a label too hastily given. It has a tendency to follow a child through life, even though it is later proved wrong. It can have a detrimental influence on his educational acceptance for years to come.

SOCIAL DEVELOPMENT

Our ultimate goal, as in any therapy, is normalcy, or as nearly normal development as possible. We realize that full normalcy can seldom be reached for the children in our program. Nevertheless, we are convinced that the more we can make normalcy our aim, the farther we can bring the child along this road. To this end, we begin on a normal nursery school basis, although at a younger age.

The beginning classrooms are typical nursery school classrooms, somewhat simplified to meet the needs of our children. There are the usual housekeeping toys, wheel toys, puzzles, and picture books, and structures for climbing, balancing, and other motor skills. The child with a neurological involvement is notably deficient in neuromuscular coordination. Not one of these children can run across the nursery floor without tripping over his own feet, far more often than one would normally expect. So we encourage the use of gross muscle equipment and see that every room is provided with some.

Another consistent symptom with these children is their inability to cope with social situations. The need for the nursery school environment is often difficult to explain to parents, who feel that the home should provide adequate play situations and that so-called "play" time for the children at school is time wasted for education.

Quite the converse is true. The most immediate value our program can offer these children is the training in adequate social adjustment.

By beginning this training early, while we can still move slowly and pace the child's normal developmental rate, the well-known distractibility and disinhibition exhibited by these children is greatly reduced. By the time they reach the usual age for educational therapy, the usual problems in attention, response, and conformity have become minimal. We have, instead, a cooperative, responsive child, who is ready for the now familiar situation of lessons and learning.

Much teaching time is gained in this way. In addition, the child has developed habits of social adjustment that he also carries into his home, thus easing greatly the pressures there and creating a more wholesome climate for his own growth as well as for the happiness of his family.

No one but the parents of a deviant child can know fully the constant tensions of living with such a child. He is demanding, hyperactive, and uncontrollable. He responds neither to the same forms of discipline by which his parents learned nor to the methods by which they have successfully taught their other children. For the sake of temporary peace, they will often surrender to the child's demands, against their own better judgment, reinforcing the already undesirable behavior.

In the nursery school, the child has the impact of association with his peers, rather than mainly older siblings and adults. He has also the objective and trained guidance of his teachers. They have seen many of these children and can, therefore, have a more realistic perspective concerning his problems than is possible for parents, who are having their first encounter and who are emotionally involved as well.

This environment is also invaluable for the child who expresses his disability by withdrawal from social contact. The typical "loner" spends much time in solitary play when he is first introduced to the nursery situation. Gradually, this becomes parallel play

and finally cooperative interchange with his classmates and his teachers. Daily constant association finally will wear away this most difficult of barriers. This is most important. Without the wish for communication, it is useless to attempt to teach the skills for communication.

For these reasons we prefer a small group situation rather than individual sessions for the initial program. These classes are held for 1½ or 2 hours, at least four days a week, preferably in succession. From six to eight children are assigned to each class. Parent observation of the work, coordinated with professional counseling, individual as well as group, is an imperative part of the program.

RECEPTIVE LEARNING

The more formal aspects of the program are begun as soon as a child's adjustment makes him amenable to such routines. When possible, the admission dates of the new children are staggered among the older ones, so that each new child may have the benefit of seeing teaching routines already established among his colleagues. When this is not possible, since there must always be a beginning somewhere, there is always a child or two more receptive than most who will consent to lead the way.

Initial lessons are familiar to all teachers of both deaf and aphasic children. Mingled with the undirected (but supervised) play are many materials and lessons that alert the child's perception, encourage development of concept, and train the child in organization.

Because our ultimate goal is words, most of these activities are accompanied by words on the part of a teacher. This is not random chatter, but carefully structured language, in full, normal sentences, repeated over and over and over.

The children are encouraged to lipread, but if a child finds two sense modalities confusing, one may be temporarily withdrawn. If he finds the environment of the playroom too stimulating, there is always a quiet little room adjacent where he may go alone with a teacher for as long as necessary. Gradually his attention is focused, and his ability to attend is extended, until he can apply himself to his lessons in a useful life situation.

The first verbal lessons consist of lipreading nouns related to realistic objects. These are gradually combined with and transferred to pictures and other symbolic representations. The first verbs are taught by dramatization and combined immediately with the nouns. Other parts of speech follow the same pattern: i.e., color matching, color words, and color and noun phrases.

Toy animals and a doll family with

matching furniture are utilized early for use of sentences. A special effort is made to maintain the sentence structure that a child must learn before he can use his own speech adequately. We do not say:
"Put Daddy on the chair."
"Put the boy in the bathtub."
That comes much later, with the meaningful presentation of the verb "to put." Now we say:
"Daddy sat on a chair."
"The boy took a bath in the bathtub."

The children are soon eagerly arranging the materials to illustrate the sentences. Meanwhile, they are absorbing not only vocabulary but sentence order and sentence structure from the very beginning of their verbal consciousness.

AUDITORY TRAINING

Auditory training is a constant part of the program. Much of this is the development of interest in listening. Music on records is used with earphones, with special attention to amplification. The piano is used for rhythm, for fun, and for training specific response to sound. Noisemakers and speech are used to train discrimination. Amplification and attention to vibration of sound by touch are also invaluable in bringing out the children's voices.

LANGUAGE

Both deaf and aphasic children respond to these techniques, although with different degrees of learning. The deaf are more ready and consistent in sound discrimination than the aphasic. They also retain verbal language more firmly, although the language-disordered children frequently show a surprising grasp of quite complicated language concepts. Their response to such language is usually fleeting and may not be elicited again for a long time. But it gives us a brief, tantalizing glimpse into the unrealized potentials many of these children may have.

So far, our approach to language has been the familiar gestalt pattern, by means of which we teach language with as much of a normal, whole structure as possible. It is when we reach the area of developing speech that the differentiation between deaf and aphasic children becomes sharp.

SPEECH

For the deaf child who has no problem in language organization, speech is at first simple imitation. As words in lipreading take on meaning, the child shapes the same speech movements that he sees on his teacher's lips, but often soundlessly. Any attempt the child makes at speech imitation is accepted and encouraged. With constant repetition, the words become more accurate and intelligible, without sacrificing spontaneity and eagerness. Normal tempo and inflection are maintained at all times. It is surprising how well they also are imitated by the child.

For the deaf child, specific analysis and correction of speech sounds come much later. For now, the goal is spontaneous, functional use of imitative speech and the habit of speech expression.

SPEECH ELEMENTS

For the child with an aphasic involvement, the problem is very different. Very seldom does this child give back spontaneous word imitation. If he does try, it is almost always garbled, formless movement and sound. Not only is this useless for functional speech, it seems to confuse and hinder the child in acquiring and retaining his receptive language, especially when it is used simultaneously.

Hard as it may seem, we have found it best to firmly discourage this type of response. (This is a very different production from the sentence-length, imitative jargon that is encouraged in the deaf child.) It is still more difficult to dissuade parents from rewarding this behavior, because they feel they are stimulating "speech" in their deaf child.

However, the major deficiency these children exhibit is lack of speech. Therefore, our most urgent goal is the development of speech. So we must begin as soon as possible to develop speech, by whatever techniques will accomplish this purpose.

It is evident that the reservoir of receptive language these children are acquiring from the beginning must be of help, for thought, for concept, and for further use of language, both in comprehension and in expression. So we will not wait for the slow training of speech before enlarging, by every means we can devise, the child's pool of words and language for reception and comprehension.

This means that, for the time being, the training of speech and the development of language are far apart. They will converge, in a year or two, depending upon many things, chief of which is probably the degree of organizational involvement in the language area for each individual child.

We begin, as simply as possible, by trying to stimulate precise imitation of a single speech sound. This is attempted again and again with each child. We seldom succeed before the child is a mature 2½ or 3 years old.

At the beginning, this lesson is individual. A child may be taken to a quiet corner of the playroom, where other children may observe and be stimulated to imitation. He may go to the adjacent tutoring room. Or the therapist may elect to take the child to her own therapy room, farther removed from the distractions of the playroom.

Whatever technique is successful is approved. Often a combination of techniques gives the best results. This means that a sensitive, highly skilled teacher must make constant judgment as to the child's progress and adapt her methods to his needs.

Because this is basically an arbitrary, meaningless exercise to the child, an arbitrary, meaningless reward is used to encourage response. One of the simplest is a marble rolled across the bench toward the child, as the teacher produces clearly a single speech element; for example, *ah*. If the child responds with an attempt at imitation, he receives the marble and drops it into a tin can, with a satisfying clatter. If he does not respond, the marble goes into the teacher's can. (Any teacher can invent any number of variations on the idea of a simple immediate reward.)

A child may watch this procedure silently, or he may struggle with an unsuccessful attempt at response, for many days. Eventually a clear vocal imitation will break through.

When this occurs, the teacher is highly pleased. She expresses her approval in whatever way is best suited to the child—an especially warm smile, a nod, a gentle pat. It is usually best to be not too dramatic with these highly sensitive children. Even approval, too forcefully expressed, may startle them and delay their first tentative progress.

When this first success occurs, the child is pleased too. Strangely, his delight will often go quite beyond the fun of the marble in the can or the teacher's approval. There seems to be an exhilarating awakening to the knowledge that he has exercised conscious control over a skill that was previously beyond his reach. For the moment, a bit of his frustration against his handicap begins to seep away.

These simple imitative games continue daily until the correct vocal response can be obtained readily and without fail. Then the teacher shifts to a second sound element, perhaps another vowel, such as *oo*. She may find that the child perseverates on the first sound. With persistence, he will come to imitate the second. Then he may find it difficult to return to the first. This will eventually be accomplished, also. As his skill increases with practice, each new element presented will be mastered more readily, until he can imitate any of the easier sounds upon request.

By this time arbitrary rewards are largely discarded in favor of just fun and games between child and teacher. As soon as they can do so profitably, several children are included in a small group to practice their vocal imitations.

When imitation comes easily enough, a child is given two or three elements to remember and repeat in succession. There is no sense of haste to blend (or smooth, as McGinnis [1] calls it) these elements together. If a child's vocal imitation is coming easily and surely, the teacher may present her vocal patterns smoothly. The child who is ready will, as a rule, follow without conscious effort. If he is confused by the attempt, his teacher merely smiles and tries again another day.

The stimulation for these vocal efforts is given, at first, with both visual and auditory cues. When the child seems ready, every effort is made to achieve the proper response by means of the auditory cue alone.

There should never be any occasion, either in lipreading or in this early speech training, when only a visual cue is used (i.e., unvoiced lipreading). Audition is the normal sense modality for oral language. Emphasis on visual cues is necessary for these children because their audition is defective. But they should never be denied any possible association with the sound of language.

Artificial lipreading is useful only for those who already know audible language, but must be trained to give attention to visual cues because they are losing their hearing. The greater danger is that we train the child so thoroughly in his lipreading skills that we neglect to call to his attention his ability in understanding by hearing.

Up to this point, there is not the remotest connection between the child's speech lessons and his ongoing progress in receptive language. If, because he has begun his training early, or because his problems in organization are minimal, he begins to use functional imitation of speech, so much the better. He is encouraged to do so, by all means. But he should never be denied the contact with the highly structured speech training embodied in the Element Association Method,[1] although he may move through it more rapidly than another child.

It is this borderline child who is often too quickly handed over to the more natural methods of teaching speech. It is very hard to realize that his tentative beginnings of speech will not continue to expand and develop. This is especially true if he is passed from one teacher to another year after year.

Each teacher will try hard with this promising child, who is still so disappointing in his actual progress. By the end of her year with him, she will say to herself, with a sigh of relief, that now he really shows signs of breaking through in speech and language, and by next year he will surely build on what he has learned last year.

Unfortunately, next year's teacher may repeat the same routine, and the next year's as well. It may be some time before someone realizes that this child is always on the verge of beginning but is never really talking.

By this time, much time and effort

have been wasted, and we must still go back to the beginning of speech training, with a child who is now older, more frustrated, and unhappily accustomed to failure.

Whether we like it or not, there are nonverbal children who need very special training before they can put together and maintain the sequence of sound elements that make up human speech. The earlier this basic training can be established, the sooner the child is freed to go forward in his use of speech.

The goal of the speech element imitation is, of course, eventual words with meaning. If a child can move into this step while he is still in these early stages, his teacher will take every advantage of his ability. Every word that he can use for functional communication will reinforce his growing interest and skill in this symbolic form of living. He must be aware by now (many of these children are acutely aware) that there is in his human environment a dimension of communication from which he is shut out. Every crack he can make in this barrier will be a tremendous step forward.

However, this is an ambiguous area. The teacher must be prepared to retreat and reteach, again and again, long after she had thought the child was ready to move forward on his own. He still cannot retain the sequence of sounds necessary to produce a word, even though he has grasped the sound elements involved.

It once took 6 weeks for a teacher and a little boy to establish and maintain for functional use the simple word "nut." This was a very bright boy, with a good deal of functional speech to his credit. But the new word still needed careful structured building and much repetitive drill before it was useful in his speech vocabulary.

THE ELEMENT ASSOCIATION METHOD

As soon as the child's maturity warrants it (preferably not before 4), the individual therapist periodically removes the child from his group or schedules him for individual sessions at other times. She then proceeds to lead him into the carefully structured Element Association Method, using reading and then writing of speech symbols as visual and motor association with speech. (These procedures have been too well documented elsewhere to need repetition here.) The teacher is free to adhere to the Method as closely as she feels necessary for each individual child, and to deviate when she finds this more profitable for a particular child. Each teacher understands thoroughly, however, the need for rigid, consistent structure in these lessons.

Structure and consistency is the security to which these children cling and

the basic foundation upon which they can step up to reach for more complicated learning. But they are still children, beneath the psychologically disfiguring handicap, and monotony and repetition becomes boring to them, as to other children. It is a wise teacher who can successfully mingle consistent structure and interesting variations in her lessons. Still, it can be done and it must be done.

We make a few exceptions in the Element Association Method, as described by McGinnis,[1] in the interests of normalcy, and have found them in no way delaying the children in the learning of speech and language.

Instead of cursive, we use manuscript writing, from the beginning. We use it for the same reasons it has become standard in schools for normal children: ease of production, ease of recognition, basic form for each individual letter, and minimal need for transfer in printed forms of reading. In addition, it puts our children into step with the work in the public school special classes to which they will soon be transferred.

The use of manuscript writing presents no deterrent in any way, but rather contributes to clarity and rapidity of progress. The argument that adult aphasics are often assisted in language recall by the motor tracing of cursive writing does not apply. In his case, the adult aphasic is using previously learned patterns to revive old memories. For our child, we are in the process of setting up memory patterns. So we may as well establish the clearest and most functional patterns at hand, from the very beginning. Properly written, a manuscript word is a compact unit, without the ambiguity of the flowing connections and with the added value of discrete form.

ELEMENT CHARTS

As the sounds to be remembered multiply, the children need visual clues for reference and drill. These are provided by element charts, which are on permanent display on the classroom walls.

For consonant sounds, we use the Northampton Consonant Chart,[2] much as it has been used for many years with deaf children. The relation of the position of a sound on the chart and its speech production is simple and accurate and all but self-evident.

A satisfactory vowel chart presented a different problem. After exploratory use of several forms, we decided upon a modified version of the Judson-Weaver Vowel Curve[3] as most suitable for our purpose. It is simple in form and presents a usable diagrammatic picture of jaw position and sound production for each vowel.

We have retained the Northampton Chart spellings, for the most part, on

both charts, as most closely related to the pronunciation of words in the reading of English. However, we have discarded artificial and bizarre spellings, because these created confusion in the child's normal use of reading and writing. Thus, for example, we no longer use the small *1* and *2* figures over identical spellings in two columns, nor do we use the spellings *o* (*r*) or (*r*) *u–e.*

The children learn readily by use of the word, as do other children, which pronunciation is required. Because a new word, when encountered in reading, will not have these designations in any case, little seems to be lost in guidance to speech.

For diphthongs and short vowels, the use of the dash is retained. It can be justified by the insertion of the proper consonant in a word, and the influence on the quality of the vowel is evident: for example, *a–e, ate; –a–, cat.*

LANGUAGE AND SPEECH

Much individual drill on speech is maintained throughout the day. By this time, these children are 5 or 6 years old and work in a day-long class group consistently. We have been so fortunate as to have a rotating staff of student teachers as assistants to the head teacher. The student teachers are a dedicated and skillful corps, inventing to a large extent their own materials and devices according to their individual talents. Much of their time is spent in individual speech work, thus multiplying greatly the contacts provided for speech. To them must go much of the credit for the children's progress.

Now, at last, the speech work and language work for these children are about to converge. In our exploratory teaching, trying to find the most effective way to intermesh the two, we set up a parallel series of lessons.

A teacher especially skilled in the Element Association Method and a language teacher were given equal time with a class of aphasic children. We wanted to explore the validity of the theory that a word once learned by a child through the intensive Element Association Method was his forever.

The results indicated that functional use was still the strongest factor in the overlearning and retention of vocabulary. So we have correlated the speech and language teaching under the guidance of one teacher, in each class.

Because the children have now mastered the ability to sound out words by speech elements, many short cuts are possible in the acquisition of new words. Briefly separating the new word into elements, later into syllables, is usually sufficient to establish pronunciation.

The children delighted in developing this game on their own. One child, in particular, would work on the articulation of a new word he met in reading, quite without direction. When he thought he had it mastered, he would then bring it to his teacher and ask for the meaning.

LANGUAGE AND READING

Throughout each child's school career, while his speech ability was building slowly, his receptive language has been increasing rapidly. With the advent of reading, he now seems ready for sentence-length speech (a skill his deaf brother has mastered long before).

The techniques of teaching reading are too familiar to need space in an article of this length. The principles applied with these children are the same as those used with deaf children, and the response is as ready.

Writing, in manuscript form, has been already begun in the teaching of speech elements. It is now expanded to include, as needed, all reading material.

The expansion of language is now the most important factor in the child's education. But the teacher must keep constantly in mind that the most important medium for this language is the use of functional speech. This is the normal means of communication for all humanity and for our children as well. This is also the area of their greatest weakness. Therefore this must be the area of unremitting emphasis in their school day. All other media of instruction and expression are made to contribute to the ability to use and the habit of using functional speech.

The language presentation now follows much the same pattern as that used for developing language with deaf children. There is no need to resort to a more rigid structure than the constant use of a normal sentence.

Nouns are presented in reading, with simultaneous use in lipreading, speech, and writing. The children have long been familiar with this form of vocabulary through their speech association lessons. No limits are set, except the usual ones of maturity and readiness for reading.

Verbs are also presented at once, linked to familiar lipreading use, but, at this point, always in the past tense. This is the form in which a child first needs a verb to use for expression, in both speech and writing. He is not yet concerned with tense or mood, only with basic meaning. It is also the most common form he will encounter in early reading (excepting only some pre-primers, which are, in any case, not functional for the child who does not have adequate previous ability in oral language).

The pattern of the Fitzgerald Key [4] is followed, with the simple question words written at the top of the chalk board. Noun and verb modifiers and prepositional phrases are taught as needed, by incidental use, by formal presentation, and by repetitive functional use, until the children are using them in spontaneous speech.

Every effort is made to retain the unity and continuity of sentence structure. A sentence is never written in disconnected fashion, either on the board or the children's papers. When a child makes a comment in the telegraphic speech typical of these children, space is left for the omitted word, as the teacher writes it for him, so that he may see his omission and supply it.

"John   a penny."
"John found a penny."

The significance of sentence sequence is important in any language, and is absorbed for each particular language by constant functional, repetitive use. It can become significant early, even for these confused children, if it is consistently presented in this unified way.

This was illustrated by the boy who, in an action lesson, chose the word "caught" for his sentence. Then he asked a classmate to chase and catch him. Since the children preferred the initial position in the sentence as the status position for their own names, the teacher prepared for an argument with the child on his resulting sentence. He began eagerly, "I caught Su——," then, with a look of dawning comprehension, he said, "No! Susie caught I."

This child had developed the all-important feeling of the significance of sentence sequence. The form of the pronoun was easily corrected by means of the pronoun chart.

Charts with words in fixed position are used only when the position of the word on the chart is significant. These charts would include a pronoun paradigm chart and verb charts illustrative of tense forms, once these are taught. All charts on permanent display are in constant use for reference.

All other forms of visual display are on flash cards and presented in pocket charts, which allows the necessary flexibility for functional use and prevents the habit of remembering position instead of form, in learning words.

Experiences and experience charts are very much a part of the curriculum. But little time is spent in stereotyped repetition of language that has once been worked out and understood. The experience charts are hung one on top of the other and left for the children to reread as stories for pleasure. They also use them, quite spontaneously, as reference works, for recall and verification of vocabulary and language principles that they need for current use.

Number work does not present any particular problem for these children. It is taught first by means of such concrete materials as small cube blocks and jackstraw sticks. As soon as possible, the children use the number workbooks designed for normal children.

Reading workbooks are also presented as early as possible. Those that are designed around simple stories with varied forms of question-and-answer following proved particularly helpful for our children.

All workbook lessons demand a great deal of supervision and attention from the teacher. Each child moves at his own rate. Often no two children are working on the same page of copies of the same workbook. But they are worth the effort for a number of reasons.

They introduce the children gradually to increasingly complicated language in a normal way. This is almost impossible to achieve with only teacher-made materials, especially if the teacher has been trained only in special education.

The library corner is an invaluable asset to the classroom. It is furnished with well-illustrated children's books of all descriptions. The emphasis, at this time, is on an abundance of illustrations. The children, however, are soon finding words and phrases they recognize and sharing the discovery gleefully with classmates and teacher.

This should be an area that is left to the children to use spontaneously and for their own pleasure. We can give them no greater gift than the desire for books.

It is a temptation, because it is easy, to forge ahead in language development by means of reading as the chief medium. This is not, however, the chief means of communication in the children's world. Nor is it the area of their greatest weakness. This knowledge brings us back sharply, again, to the major goal of this whole educational process—the functional use of speech.

LANGUAGE, READING AND SPEECH

The children can still comprehend more complicated language for reception than they can handle for expression. But they must know the language before they can use it. So we continue to devise a variety of oral games and drills.

They particularly enjoy imaginative games and like nothing better than to dramatize themselves as animals, etc. They understand perfectly well when to say, "I am a boy," or "I am a dog."

During one such game, a 5-year-old stated, with a twinkle: "I have five baby elephants at home."

At her teacher's startled look, she added pleadingly: "Not big. Small baby elephants."

Both the child and her teacher understood that this was an imaginative game. But her classmates were disappointed and a bit indignant to be told it was all pretend. They would much have preferred a small zoo in Susie's backyard.

Such games are encouraged. They are normal, they are fun, and they stimulate the development of language, speech, social communication, personality, and mental alertness. There is no child so pathetic as the one who is denied the expression of his full potential because of environmental deprivation.

However, we are most careful not to distort the symbolism that words are meant to express. For instance, we would never say, as has been done, "Throw five babies," even though the tiny dolls in the lesson box would lend themselves to such a weird action. One does not throw babies, even in imagination. Many more realistic objects are at hand to illustrate the same language structure, but with functional language.

Many of these drills and exercises grow from and center around the first lesson of the day. This is a combination of what used to be called "action work" and "news."

Most of it is initiated by the children. In the belief that a child will talk most readily when he has something that he wants to say, the children are encouraged to express their first exuberant communications each day as best they can. They use words, as far as possible, and when these fail they may resort to dramatization, drawing, or whatever is necessary to have their message understood. They may bring prized possessions to display and describe. They may recall a previous experience they enjoyed or tell of one anticipated.

As each child takes his turn, the teacher and children center their attention on understanding him and helping him express what he has to say. The teacher cheerfully supplies vocabulary and language structure he needs. Eventually she writes the completed sentences on the board, and the class take turns at reading or retelling them in a variety of ways.

It is encouraging to see how quickly this approach to language leads the children to spontaneous efforts at oral communication. As all children do, they want to tell each other and their teachers what is important to them, at home, at play with their neighbors, on weekend trips, etc. Instead of these communications being relegated to meager gesture language at free or stolen moments, they are welcomed as an important part of classroom living.

This type of teaching is particularly beneficial for the teacher. There is no possibility for her to retreat into a rut of monotonous classroom language. Nor can she lose sight of the children's ever-expanding language needs. Each day she is forced to use new vocabulary and new language, as the children demand it.

This "morning news" then forms the basis for the day's writing lesson. Sometimes, if the language is particularly complicated or there are too many unfamiliar items, the children are allowed to copy. It has been our consistent experience, however, that copied language results in more mistakes and less understanding than when each child must reconstruct it on his own.

Naturally, the children have not memorized the spelling of all newly presented vocabulary. In many instances, they know where to go to help themselves—to flash cards in the pocket charts, a particular drawer or box, to old experience charts, to picture dictionaries in the book corner. If none of these is sufficient for a child, he asks his teacher. He need only be able to make his request clear, in whatever way he can, and she will write the word on the board for him. She allows him to study it for a few moments, then erases it. Even though this must be repeated several times, it is usually better than letting him expect to copy.

These written lessons take a great deal of supervision. All allowances are made for individual ability as to length and complexity of each child's paper. But eventually each paper, within itself, must be perfect. There is no benefit in practicing mistakes.

Sometime during the day, each child has an individual session with his teacher, reading his own paper aloud. Meticulous attention is paid to articulation and phrasing. Finally, this is the paper each child takes home at the end of the day to share with his family.

In this article much has been omitted and more has been condensed, as any classroom teacher will know. In the interest of brevity, illustrations have been kept at a minimum and no lesson plans have been included.

We have presented the philosophy and progression of lesson structures by which, in our experience, children with a central auditory disorder can most quickly and effectively learn to use functional speech.

What is the eventual goal of a child who comes through such a program?

At present, we feel that he is equipped to handle the program in any good oral school for deaf children. Only the future will tell whether he can eventually go farther or do better than his deaf brother. But one thing is certain: He can develop oral communication skills adequate for daily living and for continued education.

To summarize briefly what we have attempted to say, we have described in condensed form our experience in developing a program of combined techniques in teaching language to young children with central auditory disorders, either with or without an accompanying peripheral hearing loss. This program includes techniques used in the gestalt form of teaching deaf children and aphasic children, and also some of the techniques of the Element Association Method. In all these varying and sometimes conflicting methods, we have made variations as well as combinations that seem to serve best the needs of our children. Other schools are doing the same type of exploratory teaching. Because there is really nothing new under the sun, and language is language from time unknown, we can only attempt to establish some guidelines that in our program have proved to be useful.

REFERENCES

1. MILDRED A. McGINNIS, *Aphasic Children*. Washington, D.C.: Alexander Graham Bell Association for the Deaf, 1963.
2. *Northampton Charts*. Northampton, Mass.: Clarke School.
3. L. S. JUDSON AND A. T. WEAVER, *Voice Science*. New York: Crofts & Company, 1942.
4. EDITH FITZGERALD, *Straight Language for the Deaf*. Washington, D.C.: Alexander Graham Bell Association for the Deaf, 1957.

BIBLIOGRAPHY

ALDER, SOL, *The Non-verbal Child*. Springfield, Ill.: Charles C Thomas, 1964.
BARRY, HORTENSE, *The Young Aphasic Child*. Washington, D.C.: Alexander Graham Bell Association for the Deaf, 1961.
GROHT, MILDRED A., *Natural Language for Deaf Children*. Washington, D.C.: Alexander Graham Bell Association for the Deaf, 1958.
HARRIS, GRACE MARGARET, *Language for the Preschool Deaf Child*. New York: Grune and Stratton, 1950.
MYKLEBUST, HELMER, *Auditory Disorders in Children*. New York: Grune and Stratton, 1954.
SIMMONS, AUDREY A., "Language Growth for the Pre-nursery Deaf Child," *The Volta Review*, March 1966, p. 291.

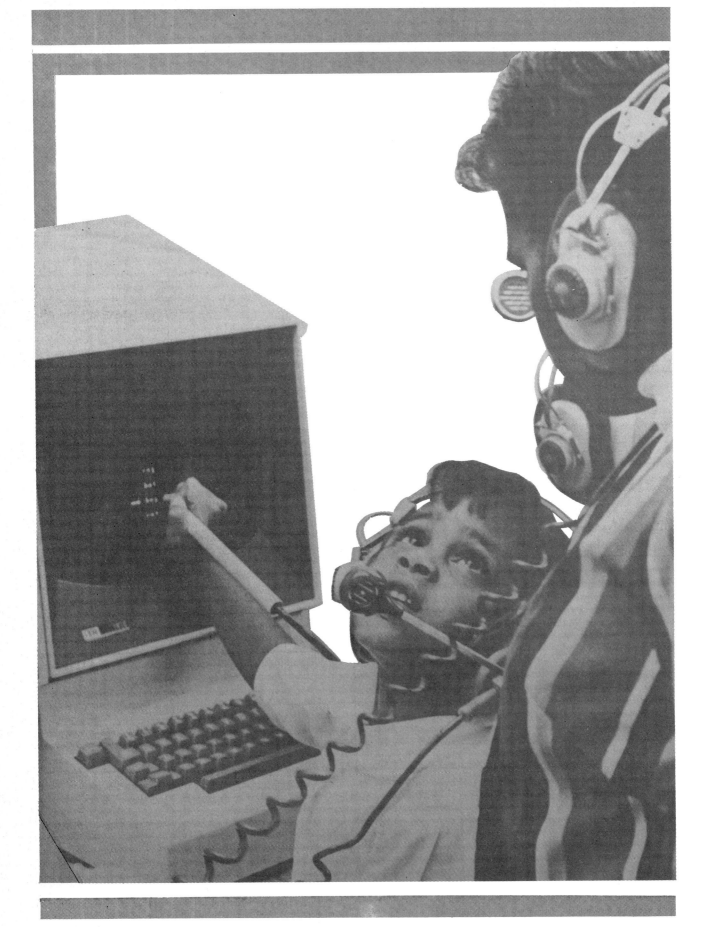

Medical, Technological and Psychological Rehabilitation

There are no basic organs of speech as there are ears for hearing. Each of the organs utilized for speech serves another function with which speech competes. The lips, the teeth and cheek muscles, soft palate and muscles of the throat are all designed primarily for speech.

For these reasons speech is considered a learned behavior. Normal channels of speech have been found to be automatic in nature, though achieved indirectly through unregulated articulatory movement. However, medically speaking, impaired speech tends to decrease a persons confidence and self-esteem, their enthusiasm, happiness, acceptance of themselves and others. They become disappointed and discouraged members of society, who experience unworthiness, feelings of apathy, discouragement, and often withdraw into loneliness.

Through educational intervention, medical assessment and special services we can begin to correct some of these deficits. Methods of personality development and acceptance have been designed to meet individual needs. Articulatory skills have been perfected to correct deviations. Emotional, intellectual and pathological corrective measures have been implemented to aid in the care and correction of disorders.

Many of these same tools of remediation can be utilized in working with the hearing impaired by the pathologist. With the addition of hearing aids, otologists can aid the pathologist in remedial measures designed to integrate and assist in the development of speech and speech reading for the hearing impaired child.

The deaf can also gain speech reading skills through specially designed programs of instruction and education. Physical equipment such as hearing aids and audiometers have been made available for the education of the deaf in order that rehabilitation will certainly be an obtainable goal.

The speech and hearing impaired have optimum goals for success both educationally and vocationally through established programs which have been formulated to meet their rehabilitative needs for worthy and productive lives, making their inborn potentialities a part of their assets and not liabilities as had been previously been thought. Objective self-realization is strikingly real and available to those who believe in the old addage:

"Where there is a will, there is a way . . ."

. . . and so it is for those who experience disorders in speech or hearing.

Hearing Aids Children Wear:

A Longitudinal Study of Performance

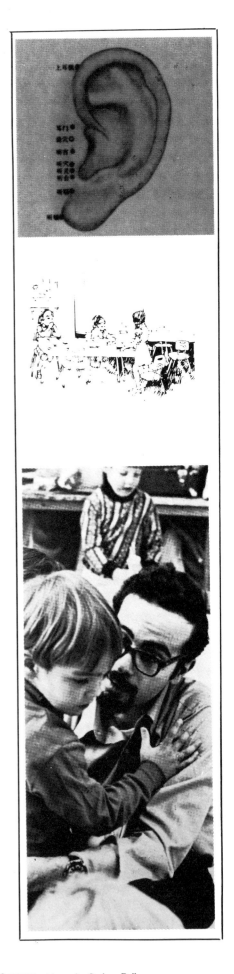

G. David Zink, M.A.

Procedures for examination of electroacoustic response characteristics of hearing aids have provided additional objective data for hearing aid evaluation and selection. Harris (1961), Jerger, Speaks and Malmquist (1966), Kasten (1965-1967), Lotterman (1965-1967), Olsen and Wilbur (1968), and Mazor (1967) have reported on the variables of hearing aid performance. Harris (1961), Bode (1968), Jerger (1966), Kasten (1967), and Lotterman (1967) have supplied evidence of decrements in speech intelligibility when excessive distortion products are present in low fidelity circuitry. Olsen (1967) reported on the importance of the width of frequency response relating to hearing aid intelligibility.

Sung and Hodgston (1969) discussed the importance of the upper frequency limits of hearing aid band width. Lotterman (1967) and Kasten (1969) reported the influence of gain control rotation on acoustic gain and nonlinear distortion. Cooper (1969) described the importance of acoustic gain in aided discrimination. Gaeth and Lounsburg (1966), in their study of children wearing hearing aids in elementary schools, utilized electroacoustic instrumentation in analyzing the aids, but found much of the data meaningless because of a multitude of defective components present in the aids. Generally, the findings have described variables in hearing aid performance and indicated the need for clinicians to have accurate knowledge of those variables.

Our program attempts to provide optimum functioning amplification for acoustically handicapped students and preschool children. New, used, and donated hearing aids are screened for suitability of acoustic response characteristics by electroacoustic measurement.

purpose of the study

The purpose of this two-year study was to evaluate and monitor electroacoustic performance characteristics of hearing aids worn by children. Areas of investigation include: study of repaired hearing aids, study of instruments in use, study of new hearing aids, and study of donated hearing aids.

Hearing aids were evaluated with Bruel and Kjaer electroacoustic instrumentation. This included a hearing aid test box type 4212, a level recorder type 2305, a random sine generator type 1024, two microphone amplifiers type 2604, a band pass filter type 1612, and a band rejection filter type 1607. Four parameters of hearing aid performance were tested during the study, viz., frequency response, acoustic gain/saturation, harmonic distortion, and gain control variability. Aids were evaluated by manufacturers' procedures when these were obtainable. Otherwise, appropriate American National Standards Institute methods were utilized (S3.3-1960, S3.8-1967). In addition, the following measures were incorporated as part of the evaluation criteria. An acceptable hearing aid meets the following criteria:

Frequency response. The fundamental frequency response curve is analyzed for transient increases or decreases appearing through the amplifying range of the instrument. One increase or decrease larger than 15 dB and/or two or more increases or decreases greater than 6 dB are unacceptable.

Gain/saturation. For new aids the instrument must be within plus or minus 6 dB of the manufacturer's specification for acoustic gain or saturation levels. For used aids the instrument must meet the wearer's gain requirements.

Distortion. In addition to the routinely measured discrete frequencies of 500 Hz, 700 Hz, and 900 Hz, a one-third octave band analysis through the maximum number of plottable harmonic components (second, third, etc.) is performed. All frequencies demonstrating distortion are also measured discretely. Nonacceptance results when measurements indicate an excess of 17 percent distortion at any one frequency.

Gain control taper. The range of gain control is divided into quarters. Output is measured at each of the four settings for an input level of 60 dB. Percentage of acoustic gain is plotted as a function of gain control rotation. Nonacceptance results when non-linearity interferes with user performance. Dearth of reserve gain, or an excessive gain increase with gain rotation are examples of nonacceptability.

Through electroacoustic hearing aid analysis, a comparison of the instrument can be made with the available specifications. In addition an objective comparison can be made between hearing aids.

The age range of the children wearing the aids was 15 months to 19.4 years. Twenty-two of the children were within the 15 months to 36 months group. Twelve were in the 36 to 72 months group with the remainder falling in the higher age categories. Hearing levels ranged from mild to profound.

repaired hearing aids

Upon completion of electroacoustic analysis hearing aids not meet-

5. REHABILITATION

ing criteria requirements are recommended for repair. When repair has been completed the aids are re-examined electroacoustically for adequacy of acoustic response. During the past school year, of 103 hearing aids evaluated, 43 (42 percent) were found acceptable, and 60 (58 percent) were rejected as not meeting criteria requirements. Table 1 shows classification of aids not meeting requirements. Any

TABLE 1. USED HEARING AIDS REJECTED
BY ONE OR MORE CRITERIA COMBINATIONS
(FIRST YEAR)

CONDITION	#AIDS	%TOTALS
GAIN VARIABILITY	19	32
GAIN / MPO	22	37
FREQ. RESPONSE	44	73
DISTORTION	50	83

of the aids may have been rejected for more than one reason and therefore can fall within more than one category. Fifty (83 percent) were not acceptable due to excessive distortion levels. Forty-four (73 percent) of the instruments were unacceptable because of frequency response limitations. Twenty-two (37 percent) were unacceptable because of acoustic gain limitations and 19 (32 percent) were unacceptable because of gain control variability.

Of the 60 rejected hearing aids 52 were re-examined after repair. Thirty-four (65 percent) were found acceptable and 18 (35 percent) were rejected. Detailed individual study of the 18 rejected instruments revealed the specific reasons for nonacceptance (Figure 1). Seven (39 percent) hearing aids did not meet the requirements for frequency response. Four (22 percent) did not meet the requirements for gain. Of these four aids, three demonstrated insufficient gain and the other demonstrated rotation variability and distortion limitations. One (6 percent) did not meet the requirements for distortion. However, six (33 percent) did not meet the combined requirements for frequency response and distortion.

hearing aids in use

During the current year 92 hearing aids were evaluated. Fifty-one (55 percent) were found to be acceptable and 41 (45 percent) were unacceptable. Any of the aids may have been rejected for more than one reason and fall within more than one category. Table 2 classifies aids not found acceptable. Twenty-four aids (59 percent) were characterized by excessive distortion. Fourteen aids (44 percent) did not meet frequency response requirements. Ten aids (24 percent) were nonacceptable because of acoustic gain/MPO limitations. Ten aids (24 percent) were nonacceptable because of physical reasons such as defective cords, defective receivers, and defective gain controls, or were completely inoperative.

A two-year comparison of aids found to be acceptable revealed that an additional 13 percent were functioning satisfactorily during the current year. The 13 percent improvement may be indicative of an increased awareness toward care of the instrument through the residual effects of the periodic electroacoustic hearing aid evaluation program now in its second year. Through interview techniques with parents, teachers, and the wearers, an attempt was made to establish plausible reasons for hearing aid malfunction. The majority of parents and teachers proved to be unaware of any reasons for malfunction with the exception of a few reports of having seen the aid dropped. From the children who could supply information, dropping of the instrument or receiver was the only reason indicated. The ma-

TABLE 2. USED HEARING AIDS REJECTED
BY ONE OR MORE CRITERIA COMBINATIONS
(SECOND YEAR)

CONDITION	#AIDS	%TOTALS
PHYSICAL REASONS	10	24
GAIN / MPO	10	24
FREQ. RESPONSE	14	44
DISTORTION	24	59

NUMBER OF AIDS
TOTALS: EVALUATED N=92 REJECTED N=41

jority were not aware of any other possible reason for malfunction. Teachers were found to have limited background information regarding care and operation of hearing aids. As long as the child wore the aid, teachers did not question the adequacy of the aid. The responsibility for continued successful operation appeared to fall primarily with the child, regardless of age. In most instances extra cords and batteries were not available at the school. Earmold fit was an area discovered to be in need of increased teacher awareness. Most responses indicated that the remedy for hearing aid feedback has been to rotate the gain control to a lower setting rather than to investigate the earmold fit or to refer the child to the appropriate resource where the service could be performed. In the past parents and teachers have had only an informal acquaintance with hearing aid management procedures. A supervised structured hearing aid indoctrination and follow-up program is necessary for effective hearing aid management.

new hearing aids

Analysis of new hearing aids obtained through local dealers was the final phase of study. This phase was designed as a preselection tool to identify hearing aids that are acceptable for use in hearing aid selection procedures. The same criteria are employed in screening new aids. Twenty-six new hearing aids were evaluated during the current school year. Nineteen (73 percent) were acceptable and seven (27 percent) were unacceptable. Of the seven nonacceptable aids, two (29 percent) were unacceptable because of frequency response limitations, two (29 percent) were unacceptable because of gain/MPO limitations, two (29 percent) were unacceptable because of frequency and gain limitations, and one aid (14 percent) was unacceptable because of distortion. The sample for the current year is smaller than that for the previous year, when 75 hearing aids were

5. REHABILITATION

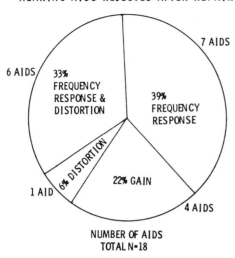

HEARING AIDS REJECTED AFTER REPAIR

7 AIDS

6 AIDS / 33% FREQUENCY RESPONSE & DISTORTION

39% FREQUENCY RESPONSE

6% DISTORTION

1 AID

22% GAIN

4 AIDS

NUMBER OF AIDS
TOTAL N=18

analyzed, with 40 (53 percent) having been classed as acceptable and 35 (47 percent) as unacceptable. Distortion was the primary reason for unacceptability, affecting 32 aids (91 percent). Frequency response was next (19 aids or 54 percent), followed by gain/MPO (8 aids or 23 percent), and gain control variability (two aids or 6 percent). An increased acceptance rate of 20 percent is noted for the current year's sample. It is our impression that during the current year dealers were more selective when supplying aids and the aids were from more current inventories.

donated hearing aids

Thirty-five used hearing aids were donated for use during the current year. The criterion for acceptance was that the aid demonstrate a usable fundamental acoustic response. Therefore, a high gain aid demonstrating low gain characteristics could be acceptable, as could an aid deviating markedly from manufacturers' specifications. Of the 35 hearing aids, three (8 percent) were found acceptable, and 32 (92 percent) were found unacceptable. Electroacoustic analysis revealed that the 32 aids were characterized by a multitude of defects and were functioning so inadequately that it was pointless to categorize the defects. Clinicians should be cautious when accepting or using donated hearing aids. Observations from this study suggest that despite good intentions, donated hearing aids may be, in fact, a detriment to the hearing impaired child.

discussion of the findings

The assumption cannot be made that because a child is wearing a hearing aid the instrument is functioning optimally or even minimally. Our findings suggest that a significant number of hearing aids worn by children are functioning inefficiently. Frequently young acoustically handicapped children are fitted with expensive individual hearing aids. If we depend upon manufacturers' specification sheets, master hearing aid information, or results obtainable through traditional hearing aid evaluation procedures, we will have limited information regarding the individual hearing aid the child will be wearing. Further, we will have only limited knowledge of the optimum function that can be expected for the individual child, based on the acoustic response characteristics of the aid that has been selected for him. Special learning environments are designed to be compatible with the characteristics of individual children. The effects of the educational program should be assessed. Because the results of the assessment should reflect the effectiveness of the educational programming, it is of critical importance that an aid function optimally. The results of this study indicate that measured behaviors may be confounded by amplification which is not functioning properly or has been improperly selected. This variable can be ameliorated by combining the available objective data in hearing aid selection with electroacoustic hearing aid study. Evaluation of electroacoustic response characteristics of hearing aids is an efficient and effective method for detection of faulty functioning. This evaluation is beneficial in selecting and maintaining optimum amplification, and ensures that the instrument is meeting basic requirements. It is recommended that each amplifying unit in use receive regular longitudinal assessment.

Clearly, there is a need for the development of standards that are applicable to clinical use. Current standards were developed primarily for design or engineering purposes, and therefore do not easily adapt to clinical variables. These variables include an individual's requirements and limitations relating to acoustic gain, reserve gain, frequency response, gain control variability, signal to noise ratio distortion, and earmold acoustics.

With a hearing aid, speech can be made audible or intelligible, as well as tolerable, if the limitations of the auditory system are not too great. It is essential to select a hearing aid that has low distortion—ample gain, and also a maximum power output and frequency response characteristic that will adequately amplify the speech signal without exceeding limits of tolerability. These factors can be elucidated for the audiologist through electroacoustic evaluation.

It has been observed that when a child is having difficulty adjusting to amplification, one of the first areas of investigation should be analysis of the hearing aid. This may yield important considerations for continuing hearing aid use (Zink & Alpiner, 1968). In addition, our findings suggest that knowledge of an instrument's acoustic response is a highly efficient initial fitting procedure. By eliminating unsuitable hearing aids from the selection, time is conserved for both audiologist and patient. Through traditional examination procedures it is not easy, in most cases, to identify hearing aids which are performing unsatisfactorily.

In some situations, children are supplied with new, reconditioned, or donated hearing aids which they are faithfully wearing. This study demonstrated that many of these aids are inappropriate for the children. This can be due to factors such as excessive distortion in the instrument, or response characteristics that are inappropriate for the wearer. Examples are: an aid with limited frequency response and limited acoustic gain; or a low frequency emphasis hearing aid selected for a patient with normal hearing through the low frequencies, but with a precipitous loss in the high frequencies. Also, problems relating to gain control variability or linearity may exist. Multiple tone control settings can be confusing, with each different setting changing the response characteristics of the aid. It is not uncommon to find only one tone control setting functioning satisfactorily. Student rejection of the aid and complaints regarding its use are indications that possibly the hearing aid has changed detrimentally in acoustic characteristics. It is recommended that the aid be examined electroacoustically for possible inoperative conditions requiring reconditioning or repair which may encourage continued use of the hearing aid. In these instances, the students are able to communicate

5. REHABILITATION

their complaints. Many children, however, because of their age or the severity of their hearing loss, cannot communicate their feelings regarding the hearing aid. For the audiologist, this stresses the importance of knowing the performance characteristics of the particular instrument.

It is essential, for several additional reasons, to have acoustic characteristic data for the hearing aids children wear. First, unless the, hearing aid is grossly malfunctioning, cursory listening tests do not reveal the faulty functioning. Second, language barriers must be overcome. Children with severe hearing involvements, or very young children, are not able to perform standardized auditory discrimination tasks. In the public schools, this may constitute a rather large population, especially if the district has a preschool program. It is now possible to provide these students with hearing aids that function optimally. Finally, it is beneficial to have acoustic characteristic data when selecting and fitting binaural amplification where specific knowledge of the acoustic characteristics of the aids is desired.

A hearing aid can mean the difference between adequate or poor reception of auditory signals. Educational delay often results from partially received or distorted auditory messages. If the full potential of the acoustically handicapped child's auditory channel is to be utilized, it is imperative that the hearing aid function optimally. It is past time for us to consider the impact of inefficient amplification upon the acoustically handicapped child.

REFERENCES

American standard methods for measurement of electroacoustical characteristics of hearing aids. American National Standards Institute, S3.3—1960.

Bode, T. L. *Effects of hearing aid distortion on consonant discrimination,* ASHA Conv. 1968.

Cooper, J. C. *The effects of hearing aid frequency response on speech reception,* ASHA Conv. 1969.

Gaeth, J. H., & Lounsburg, E. Hearing aids and children in elementary schools. *Journal of Speech and Hearing Disorders,* 1966, **31**, 283-289.

Harris, J. D., Kelsey, P. A., & Clack, T. D. The relation between speech intelligibility and the electroacoustic characteristics of low fidelity circuitry. *Journal of Auditory Research,* 1961, **1**, 357-381.

Jerger, J., Speaks, C., & Malmquist, C. Hearing aid performance and hearing aid selection. *Journal of Speech and Hearing Research,* 1966, **9**, 136-149.

Kasten, R. N., & Revoile, S. G. Variability of electroacoustic characteristics of hearing aids, *ASHA,* 1965, **7**, 364.

Kasten, R. N., Lotterman, S. H., & Revoile, S. G. Variability of gain versus frequency characteristics in hearing aids. *Journal of Speech and Hearing Research,* 1967, **10**, 377-383.

Kasten, R. N., & Lotterman, S. H. A longitudinal examination of harmonic distortion in hearing aids. *Journal of Speech and Hearing Research,* 1967, **10**, 777-781.

Kasten, R. N., Lotterman, S. H., & Burnett, E. D. *Influence of non-linear distortion on hearing aid processed signals.* ASHA Conv. 1967.

Kasten, R. N., & Lotterman, S. H. The influence of hearing aid gain control rotation on acoustic gain. *Journal of Auditory Research,* 1969, **9**, 35-59.

Lotterman, S. H., & Farrar, N. R. Non-linear distortion in wearable amplification. *ASHA,* 1965, **7**, 364-365.

Lotterman, S., & Kasten, R. Non-linear distortion in modern hearing aids. *Journal of Speech and Hearing Research,* 1967, **10**, 586-592.

Lotterman, S. H., & Kasten, R. N. The influence of gain control rotation on non-linear distortion in hearing aids. *Journal of Speech and Hearing Research,* 1967, **10**, 593-599.

Lotterman, S. H., Kasten, R. N., & Revoile, S. G. Acoustic gain and threshold improvement in hearing aid selection. *Journal of Speech and Hearing Research*, 1967, **10**, 856-868.

Mazor, M., & Lang, J. *Variability of measures of acoustic performance of hearing aids as supplied by three manufacturers.* ASHA Conv. 1967.

Olsen, W. O., & Carhart, R. Development of test procedures for evaluation of binaural hearing aids. *Bulletin of Prosthetics Research*, Spring, 1967, 22-49.

Olsen, W. O., & Wilbur, S. A. *Hearing aid distortion and speech intelligibility*, ASHA Conv. 1968.

Sung, R J., & Hodgston, W. R. *Performance of individual hearing aids utilizing microphone and induction coil input.* ASHA Conv. 1969.

USA standard method of expressing hearing aid performance. American National Standards Institute, S3.8—1967.

Zink, G. D., & Alpiner, J. G. Hearing aids: One aspect of a state public school hearing conservation program. *Journal of Speech and Hearing Disorders*, 1968, **33**, 329-344.

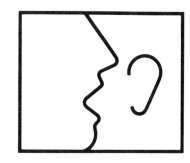

Don't Be Afraid to Wear a Hearing Aid

After all, no one laughs at your eyeglasses

BY CHARLOTTE HIMBER

YOU DON'T HAVE TO BE sixty to need a hearing aid. Millions of people in their forties and fifties would discover, if they had their hearing checked, that they've been functioning with a handicap. They get by because they "hear" what they see— facial expressions, posture, body movements. We all get clever at interpreting non-verbal messages, often developing a piercing, "mature" look.

In my case I became uncomfortably aware of a decline in my hearing when I saw people laughing and realized I'd missed the joke. Occasionally, too, people would ask me to please stop shouting—they're not deaf. But much earlier I began suspecting a problem when people's voices seemed softer and softer. Whose fault was it—theirs or mine?

Six years ago—without telling a soul—in a city far from my hometown I slinked in to one of those storefront hearing services that offers a "free hearing test." I didn't then know that this service is usually administered by dealers, not professional audiologists. I was told I needed no hearing aid.

With this reassurance I let six years pass before I went for another test, this time to an accredited hearing center and a skilled audiologist, a woman, who seated me in a quiet room where her bell-like voice felt like balm to my ears, accustomed as

I was to the grating sounds of a big city. It was a tranquilizing experience. I realized how good it felt to be able to hear every sound without straining.

Six weeks and several hearing aids later, I turned up at one of several meetings (my job keeps me hopping to them), a brand-new $350 hearing aid tucked around one ear. I was holding forth before a group of twelve when I became aware of twelve pairs of eyes widening. Absently I began to stroke something tickling my left cheek only to discover that the delicate little pink plastic arc anchored around the back

---

AFRAID OF A HEARING AID

". . . I've launched a crusade to get people to react sensibly toward hearing loss."

---

of my ear was dangling down my cheek. Quickly I put it in place, but nothing I could do or say during the rest of the meeting got through to my co-workers. In short, feelings had become so embarrassing that all communication was cut off. Why

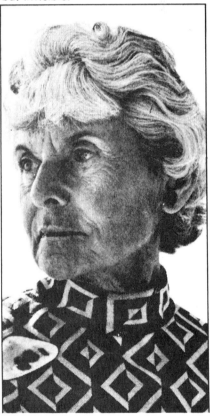

Charlotte Himber's ear mould is all but invisible.

should that have been such a catastrophe? Had I dropped an earring or my spectacles slipped, would anybody flick an eyelash?

Today I would have managed that event quite differently, for I've launched a crusade to get people to react sensibly toward hearing loss.

The phone rings. I quickly answer and say, "Just a minute, I've got to adjust my hearing aid."

Dishes are being collected and the restaurant clatter is maddening. I say to my companion, "I've got to adjust my hearing aid or I won't be able to understand you with all this noise."

I'm hanging on to a bus strap and my ear itches. Do I endure this torment? No! I calmly remove the ear mould, rub my ear, and replace the ear mould. Anybody looking? Good; he's learning something.

If you use a hearing aid or expect to, you're invited to join my crusade. Let's educate people. Hearing loss is what some of us will get. It doesn't hurt, like arthritis. It doesn't make you look different, like grey hair. It doesn't terrify you, like a heart attack. But it certainly is darned inconvenient if you must behave as if it's something sinister to be kept secret. After all, hearing aids must be handled and adjusted during the day as you move from one type of environment to another and the range of sounds changes. You can't act sneaky all day long, pretending there's a fly buzzing on one side of your head.

If you think your hearing is fine, note some of these earliest signs of diminishing hearing: You keep turning up the TV volume. You ask people to repeat what they said. You show annoyance, even anger, when someone persists in talking softly. You start scrutinizing people's faces.

They think they fascinate you, but you're getting clues from their lips and facial expressions. You act surprised when people tell you to stop shouting. ("I'm *not* shouting!")

With a different kind of hearing loss, you lower your voice. Now it's the other fellow who keeps saying, "What? What?" You put on your glasses to "hear better" (actually to get your visual clues). Your spouse says, "Stop wrinkling your brow," but you explain you're straining to hear.

Other people's reactions

I asked Ruth Green, a psychologist at the New York League for the Hard of Hearing, what happens to people when their hearing is running

down. The problems she describes from her own experience and research are familiar to you if you ever had a hearing loss. The hardest people to deal with are the members of your own family. They get angry because you don't hear, and treat you like a recalcitrant teenager ("Why don't you listen, so I won't have to keep telling you?").

Outside your family, your lack of response or slow response makes you seem stupid. So when you notice that people seem to be avoiding you, you suspect that they think you're stupid when in reality they're not aware you're having trouble hearing them. This may happen often enough to you to cause anx-

iety. Some people therefore begin to withdraw from social situations—and suffer being lonely.

Besides withdrawal, other behavior characteristics have been identified as the result of hearing loss. A man I knew had become a nuisance at dinner parties by talking loud and fast. Apparently he figured that the more he could keep everyone listening to him, the less he'd be relegated to a listening role himself. Another man reacted in the opposite way—he kept referring to his hearing problem, dragging it in irrelevantly, as if thinking, "Before they begin to suspect, I'll jump the gun and announce it." Such behavior bears the taint of aggression. It turns

---

Types of Hearing Aids

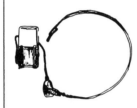

On-the-body models have larger, more powerful microphone, amplifier, and power pack. Controls may be more easy to adjust, and will let you strengthen or diminish sounds of different frequency.

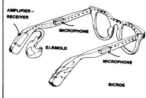

Eyeglass models are available in two forms—with microphones in one or both bows, and the amplified sound is fed to the good ear by plastic tube or through an ear mold. Both systems help to deliver sounds from all directions.

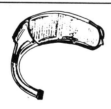

Behind-the-ear models connect with an ear mold, and can cope with loss from mild to severe. Some models have tone and volume controls, and even a telephone pick-up device.

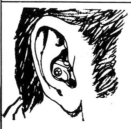

In-the-ear models are supported by the ear shell, have no external wires. They have a volume control, but may not have a tone control. Generally useful for mild hearing loss.

Source: National Bureau of Standards

AFRAID OF A HEARING AID

"Wear your hearing aid with pride—you've got hold of a gadget that wakes up the whole world for you."

---

people off, or hostile.

One woman wrote a letter to a newspaper columnist begging that one column be devoted to educating people. "On discovering that I wear a hearing aid, people speak to me as though I'm mentally deficient. Some even shout, amplifying the sound to such a high pitch I nearly faint from the thundering noise."

Isn't it ridiculous that a physical handicap should provoke so much unhappiness, just because we all persist in treating hearing loss as something to be ashamed of and to hide?

An experimental research effort involved people with normal hearing. Their ears were plugged with cotton for 24 hours, and their behavior monitored. Would you believe it—they developed the same set of neurotic behavior symptoms I've described here: withdrawal, aggression, bluffing, restlessness.

Go to a hearing specialist

Hearing should be given periodic checkups like any other part of the body. But be sure you go to an "audiologist" to test your hearing. "Otologists" are medical people who treat disease pathology — pierced eardrum, pain, etc. You go to a "dealer" to purchase your hearing aid. The audiologist is the only one who can give you a complete test, using the elaborate, necessary equipment. An audiologist gives you the prescription to be filled by a dealer.

To locate a reputable, accredited hearing clinic or center in your area, check with your local hospital. Or write to the National Association for Hearing and Speech Action, 814 Thayer Ave., Silver Spring, Md. 20910, or the American Speech and Hearing Ass'n., 9030 Old Georgetown Rd., Washington, D.C. 20014.

Of any number of hearing aids manufactured, you may react best to a certain type. At a hearing center you'll be able to try several and decide for yourself. Once you have your prescription and you've discovered, after testing several, which company's product is best for you, shop around for the best price. Dealers will usually agree to a discount. Buy an instrument on the agreement that you will rent it for one month, the rent to apply to the price if you decide to buy it, but that the charge be only the rental fee if you don't buy. Some dealers won't ask for rental fees, but will allow you a free trial period. However, ten days—the usual trial period—is not long enough; try to get it extended another two weeks.

The cost of a hearing test is nominal—about $30. Most clinics make fee adjustments in hardship cases. They can also arrange for reduced prices on hearing aids for low-income clients. Inquire of your local health department whether it has a mobile audiological diagnostic unit, or has any suggestions for hearing tests or financial problems.

Insure your hearing aid against loss or theft, especially since you'll be tempted to remove it in the beginning, or leave it home now and then. You will be advised, however, to try to get accustomed to wearing it throughout the day. Get your hearing device checked annually, as well as your hearing.

Don't resist an annual checkup just because you want to avoid bad news. Sometimes it isn't. I noted a change in my hearing after a three-month winter vacation in Florida. That's when I learned that good health, relaxation, and freedom from emotional strain will let your ears give you the best performance of which they're structurally capable.

Life is becoming so noisy it behooves us all to help shut out some of the raucousness. Audiologist Ms. Ashley Baker wears earplugs on subways. You might also try earplugs when construction workers are drilling through sidewalks near your home or business.

People weren't always embarrassed by hearing aids. Think of those ear horns and trumpets the 19th century socialites conspicuously carted around. Today it's the young who wear a modern version on streets, wires dangling from both ears to pick up each decibel of their favorite rock band. Astronauts, radar and sonar operators, and movie crewmen depend upon these amplifiers. Latest innovation is a "Stick-it-in-your-Ear" radio that plugs into any ear, in private or public. Take a cue from the kids. Wear your hearing aid with pride—you've got hold of a gadget that wakes up the whole world for you. To hear the fullness of sound in all its richness and variety is one of life's great miracles. Don't hesitate to enjoy all that's coming to you, through the instrument in your ears.

Recognition of Verbal Labels of Pictured Objects and Events by 17- to 30-Month -Old Infants

LEILA BECKWITH

University of California, Los Angeles

SPENCER K. THOMPSON

University of Texas, Odessa

Learning to understand language is as important for social communication and cognitive growth as learning to talk. The main interest of psychologists and linguists, however, has been the process by which children acquire speaking language, particularly syntax. Only recently has there been a growing interest in the processes by which children acquire semantic and syntactic comprehension (Bloom, 1974; Huttenlocher, 1974).

Investigation has been limited by the available methods of assessing vocabulary comprehension. Clinical language scales, in general, have been designed and standardized for children older than two years (Buros, 1965). Standardized infant tests contain too few language items for adequate sampling. The administration of even the few items is subject to problems, as are the more extensive measurements used in research. Essentially two procedures have been used: those that require a child to follow verbal directions in manipulating objects and those that require a child to match an examiner's verbal label with an object or picture.

"Recognition of Verbal Labels of Pictured Objects and Events By 17 to 30 Month-old Infants," Leila Beckwith, Spencer K. Thompson, *Journal of Speech and Hearing Research,* Vol. 19 No. 4, December 1976. ©1976 Journal of Speech and Hearing Research.

5. REHABILITATION

Structured situations that require a child to manipulate objects may confound vocabulary comprehension with either contextual cues, prelinguistic behavior patterns, or motivational factors, or all three. Two examples illustrate the difficulties. Nelson (1973) found that infants were more accurate in responding to the command to *give the ball to your mommy* than to the command to *give the ball to me* (that is, the observer). In that situation, differential vocabulary comprehension cannot be separated from reluctance to share with the stranger. Clark (1973) found that children were predisposed to put an object in a container but not under it—regardless of the examiner's verbal cues. On the other hand, procedures that require a child to match an examiner's verbal label to a picture depend even more on the child's cooperation with a strange examiner and often do not evoke or maintain the child's interest.

The present study describes an apparatus and procedure designed to elicit interpretable responses to an extensive sampling of the child's receptive vocabulary. The method was an adaptation of those techniques that require the child to match a verbal label with a picture. The adaptations provided the following advantages: (1) the method minimized the manipulation of materials to diminish distraction caused by the child's own actions as well as to reduce contextual cues; (2) the child's attention was focused away from the strange examiner so that social wariness was not confounded with language skill; (3) a shaping procedure was introduced so that performance was not haphazard, (4) reinforcement was included to maintain the child's attention over a large number of presentations; and (5) test stimuli were presented by colored slides of real objects, rather than black-and-white line drawings, to increase the child's intrinsic interest in the test. The method, then, was used to explore the following questions: Is the understanding of names of entities and attributes acquired in the same order as they are produced? Do environmental factors, such as parental attitudes and peer interaction, influence the acquisition of receptive vocabulary in the same ways as productive language?

METHOD

Apparatus, Procedure, and Test Stimuli

The child sat either on a small chair, or on his mother's lap facing a wooden box with a 92-cm wide × 76-cm high mahogany front. The front had two 25-cm square rearview screens onto which 35-mm slides of real objects or events were projected. Above each screen there was a 15-cm rabbit face. The examiner sat next to and slightly behind the child and operated a hand-held remote control that enabled him to change the pairs of pictures appearing on the screens and to illuminate the eyes and mouth of the rabbit faces. The initial 13 trials were used for an operant training procedure during which the child learned to touch that picture verbally labeled by the experimenter: illumination of the rabbit served as reinforcement. The next 34 paired pictures contained the test stimuli proper.

Two rules governed the selection of test stimuli. The pictured objects and events were selected from the everyday meaningful experience of most 17- to 30-month-old children. The selections were consistent with empirical findings concerning the acquisition of productive language. That is, the specific objects or events and the functional categories to which they belong (food, animals, toys, vehicles, household objects, clothing, parts of the body, people in action) predominate in the first 50 words children speak; the vocabulary consisted of names and action words in proportions roughly equivalent to that found in children's initially spoken 50 words (Nelson, 1973). Modifiers correspondent to adult classifications of adjectives, adverbs, and prepositions were included at a higher ratio in order to extend the level of difficulty to older and more skilled children. Pictures were paired so that the test items (italicized in the following examples) and the foils sometimes belonged to the same functional category (for example, foot-*hand*) and sometimes not (for example, cracker-*boat*).

Difficult items were interspersed with easier ones to facilitate completion of the entire test by every child regardless of skill. Correct choices were randomly arranged between the right and left screens. The order of presentation and the position of each stimulus were predetermined and invariant for all subjects. The Appendix describes the visual and verbal stimuli. Both English and Spanish versions were made. Both versions used the same pictures. Verbal descriptions for the Spanish version were Mexican-Spanish translations of the English version. Administration of the test lasted approximately 15 minutes.

Subjects

The procedure was administered to 106 children, six of whom did not learn a discriminatory response and were excluded. Subject loss was haphazardly distributed across age, sex, and groups. In the final samples, 48 males and 52 females ranging in age from 17 to 30 months of age were tested. Six groups of children were formed to sample different social status levels, ethnic groups, and birth order positions. The six groups are described in Table 1.

Children in Groups A and B were drawn from middle-class families from a university community. Children in Group A were reared by their mothers at home; children in Group B were enrolled in group day care at the university day care center. Groups C and D were drawn from families who were receiving medical care at a county well-baby clinic for low-income persons. Group C comprised English-speaking families; Group D, Spanish. Group D had a lower educational and occupational level than all other groups. Groups A-D were selected regardless of parity. Children in Groups E and F were first borns from middle-class families, reared by their mothers at home.

TABLE 1. Subject description, test score means, and standard deviations for six groups. Each group had an equal number of males and females except Group C which had five males and seven females. A maximum score of 34 was possible.

Group	Description	N	Age in Months Range	Age in Months Mean	Test Scores Mean	Test Scores SD
A	Middle class, English language, home reared, first and later born.	18	17-25	21.1	22	16.0
B	Middle class, English language, day care, first and later born.	14	18-26	22.4	23	16.0
C	Working class, English language, first and later born.	12	17-26	22.9	24	11.0
D	Working class, Spanish language, first and later born.	12	17-26	22.6	22	12.0
E	Middle class, English language, home reared, firstborn.	22	24-25	24.6	29	5.3
F	Middle class, English language, home reared, firstborn.	22	30-31	30.0	32	1.6

RESULTS

Reliability of Measurement

Test-Retest Reliability. Groups A and B were each tested twice with one week elapsing between the tests. Test-retest reliability was high as shown by the correlations for Group A ($r = 0.87$, $p < 0.001$) and Group B ($r = 0.94$, $p < 0.001$). Furthermore, changes over time were not haphazard; test scores improved significantly in the second testing ($t[31] = 2.01$, $p < 0.05$, for Groups A and B combined).

Item Reliability. The Kuder-Richardson coefficient obtained for test items for all 100 subjects, regardless of group, was 0.91. The high coefficient suggested that the items were homogeneous, and that individual items produced similar patterns of responding in different children. That is, item difficulty is believed to have been consistent across subjects, and those subjects who earned the higher scores were successful on the more difficult items.

Construct Validity

Relationship of Test Scores to Age. Scores were significantly related to children's ages for Groups A-D; correlations ranged from 0.64 to 0.70, $p < 0.01$. Furthermore, the 30 month olds, Group F, performed significantly better than the comparison group for 24 month olds, Group E, $t(42) = 3.4$, $p < 0.01$.

Comparability of English and Spanish Versions. The 12 subjects from Spanish language families, Group D, were matched by age and sex to 12 children from English language families, selected from Groups A-C. An analysis of variance revealed no main language or sex differences ($F[1,20] = 0.98$, $p > 0.10$; $F[1,20] = 0.45$, $p > 0.10$). Nor did the language groups differ significantly on any individual items, as assessed by t tests. However, there was a significant sex-by-language interaction ($F[1,20] = 7.18$, $p < 0.05$) which indicated that boys from English language homes were significantly more skillful than all others ($p < 0.05$, Duncan's multiple range test). The findings indicated moderate success in the choice of test stimuli which would sample vocabulary common to most children regardless of ethnic or social status group.

Relationship of Test Scores to Maternal Report. Mothers of subjects in Groups A-D made pretest estimates of their children's comprehension of the test words. Groups A-C marked checklists of the test words; mothers in Group D, many of whom were illiterate, answered verbally. In general, with the exception of Group D, maternal reports correlated significantly with test scores. The correlations for Groups A-D were, respectively, 0.85, $p < 0.01$; 0.75, $p < 0.01$; 0.49, $p < 0.05$; and 0.21, $p > 0.05$. The results from Groups A-C were interpreted as providing evidence of construct validity, whereas the results from Group D suggested the limitation of maternal report. Social status or education, or both have been found to modify the validity of questionnaire data (Tulkin and Cohler, 1973). We, therefore, considered that mothers of subjects in Group D were less accurate in reporting their children's skills.

Content Analysis

Grammatical Classes. For purposes of analysis, the test items were grouped in four grammatical classes: nominals (for example, *cup, scissors, cat*), action words (for example, *eat, drink, kiss*), locatives (for example, *in, on, under*) and modifiers (for example, *wet, broken, closed*). A treatments × subjects analysis of variance was performed on the percentage of success within the four categories for subjects from Groups A-F. Significant differences among the four grammatical categories were shown, $F(3,249) = 41.7$, $p < 0.01$. All means differed significantly from each other except modifiers and locatives, (Tukey HSD, $p < 0.05$). Children were most successful in understanding names of objects; action words were more difficult; and modifiers and locatives were the most difficult. The results were consistent with the order of acquisition of productive language reported by Nelson (1973). It is possible, however, that the order of success in our technique may have been confounded by word selection or by picture adequacy. Action words, locatives, and modifiers may be better understood through film or video presentations than through still life photographs.

Influence of Environment

Parental Attitudes. Parents of subjects in Groups E and F completed a ques-

TABLE 2. Correlations of test scores with number, sex, and age of playmates and parental attitudes in two groups.

Groups	Variables					
	1	*2*	*3*	*4*	*5*	*6*
E						
1. SES						
2. Mother's acceptance of sex role	−0.43°					
3. Father's acceptance of sex role	−0.21	0.66°°				
4. Average age of male playmates	−0.13	0.17	0.26			
5. Average age of female playmates	0.40	−0.06	−0.10	−0.04		
6. Number of playmates	0.03	0.28	0.14	0.69°°	0.01	
7. Test scores	0.00	−0.37	−0.44°	0.38	0.12	0.43°
F						
1. SES						
2. Mother's acceptance of sex role	−0.32					
3. Father's acceptance of sex role	−0.39	−0.62°°				
4. Average age of male playmates	−0.04	−0.27	−0.22			
5. Average age of female playmates	−0.14	0.19	0.34	0.16		
6. Number of playmates	0.34	−0.29	−0.21	0.45°	0.49°	
7. Test scores	0.28	−0.27	−0.34	0.40	0.03	0.27

°$p < 0.05$.
°°$p < 0.01$.

tionnaire which assessed their acceptance or disapproval of traditional sex roles (Thompson, 1975). A significant negative correlation between test performance and acceptance of traditional sex roles was found in Group E ($r = -0.44$, $p < 0.05$) (see Table 2). Parents who on the inventory stated greater acceptance of traditional sex roles tended to have children who scored lower in vocabulary comprehension. The relationship was not due to parent education, parent occupation, or family socioeconomic status (a combination of education and occupational level) since the correlations of test scores with each of these measures were not significant. Although the results of the study do not suggest the specific ways in which weaker adherence to cultural stereotypes altered the children's experiences, the finding was consistent with previous research which suggested that family control systems that offer a wider range of behavioral alternatives foster language development (Bernstein, 1964; Nelson, 1973).

Peers. Group A infants, reared at home by their mothers, were not significantly better in vocabulary recognition than were Group B infants, who spent much of their waking day with peers in a day care center ($t [30] = 0.23$, $p > 0.10$). Thus, a gross measure of amount of time spent with peers was not associated adversely with vocabulary recognition. The finding was surprising since previous research has reported significant negative correlations between exposure to peers and language facility (Bates, 1975; Nelson, 1973). Since previous studies have not separated interaction with peers from birth order, it is difficult to determine whether the adverse associations that were found were due to peer influence, per se, or to the fact that later borns tend to receive less verbal input from their parents than do first borns (Cohen, 1975).

To separate peer influence from birth order, Groups E and F were constituted of firstborn children. Their mothers were asked to report the number, sex, and age of their children's playmates. In general, as indicated in Table 2, those children who had older male playmates or more playmates tended to score higher. Number of playmates correlated 0.43, $p < 0.05$, at 24 months. Average age of male playmates correlated 0.38, $p < 0.08$, at 24 months, and average age of male playmates correlated 0.40, $p < 0.06$, at 30 months. The age of female playmates was unrelated to vocabulary recognition. The differential importance of the sex of the playmates is startling but is consistent with Koch's findings (1954) that children with male siblings, in contrast to female siblings, tended to gain higher IQ scores. Koch suggests that a male's behavior is more stimulating to another child than are a female's activities. Thus, when not confounded with parity differences in mother-child interaction, playmate interaction may facilitate rather than hinder vocabulary acquisition.

DISCUSSION

The results indicate that our technique can be successfully employed to measure receptive vocabulary of 17- to 30-month-old children, from a wide range of social status groups, and from both Spanish and English language families. Only six out of 106 children would not or could not attend to the task to perform a required discriminative response. The fact that there were no main effects of language, sex, or social status suggested that the procedure did indeed sample vocabulary available to most children of this age. Further, the speed and facility with which the items could be presented allowed a relatively large item pool (34) which increased the reliability of measurement for language categories as well as for individual subjects. Individual differences in vocabulary recognition were reliably and validly distinguished. In sum, performance was highly consistent from one week to the next; test scores correlated with age; and test scores correlated with pretest estimates made by more educated mothers of their children's vocabulary.

Two aspects of the procedure should be noted. Children were required to recognize two-dimensional still-life photographs of objects and events arranged in unfamiliar ways and vocabulary comprehension was deliberately divorced from children's actions. Test performance, therefore, could be attributed to children's response to verbal cues rather than to their preferred prelinguistic schemas. However, another possible source of nonverbal cues existed. Since most of the children sat on their mother's laps, the mothers' movements might have supplied nonlinguistic cues. This potential confounding seems to be an unlikely explanation of the consistent order of difficulty that was found for nominals, action words, and modifiers. Test performance, though, was influenced by the words selected and the adequacy of the pictures chosen. During test construction, it was not easy to find words, particularly modifiers and action words, which could be unambiguously portrayed.

On the other hand, the recognition of the array of distinctive features which characterize semantic categories is an essential aspect of language acquisition. Those features may include actions, or changes in state, or end-state representations regardless of the actions taken to attain that end. The task assessed the understanding of words, even action words, used as end-state representations. For example, the child was asked to match the phrase, *up in the air,* with a picture of a boy being held by a man above the ground. The task was different than matching the phrase with one's own movements through space. Similarly, associating *dog in the box* with a picture, was different than matching an appropriate action to the phrase. Vocabulary used to accompany action in "dynamic" situations and vocabulary used to describe end-states in "static" situations are not necessarily acquired at the same time (Bem, 1970; Bloom, Lightblown, and Hood, 1975). It is likely that dynamic events are encoded before static ones.

Specific environmental factors were found to correlate with test performance. A measure of parental disagreement with cultural stereotypes was associated with more proficient vocabulary comprehension. The finding was interpreted as consistent with previous research which suggests that family control systems that offer a wider range of behavioral alternatives facilitate language development. Peer interaction was also associated with more proficient vocabulary comprehension, at least in firstborn children. Peer interaction for that group of children may facilitate rather than impede the acquisition of vocabulary. Or children with more friends may be exposed to more experiences outside the home, a factor that has been found to facilitate vocabulary production (Nelson, 1973).

The findings illustrate the utility of the method for further study of the effects of child rearing practices on the acquisition of receptive vocabulary, as well as for further study of the relationship among different aspects of vocabulary comprehension and vocabulary production.

ACKNOWLEDGMENT

This research was supported by USPHS Contract 1-HD-3-2776, "Diagnostic and Intervention Studies of High-Risk Infants," and NICHD Grant HD-04612 to the Mental Retardation Research Center, UCLA. Computing assistance was obtained from the Health Sciences Computing Facility, UCLA, sponsored by NIH Special Research Resources Grant RR-3. Requests for reprints should be sent to Leila Beckwith, 23-39 Rehabilitation Institute, UCLA Campus, Los Angeles, California 90024.

REFERENCES

BATES, E., Peer relations and the acquisition of language. In M. Lewis and L. Rosenblum (Eds.), *Friendship and Peer Relations: The Origins of Behavior.* Vol. 3. New York: Wiley and Sons (1975).
BEM, S. L., The role of comprehension in children's problem solving. *Dev. Psychol.,* **2**, 351-358 (1970).
BERNSTEIN, B., Elaborated and restricted codes: Their social origins and some consequences. *Amer. Anthropol.,* **66**, 55-69 (1964).

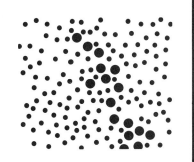

How to Protect Your Hearing

Early and regular hearing
health exams can detect hearing loss,
make treatment and correction
easier and, hopefully,
less costly

BY KEN ANDERSON

IF THE CONVERSATIONS in your own home are punctuated with "Huh?" or "What?" it may not be the fault of the other person. You may be one of an estimated 14 million Americans who suffer some degree of hearing loss.

Treatment varies with problem

Not all types of hearing loss require surgery or other corrective measures. Even a minor obstruction in the ear canal, such as a lump of ear wax, can distort what you hear by blocking a part of the sound waves. An ear cleaning may be all that's needed to restore hearing.

While hearing depends primarily upon air conduction of sound waves via the ear canal, the bony areas of the skull around the ear also transmit sound vibrations to the inner ear. The two hearing routes—through the ear canal, and vibrations of bony areas—also play an important role in the diagnosis and treatment of hearing loss.

When an examining physician finds that a patient can hear with the inner ear but cannot receive sound waves carried by air, he assumes that the defect is in the air conduction system of the ear. On the other hand, a failure of the inner ear components, termed nerve deafness, or sensori-neural loss, means that sound is no longer transmitted effectively through the bones around the ear.

In addition to ear wax obstruction, hearing loss can result from an infection that causes membranes to swell. "Catarrhal deafness" is

Ken Anderson, a former editor of To-day's Health, writes on medicine, science, psychology, recreation. His latest article for RL was "How to Save Money on Your Medications," (Feb., 1975).

a term used to describe a variety of complaints including chronic infection of the sinuses, tonsils and adenoids, infection or fluid in the middle ear, perforation of the eardrum. Any of these conditions can produce hearing loss.

Surgery can correct impairment

Generally, conduction hearing loss due to a viral or bacterial infection can be treated medically. However, an untreated ear infection can re-

---

10 Ways to Test Your Hearing

Self-diagnosis is neither safe nor sure. But you can take this simple test to help determine whether you should consult a physician.

	YES	NO
1. Can you hear speech but occasionally find it difficult to understand?	☐	☐
2. Do you prefer to sit up front during church services, lectures or public meetings?	☐	☐
3. Does it seem that you can hear better some days than others?	☐	☐
4. Do you sometimes find it difficult to understand speech in group situations or against other background noise?	☐	☐
5. Do you like to talk because you feel uncomfortable when there is silence in a room?	☐	☐
6. Can you usually tell one kind of noise from another?	☐	☐
7. Can you distinguish speech from other sounds?	☐	☐
8. Can you hear and understand another person better if he speaks loudly into one ear or the other?	☐	☐
9. Can you understand what a person says without seeing his face if he talks to you in a low voice?	☐	☐
10. Can you understand what a person says without seeing his face if he talks to you in a normal voice?	☐	☐

If your answer to the first five questions is "yes," you should ask your family physician or an ear specialist to give you a thorough exam. If you answer "no" to questions 6 through 10, you should also get a complete hearing checkup.

In self-testing, the whispered or spoken voice used in question 10 should be presented in a quiet room. And the speaker should stand 15 feet away from the person being tested. If the listener's hearing is normal, he should be able to understand a quietly spoken voice from that distance.

"How to Protect Your Hearing," Ken Anderson, *Retirement Living*, Vol. 15 No. 5, May 1975. ©1975 Retirement Living.

sult in lasting damage to the tissues. An infection can, for example, invade the bony tissue of the ear, requiring delicate surgery to rebuild the eardrum or the ossicles, those three tiny ear bones known as hammer, anvil, stirrup.

Another cause of conduction deafness is otosclerosis, which seems to be inherited by some patients. It is caused by abnormal bone growth which spreads slowly until it immobilizes the stirrup bone of the middle ear. Otosclerosis can develop during the teenage years or build up gradually, not becoming noticeable before middle age.

Because of recent advances in ear surgery, otosclerosis and other kinds of impairment of the middle ear usually can be treated.

A punctured eardrum may be restored by plastic surgery, using a tiny flap of skin from the ear canal to fill the hole in the membrane. And, the patient is usually able to swim again.

'Nerve deafness' can be helped

Nerve deafness is most commonly caused by retarded circulation of the blood to the ears, mechanical injury, disease, or damage caused by certain drugs. Mumps, measles, and other viral infections can lead to hearing nerve damage.

Patients with normal nerve function who are treated early can expect complete restoration of hearing. Some patients who had depended upon hearing aids were able to discard them after surgery. And some patients were relatively free of hearing loss symptoms for as long as 20 years after surgery.

Another kind of inner ear deafness associated with advancing years is *presbycusis,* a Greek word combining the terms for "old" and "hearing." It usually appears among people in their sixties. Not everybody is affected by presbycusis; many individuals live into their eighties and nineties without noticeable impairment.

Not all loss is permanent

A sudden hearing loss also may be associated with Meniere's disease, an ailment marked by dizziness, nausea and vomiting, sweating and pallor. There also is a feeling of fullness and discomfort in the area and a low-frequency ringing or buzzing. The hearing loss can fluctuate, and is often greatest in the lower frequency ranges.

The effects of Meniere's disease may last only a few moments or they can persist for days or weeks at a time. The treatment includes measures to reduce the fluid in the body. Smoking must be curtailed and anti-motion sickness drugs also may be prescribed. Surgery usually is reserved only for cases that do not respond to medical treatment.

A recent study of more than 30,000 men and women by the Kaiser-Permanente Foundation of California suggests that cigaret smoking can contribute to early hearing loss, although researchers so far have found no scientific explanation for the phenomenon.

More is known about the effect of prolonged exposure to loud noise—such as daily travel on noisy subways—where the scream of wheels against rails often reaches 140 decibels—and rock music concerts. Young listeners and musicians alike think they can't "enjoy" the music unless it is so loud as to almost make them nauseous. Recent studies show that after continued exposure to the loud amplification used at rock concerts, musicians' ability to clearly hear the higher frequencies becomes impaired, a condition which can lead to progressive hearing loss.

AIR VIBRATIONS
EARDRUM
AUDITORY NERVE TO BRAIN
THROAT

How Do You Hear?

Think of the sounds you hear as little puffs of air that vibrate at certain frequencies. The higher the rate of vibration, the higher the pitch of the sound. Although most human speech falls between 300 and 2,500 vibrations, or cycles per second, the human ear is capable of hearing from 40 cycles to 20,000 cycles per second.

The vibrations move along the tube leading from the outer ear to the eardrum. On the other side of the eardrum is the middle ear, which contain three tiny bones, the hammer, anvil and stirrup, which stretch across the middle ear and relay the vibrations from the eardrum to the inner ear. Here, the vibrations are converted into impulses sped to the brain where they are interpreted as music, speech, noise and other patterns of vibrations we have learned .

In determining the extent of hearing loss, the hearing specialist may use voice tests or the watch-tick test. Most physicians will also use a vibrating tuning fork. When the stem of the vibrating tuning fork is placed firmly against the mastoid area behind the ear, the examiner can tell whether there has been any bone conduction hearing loss.

Electronic audiometry equipment produces sounds of varying frequency and intensity which the person hears through earphones. In addition to transmitting pure tones audiometers can present recorded word sounds to test the patient's ability to hear and understand speech. The results of the audiometer test help determine what kind of hearing aid, if any, will benefit the person.

Research Implications
for Communication
Deficiencies

JOHN H. HOLLIS
JOSEPH K. CARRIER, JR.

Abstract: This article traces, historically, four decades of chimpanzee research relevant to the prosthesis of communication deficiencies. The prosthetic methods reviewed include the following: (a) environment and specialized prosthetic training, (b) mechanical devices for the production of expressive speech, (c) learning of sign systems, e.g., American Sign Language, and (d) a language system based on nonspeech manipulable symbols. The knowledge and techniques resulting from the chimpanzee research have been applied to the training of retarded children. This article discusses the results of this research and its implications for the prosthesis of communication deficiencies in the retarded and deaf.

John H. Hollis *is Research Associate, Bureau of Child Research, University of Kansas, Lawrence; and* **Joseph K. Carrier, Jr.,** *is Research Associate, Parsons Research Center, Parsons State Hospital, Parsons, Kansas. Parts of this article were presented at the 1973 meeting of the American Association on Mental Deficiency at Atlanta, Georgia. The research reported herein was supported in part by funds provided under the National Institute of Child Health and Human Development grants HD 00870 and HD 02528, Bureau of Child Research, University of Kansas.*

It has long been recognized that communication deficiencies are a salient characteristic of many handicapped children. Mentally retarded individuals, for example, reveal significant deficiencies in communication skills (Matthews, 1957). These behaviors may be only slightly below norms or appear to be totally absent, but in any case they are observed to be deficient in normal human environments (Lindsley, 1964). It could be argued, however, that although these children lack speech and language, they are not retarded or deficient with respect to communication per se. Rather, many do communicate by other means such as gestures, scent marking, and role playing (nonspeech behavior that functions in a communicative fashion).

A fundamental assumption underlying the development of communicative processes is that speech and language behavior are acquired and maintained in accord with the same principles as other behavior. However, as with any behavior, the learning organism must have the physiological requisites for performance before learning is possible. Deaf children require special training to compensate for their inability to perceive and process auditory stimuli. Similarly, there are many communicatively handicapped children who may be having difficulty learning speech and language because of other impairments.

The problems in teaching children with such deficiencies may, in some ways, parallel the problems encountered by researchers who have attempted to teach subhuman species to use a human communication system. Spoken language, as used by humans, is not feasible in an organism lacking certain cognitive or physiological abilities, but certain types of prostheses, adapted to the organism, make some parameters of communication quite possible.

The purpose of this article is to trace the most significant animal research in the prosthesis of communication deficiencies and suggest areas where information from animal research might contribute to clinical management of communicatively impaired children.

Prosthetic methods and devices (Lindsley, 1964) which provide a means of circumventing deficiencies in language and speech for both handicapped children and animals can be divided into four general categories:

1. A *prosthetic environment* is one which maximizes behavioral efficiency. For example, specialized prosthetic training (contingencies and consequences relevant to language) could be provided applying conditioning procedures or behavior modification programs to enhance the acquisition of language.
2. *Phonologic prosthesis* (mechanical mode) provides devices for the production of expressive (productive) aspects of speech, e.g., an artificial larynx (mechanical device) that provides synthetic sounds.
3. *Phonologic and auditory prostheses* (gestural mode) use sign systems such as finger spelling or American Sign Language.
4. *Phonologic and auditory prostheses* (synthetic mode) use a language system based on nonspeech manipulable symbols (physical objects) analogous to Chinese characters.

It should be apparent from the foregoing that the four techniques suggested for the prosthesis of communication deficiencies form a hierarchy ranging from the extremely complex to the relatively simple.

Environmental Prosthesis: Acculturation Mode

Four decades have passed since Kellogg (1931) discussed humanizing the ape. Kellogg's idea was to take an ape and rear it in a *prosthetic environment,* a human environment. Relevant to this he stated:

> The opinion seems to persist among certain contemporary psychologists that a sharp qualitative demarcation between the behavior of man on the one hand and the behavior of infrahumans including the anthropoid apes, on the other hand, is an established fact. (p. 160)

It would appear from the writings of Kellogg that he was suggesting that the ape had the capacity for development of language and human speech or for at least acquiring some aspects of human culture.

At the time Kellogg proposed his study for humanizing the ape, it was believed that the anatomy and vocal mechanism of the ape was such that it did not preclude the possibility of human speech (Traill, 1821). Although Kellogg and Kellogg (1933) and Hayes and Hayes (1954) have reported limited success in human speech development in the chimpanzee (i.e., three to four words), for the most part this hypothesis is untenable today.

Prosthetic Training

Phonologic Prosthesis: Mechanical Mode

Disease and injury may cause damage to the vocal, articulatory, or auditory system. Compensatory prosthetic devices include a variety of types of artifical larynges and hearing aids. Artificial larynges are most commonly used by adults who have already learned speech and language, although there is at least one report of teaching speech and language to a child laryngectomized at 20 months of age (Peterson, 1973). Hearing aids have been helpful prostheses for all age groups—prior to, during, and after speech and language development.

Bryan (1963) has suggested, contrary to an earlier point made in this article, that the vocal apparatus of the chimpanzee differs from that of man to an extent that mitigates against the development of human speech. However, there appears to be sufficient evidence to substantiate the ability of the chimpanzee to learn to respond to human speech (receptive auditory mode) (Hayes, 1951). The chimpanzee ranks high enough on the phylogenetic scale with respect to sociability and intellectual potentiality (Yerkes, 1943), that he has frequently been selected as the subject for the study of higher mental processes.

Premack and Schwartz (1966), believing that the chimpanzee's major deficiency lay in the expressive area of speech, embarked on a project to develop a synthetic (mechanical) device capable of producing complex auditory stimuli. The production of auditory signals was to be controlled by a joy stick apparatus with the sound produced by a device similar to an electric organ. It was proposed that the chimpanzee would be taught grammar, having context free rules, minimal nesting, no self embedding, and no recursiveness. It should be noted that the authors and others were generally pessimistic as to the outcome of this line of research. This system was eventually discarded, perhaps because of its complexity. There remained, however, good reason to use the chimpanzee as a "drawing board" for deline-

5. REHABILITATION

ating strategies and tactics relevant to communication problems. In another article, Premack (1970) presents a study that was successful in establishing a continuity between human language and animal communication.

Phonologic and Auditory Prosthesis: Gestural Mode

There is little doubt that the laboratory and home reared chimpanzee still displays many of the characteristics of a wild animal (Hayes, 1951). However, chimpanzees are highly social animals and do respond differentially to social roles, even those played by humans (Mason, Hollis, & Sharpe, 1962). Moreover, the chimpanzee finds manipulatory mechanical problems his forte, and even laboratory chimps have been frequently observed to spontaneously emit gestures (Yerkes, 1943).

Fingerspelling and the American Sign Language (ASL) are standardized systems for two way communication for deaf exceptional children. Training a chimpanzee to use ASL would provide a linguistic environment independent of spoken responses.

The Experiment with Washoe. The Gardners (Gardner & Gardner, 1969) undertook the task of training Washoe, a chimpanzee, to use ASL. The strategy was to take advantage of two chimpanzee characteristics: (a) the ability to make complex hand movements and (b) the frequency with which chimpanzees have been observed to imitate human acts. The tactic for training was to provide an environment conducive to the development of chimpanzee human social interactions, while applying shaping and operant conditioning techniques to develop sign language in the chimpanzee.

The Gardners maintained records indicating that 30 signs had been learned by the 22nd training month. Washoe's rate of acquisition for the first 21 months of training clearly indicates the phenomenon of "learning to learn" or "learning sets" (Harlow, 1949). The Gardners suggest that the equivalence between Washoe's signs and English is only approximate but this is true for any two different languages. From the reports on Washoe's use of ASL, there is some evidence that on some occasions the signs were context dependent and on other occasions they were inappropriate for the context.

The Gardners were cognizant of a context problem and viewed it in terms of sign transfer, i.e., from a specific referent in initial training to new members of each class of referents. Thus, in initial training, Washoe learned *open* for a specific door and *hat* for a specific hat, and transfer occurred spontaneously to new members of each class of referents. In their article the Gardners gave several examples of this class of behavior. They pointed out in their discussion of key use (to open locks) that Washoe learned to ask for keys (emitted key sign) when no key was in sight. In addition, Washoe was observed to emit strings of two or more signs without specific stimuli. It can be asked, "Did Washoe develop a functional language?" The results of the experiment show that Washoe demonstrated (a) spontaneous naming, (b) spontaneous transfer to new referents, and (c) spontaneous combinations and recombinations of signs. Fouts (1973) has, in essence, replicated the ASL study of Gardner using 4 young chimpanzees. Thus, the learning of ASL in the chimpanzee population is not unique, and it can be concluded that Washoe was not an exceptional chimpanzee in her ability to acquire signs.

Teaching signs to retarded deaf children. Berger (1972) reported a clinical program for the development of language in multi-handicapped children. Retarded deaf children were taught to use manual signs with procedures similar to those used with the chimp, Washoe. Imitation and handshaping techniques were used to develop appropriate matching, selecting, or pointing motor responses. The 9 children who participated in the program received 18 to 24 months of training. They had some degree of success encoding and decoding with fingerspelling. They learned to imitate signed phrases or sentences and to initiate some signs.

Phonologic and Auditory Prosthesis: Synthetic Mode

Up to this point, we have seen the contribution of linguistics, programing, and logic to teaching language to the chimpanzee and language deficient child. The limiting factor for language development by the chimpanzee or language deficient child may not be language per se, but the complexity of the response, i.e., its topography. For example, the response mode most commonly associated with language is oral speech, which can be defined as various phonemic responses arranged to create morphemes—which, in turn, may be arranged to create grammatical utterances (Carrier, 1973). Premack (1971) has reversed himself and moved from the complex topography required by a mechanical device for phonologic prosthesis, to a simple synthetic (plastic word) system. Again, Premack is asking the question, "Can the chimpanzee be taught language?" The determiner of the answer to this question is, "What is language?"

Premack's system. In Premack's system, one must first provide a list of exemplars, things the chimp (or child) must be able to do in order to demonstrate a functional language. Second, a method of training must be provided so that the chimp can be taught those exemplars. As a beginning list of exemplars, Premack suggested:(a) words, (b) sentences, (c) questions, (d) metalinguistics (using language to teach language), (e) class concepts, (f) the copula, (g) quantifiers, and (h) the logical connective, if-then.

The word stimuli in this system are pieces of plastic backed with metal so that they will adhere to a magnetized slate. The plastic words are abstract in configuration and are analogous to Chinese characters. The placing of the plastic words on the slate requires only gross motor movements. This is a great simplification when compared to the complex motor behavior and auditory discriminations required for spoken and gestural communication. A second advantage derives from the fact that the sentence made by the chimp is permanent, thus circumventing the memory problem. Third, the experimenter can modulate the difficulty of any task by controlling the number and kinds of words available to the subject at a given time. It should be evident that the phonologic problem has been *prosthetized* and that the basic unit is the *word* (Premack, 1971). No attempt will be made to present the details of the training procedure here, since it has been made explicit elsewhere (Premack, 1970, 1971; Premack & Premack, 1972).

Sarah's achievements. Sarah, Premack's chimpanzee, is now able to read and write (using the plastic words) over 130 words. But more importantly, she has learned the use of (a) the interrogative, (b) metalinguistics, (c) class concepts, (d) simple and compound sentences, (e) pluralization, (f) quantifiers, (g) the logical connective, if-then, and (h) the conjunctive *and*. What Premack, in fact, has accomplished is to provide a functional analysis of language. This approach to analyzing and teaching language has reduced the cognitive parameters of language to discrete events that can be defined and manipulated. This strategy coupled with the tactic of a simple response topography provides a powerful technique for training communication deficient children.

Teaching Language to the Severely Retarded

It is a foregone conclusion that there is a significant relationship between language development and measured intelligence. The traditional intelligence tests contain both verbal and performance scales. It is the verbal scale (language) that proves most difficult for the severely retarded child and places him in the category of untestable. Are these children severely retarded (with respect to measured intelligence) because of their failure to learn language or because of some yet undetected factor?

Interactions between Language and Nonlanguage Learning

It would appear that the interactions between language and nonlanguage learning is so strong that it is doubtful that a child can make much progress in learning one without acquiring skills in the other (see Kellogg & Kellogg, 1933). In an attempt to answer these questions, Carrier (1973) has begun a replication of Premack's experiment with Sarah, using severely retarded children as subjects.

Carrier (1973) clearly differentiated between demonstrating linguistic function in a chimpanzee and teaching communication skills to a child. Using the chimpanzee as subject, it was only necessary to demonstrate linguistic functions; however, the task of teaching children to communicate does not permit such latitude. The language system of a child's environment is a fact of life, and however inefficient it may be, it is the one the child must learn. Thus, the process of determining program goals for children requires not only a consideration of language function but also a consideration of semantics and syntax as they actually exist. In other words, the programer must select from the corpus of acceptable linguistic responses a set that will serve the communication needs of the child.

Model for Language Development

Carrier (1973) outlined a model for language development in the child. Since it is quite complex, only a brief outline of the initial steps will be presented.

Rules and principles. The first step in the development of this model was an attempt to define operationally two sets of rules and principles, each of which is an integral part of language. One set of rules consists of those used for the selection of symbols to represent different meanings. In writing, the

5. REHABILITATION

written symbol *boy* may be used to represent a young male human. Such rules and principles relate to what we may refer to as the *semantic* parameter of language. The other set of rules or principles, relating to what we call the *syntactic* parameter of language, consists of those which determine the sequential arrangement of symbols in a standard grammatical response. For example, in an active declarative sentence, the subject noun precedes the verb, articles precede nouns—the order of words is a constant "standardized" through usage. In carrier's (1973) analysis, semantic and syntactic systems are treated separately, although each is certainly dependent on the other for ultimate linguistic performance. The purpose of the syntax parameter of the model was to define operations that would result in correctly arranged sequences of symbols. The function of the semantic model was to delineate operations necessary to appropriately select symbols. Because there are many functionally determined classes of symbols, the semantic model consists of several different parts. Each part defines the operations necessary for selecting a specific member from that class. The operations are nothing more than a series of binary discriminations, performed in specific sequences.

The programs. Procedures for teaching communication behavior to retarded individuals in the nonspeech response mode include a series of programs, each designed to teach some specific parameter of the model, and each carefully integrated into the total goals of the training (these programs are presented in detail in Carrier, 1973). The programs in this series all have certain features in common:

1. They are all written in step by step sequences. Every operation performed by the teacher is carefully described, and every decision to be made is presented in the form of a binary decision question, i.e., a yes or no answer. Such a format not only simplifies the job of the teacher but expedites the option of direction adaptation of the programs to relatively simple programing equipment.

2. Rather than spoken words, the symbols for various morphemes to be taught are geometric forms of different shapes cut from 3 inch squares of masonite. Each form is marked on its face with colored tape to indicate the grammatical class of the linguistic constituent it is to represent (noun, verb, article, plural marker, etc.). The shape of the form (triangle, square, etc.) indicates the specific morpheme to be represented.

3. The response board is a simple plywood tray similar to the tray of a chalkboard.

4. The child's response consists of arranging appropriate symbols on the tray in a left to right sequence as if he were writing sentences.

5. In all program steps, the child is seated at a table with the response tray directly in front of him. Prior to eliciting the child's response, the teacher places between the child and the tray those geometric forms designated by the appropriate step of the program.

6. In all programs, the children receive positive reinforcement for correct responses. Reinforcers are selected on the basis of child preference prior to each session. The most common reinforcers have been pieces of candy, cereal, a few drops of pop, or water. No attempt is made to provide consequences for incorrect responses.

7. The data recorded includes pretest and posttest responses, records of every response in each step of the program, and, where appropriate, a probe test performance indicating stimulus and/or response generalization. Records also include precise identifying information about stimuli (geometric forms and, where appropriate, pictures) and reinforcers. Time measures include the child's rate of responding (responses/unit of time) and a measure of the time required for the clinician to perform various operations.

Results. Presently, data is available for 50 subjects who have gone through at least some part of the training sequence. These subjects are all institutionalized and classified as severely or profoundly retarded (Heber, 1961). Many of the subjects have mild sensory and/or motor involvement, but none are so impaired as to be physically unable to perform the required tasks. None of the subjects initially used speech for communication. (Preliminary results are summarized in Table 2.) The results may briefly be summarized as follows:

1. The acquisition of the first two verbs and prepositions are the most difficult.

2. Session times required to learn various constituents become shorter and shorter as subjects progress through the programs.

3. The data suggests that semantic features of the symbols are becoming cues for syntactic sequences.

4. Teaching additional sentence structures becomes easier.

5. Errors in advanced stages of the program resemble those in the grammar of speaking children.

6. The subjects become extremely proficient at constructing sentences, but as the number of alternative forms become large (50 to 100), the rate of response decreases and occasional errors occur.

Implications for Prosthesis of Children's Communication Deficiencies

Of the methods presented in this article for the prosthesis of communication deficiencies, Premack's systematic approach to teaching language appears to offer the most promise. Although his work is still in its early stages, Carrier (1973) has presented rather impressive evidence which substantiates this conclusion.

The Severely Retarded Child

Perhaps most significantly Carrier has obtained conclusive evidence that many severely and profoundly retarded children can and do learn at least parts of a communication system when using Premack's nonspeech response mode. The fact that these subjects are able to learn the necessary concepts to use the geometric forms (plastic words) is extremely encouraging and a great step forward in training those at this level. The next step visualized would be to have two subjects communicating with each other over closed circuit TV using plastic words. Certainly this would demonstrate that it is a functional language within the peer dyad.

The Young Deaf Child

The severely auditorily impaired child does not learn language on his own and only after extensive training does he learn to use language and to speak. He always appears to trail behind his peer age-mates in the academic arena. So far there has been no concerted effort to effect the transfer of learned concepts, such as in Premack's nonspeech mode, to a more functional response mode, such as speech. However, the young deaf child provides an ideal "drawing board" for the test. It seems reasonable to hypothesize that mastery of a comprehensive set of concepts (nonspeech language) should make it much easier to learn the more functional response mode such as speech. Just as the nonspeech programs eliminate the need for learning speech simultaneously with linguistic principles, the subsequent teaching of speech should eliminate the need for learning linguistic principles simultaneously with speech. Premack's language research appears to have important implications for the development of language programs for normal young children.

Prosthesis of Intelligence

Children tend to steadily improve in their performance on intelligence tests until their late teens. In addition, it has been demonstrated that retarded children can, with training, improve their performance on intelligence tests. What then is intelligence? Boring (1923) answered this succinctly with this statement, "Intelligence is what the tests test" (p. 37). A relevant point frequently overlooked is that intelligence tests (e.g., Stanford-Binet Intelligence Scale) are validated on academic, classroom performance. Although the two widely used individual intelligence tests, the Binet and Wechsler Intelligence Scales for Children, contain verbal and performance scales, they are heavily dependent on language ability. Second, neither of these tests employs a single type of mental operation. They are essentially a battery of single tests that test different abilities. Thus, in fact, they do not measure a "common factor," but if one could infer one, it would be the ability to use language. Until recently this was considered an ability ascribed only to humans. However, the successes of the Gardners and Premacks in teaching language to chimpanzees no longer makes this a valid assumption.

Let us now consider the severely or profoundly retarded child with respect to the concept of intelligence. Educators have classified him as retarded on the basis of measured intelligence, knowing full well that the tests are heavily loaded with language. Furthermore, as we have already pointed out, the interaction between language and nonlanguage learning may be so strong that it is doubtful that a child can make much progress in learning one without acquiring skills in the other. Even a cursory overview of Premack's work would suggest that he is rapidly developing procedures for demonstrating the concepts underlying language. These concepts are independent of language and are developed through the natural contingencies provided by the physical environment rather than through social contingencies as are

5. REHABILITATION

applied to language. For example, Mason (1971) has studied in detail the concepts developed by infant rhesus monkeys with respect to the physical characteristics of their mother surrogate, a nonsocial entity. It would appear that the mapping of existing environmental distinctions (one's stimulus surroundings) is a necessary prerequisite for the development of language.

For both the retarded and the young deaf child, it would appear that the prosthesis of intelligence may be a reality. That is, educators now can surmount the language barrier by providing a nonspeech response mode for communication. This eliminates the need for learning speech (or learning speech simultaneously with linguistic principles) and opens a broad new vista for teaching the language deficient. Thus, current research concerned with the prosthesis of communication deficiencies has begun a whole new chapter on the relationship between the concept of intelligence and what is measured and labeled as intelligence.

References

Berger, S. L. A clinical program for developing multimodal language responses with atypical deaf children. In J. E. McLean, D. E. Yoder, & R. L. Schiefelbusch (Eds., *Language intervention with the retarded*. Baltimore: University Park Press, 1972.

Boring, E. G. Intelligence as the tests test it. *The New Republic,* 1923, *35,* 35-37.

Bryan, A. L. The essential basis for human culture. *Current Anthropology,* 1963, *4,* 297-306.

Carrier, J. K., Jr. *Application of functional analysis and nonspeech response mode to teaching language* (Report No. 7). Parsons: Kansas Center for Research in Mental Retardation and Human Development, 1973.

Fouts, R. S. Acquisition and testing of gestural signs in four young chimpanzees. *Science,* 1973, *180,* 978-980.

Gardner, R. A., & Gardner, B. T. Teaching sign language to a chimpanzee. *Science,* 1969, *165,* 664-672.

Girardeau, F. L. Cultural-familial retardation. In N. R. Ellis (ed.), *International review of research in mental retardation.* New York: Academic Press, 1971.

Harlow, H. F. The formation of learning sets. *Psychological Review,* 1949, *56,* 51-65.

Hayes, C. *The ape in our house.* New York: Harper & Brothers, 1951.

Hayes, K. J., & Hayes, C. The cultural capacity of chimpanzee. *Human Biology,* 1954, *26,* 288-303.

Heber, R. F. A manual on terminology and classification in mental retardation. *American Journal of Mental Deficiency,* 1959, *64.* (Monograph Supplement, Rev. ed., 1961)

Kellogg, W. N. Humanizing the ape. *Psychological Review,* 1931, *38,* 106-176.

Kellogg, W. N., & Kellogg, L. A. *The ape and the child.* New York: McGraw-Hill, 1933.

Lindsley, O. R. Direct measurement and prosthesis of retarded behavior. *Journal of Education,* 1964, *147,* 62-81.

McLean, J. E., Yoder, D. E., & Schiefelbusch, R. L. (Eds.). *Language intervention with the retarded.* Baltimore: University Park Press, 1972.

McNeill, D. The development of language. In P. H. Mussen (Ed.), *Carmichael's manual of child psychology.* New York: J. Wiley & Sons, 1970.

APPLYING TECHNOLOGY TO SPECIAL EDUCATION

VIVIAN HEDRICH

Mrs. Hedrich is Publications Specialist
for Seattle Public Schools.

Advanced scientific technology and a good deal of hope are being injected this year into a Seattle Public Schools Special Education program that appears to be breaking new ground in the teaching of severely handicapped children. At its core is a team composed of a neurophysiologist, an electrical engineer, an electronics technician, and skilled persons in many other fields, and backed by $55,000 in Federal funds provided under title VI-B of the Elementary and Secondary Education Act.

The intent is to demonstrate some of the practical applications of technology and research to the critical educational problems inherent in such grievous disabilities as cerebral palsy. The evidence so far suggests that such applications are practical indeed.

Five-year-old Lori attends Seattle's Lowell Elementary School. A pretty child with strawberry blond hair and a winsome smile, she daily faces difficulties of such magnitude as to challenge the most skilled and understanding of teachers.

Since birth, cerebral palsy has cheated Lori of much of what living is all about. Faulty sensory "input" makes it difficult for her to interpret events in the world around her, and poor muscular control severely restricts her movement and ability to respond appropriately to what she does perceive. Her academic world is Room 109 in Lowell's modern orthopedic wing, cheerfully carpeted and filled with colorful toys and special equipment.

One morning recently she had an opportunity to try on a new piece of wearing apparel—a lightweight plastic prototype model helmet being field-tested as a "stabilizer" to help children such as Lori control the position of their heads. The new device includes a gravity-sensitive "pickup" and small circular vibrators positioned near the ears. When the head

tilts beyond a certain point, the vibrator emits a clicking sound on the appropriate side. The frequency of the clicking corresponds to the degree of tilt and alerts the wearer to return his head to the "neutral" position.

A few minutes after the helmet was in place, observers began to see a marked change in Lori's ability to hold her head erect. The experience will be repeated daily, with the goal of building new habit patterns that eventually will enable Lori to maintain head balance without the assistance of any device.

Among the most interested of the onlookers that morning was Francis Spelman, senior engineer at the University of Washington's Regional Primate Center. He along with neurophysiologist Fredric Harris, the chief consultant for the project, and electronics specialist John Hymer have developed a new model of the "head stabilizer" and are continuing to refine the equipment for further tests this year.

Spelman brings a unique background to the project. In his capacity as head of the primate center's instrumentation development division, he has designed over the past decade a number of electronic instruments for biological research. His experience with cardiovascular control systems is invaluable background for the sensory motor control systems study under way at Lowell School.

"My work in radiotelemetry of physiological functions in free-moving monkeys should also apply when we extend this project to freely moving children," Spelman says. "Ideas from an automatic monkey-training apparatus will lend themselves to the design of an automatic response/reward device that will be used with the children in this project."

One of the bounciest members of the special education class at Lowell Elementary School is dark-eyed Paula, who arrived in Seattle recently from the Philippine Islands specifically to participate in this program. Of above-normal intelligence, Paula seems to be everywhere at once, despite a speech problem and a birth injury that left her right arm so severely disabled that a doctor had recommended

amputation. Her parents instead decided to see what the people at Lowell could do. Barbara Harris, school district supervisor of the physically handicapped and wife of the project director, says chances look good that the child will be able to achieve reasonably normal development.

In the coming weeks she will be fitted with a new artificial sensory device—developed in the laboratory by specialists to meet her special needs, as observed in the classroom and in therapy sessions—that will help her learn to move and control the damaged arm. Meanwhile, toward dealing with her speech problem, Paula will be taught to use a microphone connected to an oscilloscope. Thus combined, the instruments convert sound into electrical "potential variations" which are made visible as a pattern on a cathode-ray tube.

As the little girl pronounces a new word she will watch the small screen carefully, trying to make "her picture" match the correct image made by normal speech. It is hoped this visual feedback will help Paula compensate for her faulty auditory monitoring of sound.

Bringing neurophysiological concepts and theory together with electronics know-how to improve the perceptual skills and mobility of handicapped children is only one of the title VI project's objectives. Another is to provide valuable inservice training to Seattle professionals who work with the neurologically impaired. These include the physically handicapped, children with learning and language disabilities, and a selected group of preschool-age children with thus far uncategorized learning problems. A special program for the latter group has been established at Stevens School, to which children are referred by community agencies, private physicians, and parents who suspect their youngsters have special problems.

In this project new diagnostic and screening tests are being developed as specialists representing many medical and paramedical disciplines contribute their expertise in identifying each youngster's problems. As those who work closely with the handicapped have long observed,

"Applying Technology to Special Education," *American Education*, February 1972. ©1972 United States Department of Health, Education and Welfare.

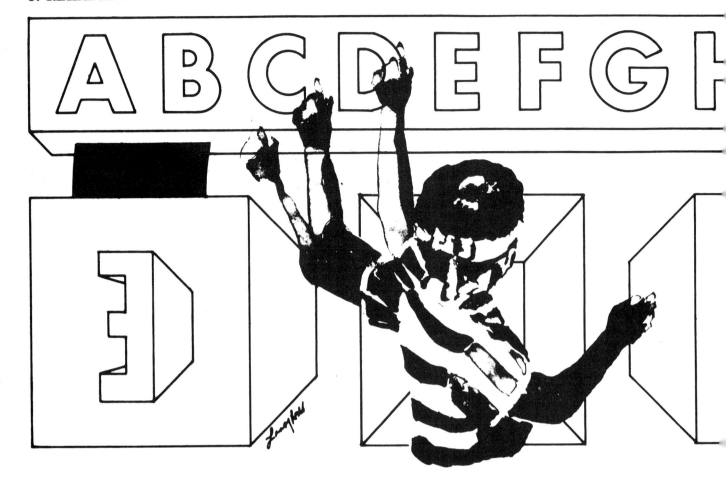

such early identification is vital if successful remedies are to be found.

Charlene Davis, who teaches the ten children assigned to Room 109, explains why:

"All children learn by doing, beginning with such basic movements as sitting up, rolling over, crawling, and walking. Children with motor handicaps such as Lori's and to a lesser extent Paula's are necessarily much slower than normal children in engaging in this kind of exploration and manipulation. And yet it is through such activity that the child begins to comprehend distance, discover which lid fits on which pan, observe that a banana feels squishy, and learn that the right shoe is somehow different from the left. Denied this essential preliminary training, the handicapped child just cannot be ready to begin his formal education at the age of five."

Susan Boll, a physical therapist who works closely with Mrs. Davis, has high hopes that new technology and the people behind it will do much to compensate for the handicapped child's inherent learning disadvantages.

"Left alone, a motor-handicapped child will do nothing and learn nothing," Mrs. Boll says. "A person with training can provide constant assistance to correct the child's movements and help build more normal muscle tone, but so far this has only been possible on a one-to-one basis. There are literally hundreds of ways that technology could help reinforce our work, such as by providing means to monitor children's movements and reactions. With each new breakthrough many more new possibilities will open up."

No matter how dedicated and expert the classroom personnel may be, however, and irrespective of what developments may come from the laboratory, Mrs. Boll says that parents have an irreplaceable role to play in the handicapped child's education.

"We only see the child for a few hours a day," she points out. "Without cooperation at home our efforts cannot really succeed. If the parent works consistently with the child and continues to reinforce what he has learned during the day, we often see progress that is amazing. It boils down to parents needing to learn more about how to handle their own children, who require special help."

One of the consequences of failure to achieve this school-home carryover is what many educators often call "therapy behavior," in which the handicapped child drops the improved habit patterns he has laboriously developed the minute he leaves school. A poignant example occurred at Lowell recently.

"After many months of effort," Mrs. Boll recalls, "I was able to bring one of the cerebral palsy children up to a nearly normal walking gait. You can imagine how dejected I felt one afternoon when I happened to observe her leaving the building and saw her walk revert to the previous pattern almost as soon as she reached the sidewalk. Later when I asked her why this happened, she told me she felt more comfortable 'the old way.' From the child's point of view, what society calls normal is in fact abnormal. These children need to be conditioned to the correct ways of doing things 24 hours a day in order to accept them."

Toward this end parents of the approximately 200 children involved have been carefully briefed on what the project is seeking to accomplish and how, and they are invited to periodic meetings for discussion and demonstration of the materials and techniques in use. At a typical session they might be alerted to such matters as the staff's efforts to counter the behavioral and emotional problems that often develop in children whose physical condition prevents them from moving about at will.

"The emotional gains that customarily accompany the 'repair' of functional defects have a significant effect on the learning process," Dr. Harris says. "The application of appropriate technology can help handicapped children escape chronic failure and begin to succeed in mastering their problems, and thus begin to build a new self-image."

As a consultant in such activities as these, Dr. Harris currently divides his time between the three project centers—Lowell, Stevens, and Surrey Downs Reading Laboratory located in suburban Bellevue—and the University of Washington Medical School. A "doer," he believes in trying the untried, whenever doing so appears theoretically sound.

"Over the years since I first offered a class for public school Special Education teachers in 1967, I have become more and more aware of the importance of moving promising theoretical concepts out into the classroom where they can be tried and the results reported back," he says. "At each of our project centers we have provided the opportunity for a high-intensity, one-to-one relationship between the child and the teacher or therapist. Throughout the year as refinement of diagnostic tests and remedial breakthroughs occur at any one of the centers, we will immediately disseminate the information to everyone involved."

It is most frequently the public school educator, Dr. Harris points out, who is in a position to bring a problem to the attention of the researcher and thus help to speed new developments. Nor should teachers be inhibited by the fact that some

of the devices emerging from the laboratory are highly sophisticated and complex, for many others are relatively simple and inexpensive.

"For example," Dr. Harris says, "we use wooden boards on which letters of the alphabet are routed with a hand tool to help children remedy such problems as letter 'reversals.' This approach is based on research showing that under certain conditions, special information gained through the senses of touch and kinesthesia dominates that gained through sight."

Some dyslexic children may reverse letters or letter combinations, Dr. Harris says, because they have accidently learned an "abnormal pattern" of eye movement, such as tracing horizontal portions of letters from right to left rather than from left to right. In the classroom a dyslexic child is blindfolded and helped to trace letters properly, using the sense of touch for guidance and obtaining kinesthetic feedback. When the blindfold is removed the child's eyes tend to continue to follow his hand in correct sequence. Correcting the eye movement habit often seems to remedy the visual perceptual problem and help "build out" the reversal tendency.

Dr. Harris believes that one of the most readily identifiable gaps in special education efforts has been the lack of a unifying conceptual framework within which to view the problems of handicapped children. There is a great need, he feels, to "educate the educators" to understand how the brain functions in relationship to such aspects of the learning process as

memory, attention, and motivation.

"Just as one needs to know about the container into which he is attempting to pack merchandise, teachers need to know something about the properties of the brain into which they are attempting to cram information," he says. "How can we get it in? How long will it stay there? In what condition will it be after various intervals of time? How can we get it out and in what forms? Every teacher should be concerned with these questions and be knowledgeable about answers that are being supplied by research."

Thus a key element in the project is in-service education for Seattle's special education teachers and for the many from outside the district who have requested to participate. Members of the staff share their experiences and observations primarily through lectures and demonstrations and make videotapes of these demonstrations available to nonparticipating local agencies.

"The many professions, interests, and backgrounds represented in this effort add up to a major resource," says Dr. Harris. "Together we hope to bring new scientific theory and instrumentation—represented at present by the balance control device, the limb position monitor, speech training apparatus, and equipment for automated visual discrimination presentation—in a way that will help to 'make it up' to children with serious physical and academic handicaps.

"We want our efforts to bring something really 'special' to special education."

Noise

Buses, subways, trucks, sirens, planes, and jackhammers
punctuate the day and night with roars, blasts, and chatters.
As a result, 1 out of 20 persons has a hearing loss

Lawrence S. Burns

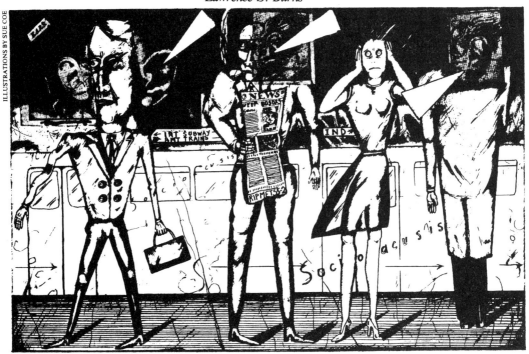

ILLUSTRATIONS BY SUE COE

N o i s e Sue Coe
(an approaching subway can be as loud as the Concorde

The Concorde controversy—why should that sleek but deafening plane be allowed to land at Dulles but not at Kennedy Airport?—has returned the subject of noise pollution to the front page. But airplane noise is only part of the larger problem defined by that newly minted word *socioacusis*.

Socioacusis means loss of hearing resulting from everyday noise. Until recently, speech and hearing experts paid it scant attention because industrial noise was the real villain. But recent tests show that hearing is damaged at noise levels much lower than previously thought, while other studies indicate that the average city soundscape rises to or exceeds those lower levels many times a day.

Some 80 million Americans, according to an Environmental Protection Agency report, live in areas in which the ambient sound gets loud enough to interfere with speech many times daily. Of these, 40 million must tolerate sound levels that clearly threaten their hearing—1 out of 20 citizens now has some hearing loss. Noise not only reduces the quality of city life; it can impair mental and physical health.

As a public problem, noise is nothing new. Julius Caesar wrote the first anti-noise ordinance in 44 B.C.—to little effect. Two centuries later Juvenal complained of Rome: "It is absolutely impossible to sleep anywhere in the city. The perpetual traffic of wagons in the surrounding streets is sufficient to

wake the dead." In a joint letter supporting an 1864 proposal to quiet London, Dickens, Tennyson, and others complained of being made "objects of persecution" by "beaters of drums, grinders of organs, and bangers of banjos." But in the United States, noise as a political issue is practically brand-new—few ordinances are more than 15 years old, and most of them deal with airplane noise.

• • •

The Concorde has attracted so much attention because it is unusually loud. A late-model jumbo 747, for example, creates 100 or more decibels of sound over a three-square-mile area. The Concorde spreads a 100-decibel-plus blanket of noise over some 54 square

"Noise," Lawrence S. Burns, *Horizon*, October 1977. ©1977 Horizon Publishing Co.

miles. "On takeoff," says Steven Starley, an aviation-noise expert at the EPA, "the Concorde sounds like four F-4 fighter jets taking off at once." Its penetrating, low-frequency rumble makes the Concorde "completely distinctive" from other jets.

What bothers noise experts is that plenty of commonplace machines are just as loud as, or even louder than, the Concorde. A sanitation truck during compaction can be noisier, and so can a heavy diesel truck pulling away from a stop sign. One expert who has gone out of his way to dramatize the prevalent obnoxiousness of the city soundscape is Dr. Thomas H. Fay, director of speech and hearing at Columbia-Presbyterian Medical Center in New York. At the height of the anti-SST demonstrations at Kennedy Airport last spring, Dr. Fay took a soundmeter into a West Side subway and proved, for the benefit of a reporter, that an approaching train can be twice as loud as the Concorde.

Since World War II, the number of high-powered noisemakers, from trucks and motorcycles to air conditioners and sirens, has increased almost geometrically. It's no wonder, as the EPA found, that in many areas of the country, especially in the suburbs, the average sound level has doubled in 20 years. R. Murray Schafer, a Canadian composer and sound expert, estimates that ambient city noises are increasing a half-decibel a year. One EPA study found that in 1971 the quietest parts of Los Angeles—thought to be a relatively quiet city—were louder than were the loudest districts of New York in 1937.

In general, the higher the population density, the louder the city. Hence Manhattan consistently turns up the highest readings of ambient noise. But in all cities, background sounds can reach 70 or 75 decibels for extended periods of time. Sanitation trucks, jet planes, pneumatic drills, buses, and heavy trucks puncture the day and night with roars, blasts, and chatters of 90 and 100 decibels. All this sound is well beyond the annoyance point; some of it is clearly dangerous.

As Dr. Fay explains, audiologists assess noise pollution according to the following rule of thumb: when speaking, background noise of 45 to 60 decibels is moderately disturbing; over 65 decibels one has to shout to be heard. When trying to sleep, 35 to 40 decibels is slightly interfering, and 50 to 70 decibels is moderately disturbing. Risk to hearing begins at 70 decibels, is moderate between 80 and 90 decibels, and severe at higher levels. Just how harmful a noise is to your hearing depends on exactly how loud it is and how long you are exposed to it.

Ordinary conversation at 12 feet is a safe 50 decibels. Freeway traffic 50 feet away is about 70 decibels, and, according to standards for environmental noise set by the National Institute of Occupational Safety and Health, 16 hours' exposure a day to that level of noise will produce noticeable hearing loss in most people in about 20 years. But the sound of a heavy truck at 50 feet is 90 decibels, which will damage hearing in the same period with only an hour of exposure a day. At 100 to 113 decibels, some subways are loud enough so that just 3 to 15 minutes' exposure daily can start hearing loss. "That's why I wear earplugs every time I ride the subway," Dr. Fay volunteers. "It's foolish not to."

• • •

An important factor in all noise-related hearing loss is that the ear, which can be an excellent judge of harmonics, is a poor arbiter of sound intensity; we expose ourselves to harmful sound levels unwittingly. Low-frequency sounds are apparently more destructive to the inner ear than high-frequency sounds, though we tolerate them much better. And the ear's own "soundmeter" is hopelessly inaccurate. An increase of 10 decibels is perceived as a doubling of sound, though it's really a tenfold rise in sound energy.

Similarly, an increase of 20 decibels is heard as a quadrupling of sound, though it represents a hundredfold rise in sound energy. It is almost tragic that pain doesn't register until 120 decibels; at 118 decibels the average discotheque produces sound energy approximately 80,000 times more intense than that at which hearing loss begins.

Hearing damage of this sort, so often found in factories that it has come to be known as boilermakers' disease, begins with loss of ability to hear higher-pitched sounds and worsens to include all soft sounds. It becomes particularly frustrating when ordinary speech cannot be distinguished from background noise. Common in old people, this syndrome is showing up more and more in teen-agers. "I see a lot of kids with middle-aged ears," says Dr. Fay. "Usually it turns out they've been to a rock 'n' roll concert every week."

Factors such as time of day, volume of ambient noise, one's mood, and even the weather can determine how irritating a sound is. Thomas O'Hare, head of the EPA's noise bureau in New York, recalls the experience of a man who bought a house not far from Kennedy Airport. Worried about noise, the man had visited the house repeatedly over a three-month period and to his surprise found the planes remarkably quiet. So he bought the place. Two days after moving in, he couldn't take the din and wanted to sell. O'Hare explains that when the man had visited the house, there was snow on the ground, dampening the sound. It melted just before he moved in.

According to Dr. Fay, who, in addition to his responsibilities at Columbia-Presbyterian, is chairman of the Committee on Noise Abatement of New York City's environmental council, "hearing loss is far less of a problem than the erosion of the quality of life for the millions of people who have to put

---

Some 80 million Americans live in areas in which the ambient sound gets loud enough to interfere with speech many times daily.

---

5. REHABILITATION

In many areas of the United States, especially in the suburbs, the average sound level has doubled in 20 years.

---

up with intolerable noise levels." Loud and ubiquitous, city noise and the stress it produces are "probably causing all kinds of physical and emotional problems we don't even know about yet."

• • •

Noise has long been known to cause sleeplessness and irritability, and now other studies are linking it to a wide range of mental and physical disturbances. In Los Angeles, researchers have found that people living near the airport have a higher rate of mental illness than people of the same socioeconomic background living just five miles away. Though other environmental factors, such as polluted air, have not been ruled out as possible causes, the Los Angeles report does confirm the findings of a similar, earlier survey conducted near London's Heathrow Airport. In Osaka, one of the loudest cities in Japan, babies born to mothers living near the airport have unusually low birth weights. And tests of children raised near expressways in the Bronx in New York City showed them to be poor readers compared with other children living slightly farther away and with children living in the same area but for a shorter time.

In industry, a correlation has been found between high noise levels and high incidence of cardiovascular disease and stress-related problems. The effect on people is borne out by experiments on rats, which show that those exposed to certain high-frequency sounds had up to 20 times the normal amount of adrenalin in their blood.

Dr. Barbara A. Bohne, a professor at Washington University in St Louis, suggests that one reason noise has become a problem is that the ear is now subjected to sounds evolution did not prepare it for. Its original function was to detect soft sounds that usually signaled danger or food and then to trigger the body's fight-or-flight mech-

anism. Today, she says, though most sounds are no longer threatening, the mechanism is part and parcel of the human body and cannot be turned off.

Thus, hearing a loud sound sets off a nervous reaction not unlike an anxiety attack. Adrenalin is injected into the blood, the heart speeds up, blood vessels constrict, muscles tense, pupils dilate, and the gut goes into brief spasms. According to Dr. Samuel Rosen, a leading ear specialist, prolonged exposure to high levels of sound can even cause fluttering of the heart. Says Dr. Fay: "Undoubtedly a lot of heart attack victims are finished off when the ambulance siren is turned on." Can long exposure to loud sounds shorten your life span? "Nothing has been proved one way or another," says Jeffrey Goldstein, an EPA bioacoustician, "but it figures that if stress shortens the life span, and noise causes stress, noise can shorten the life span."

In Ottawa, Dr. George J. Theissen set up an experiment to see whether prolonged exposure to a sound leads to physical accommodation and inadvertently found a clue as to how noise might affect mental health. Sleeping subjects were exposed to 80 or more low-level recordings of a truck passing by. In monitoring their brain waves with an electroencephalograph, Theissen found that the neurological disturbances were the same each time the sound was played, the only accommodation being a slight tendency not to wake up. More important to psychologists, however, was his finding that upon hearing the noise, the subjects slipped into a lighter level of sleep and stopped dreaming. Long-term interruption of sleeping and dreaming is known to cause serious mental and physical problems. Here was proof that low levels of noise can disturb sleep even when the sleeper does not wake up. It is possible that in a city, at least, a lot

of people who think they're getting a good night's sleep aren't.

Prolonged exposure to high ambient noise seems to make people more sensitive to sudden, loud sounds, not less, as one might expect. The National Institute of Mental Health found that people accustomed to high ambient noises have a much more pronounced physical reaction to sudden noise than do people used to quieter settings. In other words, city people are more likely to snap at hearing a loud sound. Bizarre incidents have been recorded in the news: a man upending a sanitation worker into a trash barrel, a woman threatening the foreman of a construction site with a shotgun, a man running amuck in a café in Mexico City and killing five people—all because of noise, the offenders claimed.

Noise alone may cause violent behavior, and it can certainly set off a person already disposed to it. Dr. Fay recalls a visit he made to New York's Tombs prison, which was often plagued with riots. Dr. Fay found the prison "insufferably loud—bullhorns, shouting, clanging on the bars, all reverberating on the cement walls and floors." The noise level was more than 90 decibels, he says, and surely contributed to the tension and claustrophobia that had so often led to violence.

• • •

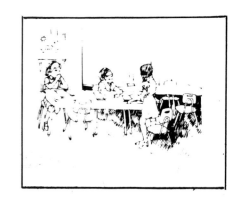

Language Training for the Severely Retarded: Five Years of Behavior Analysis Research

LEE K. SNYDER
THOMAS C. LOVITT
JAMES O. SMITH

In the past 20 years, an increasing amount of research has focused on the complex questions related to language development. This trend is reflected in both journals and texts on mental retardation, and has been documented by several thorough reviews of the literature (e.g., Schiefelbusch, 1969; Smith, 1962). Such an emphasis is not surprising in light of the high incidence of language disorders reported among the retarded and considering the central role which language plays in almost every aspect of our daily lives.

Recently, parents, professionals, and legislatures have exerted pressure on the public schools, as well as on state institutions, to provide a meaningful and appropriate education for all handicapped students, including those who are severely retarded. Certainly, language training must play an important part in any such educational program. Behavior analysis researchers have been especially prolific in their response to this new urgency. In the past few years, so many relevant and promising studies have been offered by the behavior analysts, and in such rapid succession, that it has become difficult for the educator to keep abreast of the latest developments in this area. Thus, the need has become apparent for a brief review of the most recent work in this rapidly expanding field of research.

The Focus

The research to be discussed here deals specifically with subjects who have been identified by the investigators as severely retarded, or whose reported levels of functioning and IQ would indicate such a classification. The term "severely mentally retarded," according to the 1973 American

Association of Mental Deficiency (AAMD) classification system, refers to persons whose measured intelligence is at least four standard deviations below the mean.

Although adaptive behavior criteria are somewhat more ambiguous, Dunn (1973) suggests that severely retarded individuals "have the ability (1) to walk, toilet, dress and feed themselves; (2) to speak in a very elementary fashion; and (3) to perform simple chores in the home or in a very protective environment" (p. 86). This population has been selected as the focus of concern because (a) for the first time, large numbers of these students are being enrolled in the public schools, requiring new instructional programs and techniques, and (b) it seems at least possible that these students may exhibit qualitatively, as well as quantitatively, distinctive patterns of learning and responding. Therefore, in limiting the focus of this review, it has been decided to exclude the many interesting and exciting language development studies which employed subjects who are "high level retardates" (e.g., McLean, 1970) or extremely disturbed children (e.g., Lovaas, 1968).

Additionally, the scope of this article has been limited to studies of language behavior. Specifically, only those studies dealing with language as meaningful, symbolic communication (both oral and aural) will be considered. Thus, related research in such areas as articulation, audiometry, and motor imitation are not included here.

Finally, this article covers only those studies which have employed a behavior analysis research design. Each of these studies met the following criteria: (a) the behavior under study (the dependent variable) was clearly defined in observable terms; (b) this behavior was directly and precisely measured on a continuous basis with data reported accordingly; and (c) the research analyzed the effects of systematic manipulation of specific environmental factors (the independent variables). There has been an obvious trend in recent educational research toward this methodology. This seems to be a particularly promising approach to the study of language acquisition.

So many studies of this type have appeared in the literature of the past two decades that it would be impossible to discuss all of them here. Therefore, only those studies published since 1968 are included. The 23 studies which

were found to meet the above criteria are characterized in Table 1.

The first section of this article will be a summary and comparison of the specific language behaviors investigated in these studies. Several aspects of the research methodologies employed will be considered next. Finally, the implications for classroom or clinical practice, as well as for future research will be discussed.

Target Behaviors (Dependent Variables)

In all of these studies, the behavior under analysis was the subject's performance on specific language tasks. These tasks may be classified along two dimensions—type and level. There are two main types of language: receptive (auditory perception, "input") and expressive (usually vocal production, "output"). Tasks in either of these modes may be at one of three levels—initial acquisition (if the subject lacks prior reception and/or expressive language), appropriate use of language, or, use of correct grammar or syntax.

Another feature which may be incorporated in a study of language development is the generative property of language; that is, the ability to produce and receive "an unlimited number of utterances which share a limited number of regularities" (Lahey, 1973, p. x). This concept is illustrated by the following statement by Twardosz and Baer (1973),

> Several studies have shown that when a child is taught to use specific examples of a grammatical rule, he also produces novel examples of this rule that have never been trained, i.e., the rule is generative, (p. 655).

Elsewhere, this phenomenon is referred to as "generalization to untrained stimuli" (p. 660). It has been suggested by Baer and Guess (1973) that, "So conceptualized, these rules of morphological grammar appear equivalent to the behavioral concept of response class" (p. 498). This suggestion, that "generative" and "response class" may actually be equivalent concepts, seems supportable in light of the definition of a response class as "a set of responses so organized that an operation applied to a relatively small subset of their members produces similar results in other members as well" (Garcia, Guess, & Byrnes, 1973, p. 299). Therefore, in the present discussion, those studies which dealt with the generalization of responses to untrained stimuli, or with the formation of a linguistic

"Language Training for the Severely Retarded: Five Years of Behavior Analysis Research," Lee K. Snyder, Thomas C. Lovitt, James O. Smith, *Exceptional Children*, Vol. 42 No. 1, September 1975. ©1975 The Council for Exceptional Children.

5. REHABILITATION

response class, are all considered analyses of the generative property of the language behavior under investigation.

Receptive Language

Only three of the studies under consideration dealt exclusively with receptive language. Two of these dealt with initial acquisition of the ability to receive (i.e., respond to) verbal instructions (Whitman, Zakaras, & Chardos, 1971; Striefel & Wetherby, 1973). The generative property of this ability was assessed in both studies, with very different results. In the earlier study (Whitman, et al.), the subjects learned to respond correctly to 11 specific verbal commands and generalized this ability to a set of 11 similar, but untrained, instructions. However, Striefel and Wetherby (1973), working with an older and more severely retarded subject, found no generalization to similar instructions, or even to variations of the same 20 instructions which had been successfully trained.

Baer and Guess (1971) assessed the effects of training the receptive discrimination of comparative and superlative forms of adjectives (concepts of which had been previously trained as opposites). All three of their subjects learned to point correctly to pictures representing the superlative and comparative forms of specific adjectives and generalized this ability to similar, but untrained, adjectives.

Expressive Language

Seventeen studies focused exclusively on the modification of expressive language, and nine of these were concerned with the initial acquisition of the ability to imitate and produce specific words or phonemic elements. Four studies (Sloane, Johnston, & Harris, 1968; Kircher, Pear, & Martin, 1971; Stewart, 1972; Jeffrey, 1972) simply demonstrated the effectiveness of operant conditioning in developing and maintaining verbal responses to specific stimuli (e.g., pictures or adult model). The work of Peine, Gregersen, & Sloane, (1970) and Lawrence (1971) was similar in nature, but additionally demonstrated successful manipulation of spontaneous speech through contingent reinforcement. The generative nature of imitative vocal responses was investigated by Garcia, Baer, & Firestone (1971) and by Schroeder and Baer (1972). In both these studies, subjects who had been operantly trained to imitate specific types of motor and vocal responses generalized this ability to the imitation of topographically similar, but untrained, responses. Griffiths and Craighead (1972) successfully trained a specific response class (pronunciation of 10 words with the initial phoneme /l/) which generalized across three different types of stimuli (all evoking the same 10 words), but not across two different settings.

The appropriate use of language was successfully manipulated through contingent reinforcement in three studies. Barton (1972) increased the amount of social speech (verbalization directed toward others) in four severely retarded women. In 1970, Barton reported the success of operant training techniques in increasing the number of appropriate responses made to magazine pictures by an 11 year old institutionalized boy. However, she found that this behavior did not generalize to similar, but untrained, tasks. In contrast, Twardosz and Baer (1973) succeeded in training two institutionalized adolescents to ask a specific class of questions ("What letter?") in one setting, and found that this did generalize to similar stimuli within the same setting.

Five studies in recent years dealt with the operant training of grammar or syntax in expressive language. Guess, Sailor, Rutherford, & Baer (1968), Sailor (1971) and Garcia, et al. (1973) successfully trained subjects to correctly use singular and plural forms of nouns and, through the use of probes and experimental reversals, clearly demonstrated the generative nature of these learnings. Similarly, Schumaker and Sherman (1970) trained three subjects to produce verbs of the appropriate tense (past or present progressive) in response to verbal stimuli, and demonstrated the generation of appropriate tense use in untrained verbs. Baer and Guess (1973) reported successfully teaching four severely retarded adolescents to produce noun suffixes ("__er" and "__ist") and generalize this skill to untrained words.

Receptive and Expressive Language

Finally, three studies analyzed both receptive and expressive language behaviors. MacAulay (1968) reported on her work with 11 severely retarded students, between the ages of 9 and 15, at the Rainier State School in Buckley, Washington. These studies were discussed rather informally in an article intended to give an overview of the procedures employed, and no complete list of the specific behaviors was provided. However, the data which were presented demonstrated successful operant training of vocabulary reception ("point to the ___"), phoneme production, and morpheme production in response to verbal, pictorial, and, in some cases, written stimuli.

Two more studies dealing with pluralization (Guess, 1969; Guess and Baer, 1973) explored the interrelationships, in terms of generalization, between receptive and expressive training. The earlier study demonstrated that successful training to discriminate receptively between the singular and plural forms of a noun did not generalize to the production of the appropriate form of that noun. In the followup study, four subjects were trained to receptively discriminate one class of plurals and expressively use another class. Probes revealed no generalization across modes.

Research Methodology

Subjects and Settings

The 23 studies discussed here involved a total of 64 subjects. With very few exceptions, these subjects had either been officially diagnosed as severely retarded, according to the AAMD classification system, or could be so classified on the basis of their reported functioning and IQ. Four of the studies, employing a total of 9 subjects, involved children under 8 years of age. Fifteen subjects, in 7 different studies, were over 14 years of age. The remaining 36 subjects, involved in 15 of the studies, were all between the ages of 8 and 13. (Several studies employed subjects of widely varying ages and so were counted twice in these figures.)

Nineteen studies, involving 52 of the subjects, were conducted within residential institutions for the retarded. Only 5 studies, involving 12 children, were carried out in noninstitutional settings. These included one public school, one preschool, one day care center, and two clinics.

Intervention Techniques
(Independent Variables)

Most of these studies involved more than one independent variable. Without exception, all of the studies included the use of some tangible reinforcement (12 using primaries and 11 using tokens) for desired verbal behavior. In two studies, the relative effectiveness of different reinforcers was assessed. Lawrence (1971) found that the use of social reinforcement, alone or paired with a consumable primary, was more effective with three adolescents than the use of the consumable alone. In a study with four retarded women, Barton (1972) found that token reinforcement produced dramatically greater increases in verbal behavior than did primary reinforcement.

Several of the studies placed the subject(s) on a continuous or fixed ratio schedule of reinforcement only until the verbal behavior attained a predetermined criterion level (Sloane, et al., 1968; Guess, 1969; Garcia, et al., 1971; Baer & Guess, 1971; Sailor, 1971; Schroeder & Baer, 1972; Garcia, et al., 1973; Guess & Baer, 1973; Twardosz & Baer, 1973). The behavior was then placed on a variable ratio schedule (VR) of reinforcement (usually VR 2 or VR 3) to facilitate the interjection of nonreinforced probes designed to assess generalization of learning.

In many of the studies, a time out contingency (ranging from 10 to 30 seconds in most cases) was arranged for incorrect responses or nonattending behavior (Sloane et al., 1968; Schumaker & Sherman, 1970; Barton, 1970; Baer & Guess, 1971; Kircher et al., 1971; Lawrence, 1971). No evidence is provided in any of these studies to support the effectiveness of this technique, and one might question its appropriateness with this population. As Lawrence (1971) has observed, time out from reinforcement is the usual state of affairs for most institutional residents. In fact, Kircher et al. (1971) demonstrated the relative ineffectiveness of time out, as contrasted with contingent mild shocks, in decreasing inappropriate behavior.

In 11 of these studies, antecedent modeling of desired responses was provided. Usually, if this failed to elicit the correct imitation or verbalization, the response was shaped through reinforcement of increasing approximations as physical prompts were gradually faded out. In two studies (Whitman, et al., 1971; Striefel & Wetherby, 1973), this process of shaping and fading was the central intervention technique under study.

The relative effectiveness of two different training procedures on generalization to untrained response types was assessed by Schroeder and Baer (1972) in their study of vocal imitation. Two subjects were taught to verbally imitate groups of three words (through modeling and shaping) with two

TABLE 1 Characteristics of 23 Behavior Analysis Studies of Language Training for the Severely Retarded

Author/date	Intervention Techniques					
	Target behavior		Antecedent events	Consequent events		Research design employed
	Type	Level		Reinforcement	Nonreinforcement	
Guess, Sailor, Rutherford, & Baer (1968)	Expressive [a]	Grammar, Syntax		Primary		Reversal of contingency
MacAulay (1968)	Receptive, Expressive	Initial Acquisition [b]	Shaping/fading; Modeling	Token		
Sloane, Johnston, & Harris (1968)	Expressive	Initial Acquisition [b]	Shaping/fading; Modeling	Primary	Time out	Noncontingent reinforcement
Guess (1969)	Receptive, Expressive	Grammar, Syntax		Token		Reversal of contingency
Schumaker & Sherman (1970)	Expressive [a]	Grammar, Syntax	Modeling [c]	Token	Time out	Multiple baseline
Barton (1970)	Expressive [a]	Appropriate Usage		Primary	Time out	Reversal of contingency
Peine, Gregersen & Sloane (1970)	Expressive	Initial Acquisition [b]		Token [d]		Reversal of contingency
Garcia, Baer, & Firestone (1971)	Expressive [a]	Initial Acquisition [b]	Shaping/fading; Modeling	Primary		Multiple baseline
Baer & Guess (1971)	Receptive [a]	Grammar Syntax		Token	Time out	Multiple baseline
Kircher, Pear, & Martin (1971)	Expressive	Initial Acquisition [b]	Modeling	Token	Time out	
Whitman, Zakaras, & Chardos (1971)	Receptive [a]	Initial Acquisition [b]	Shaping/fading	Primary		A-B-A design
Sailor (1971)	Expressive [a]	Grammar, Syntax	Modeling	Primary		Multiple baseline
Lawrence (1971)	Expressive	Initial Acquisition [b]		Primary [d]	Time out	A-B-A design; Pretest/posttest
Stewart (1972)	Expressive	Initial Acquisition [b]	Modeling	Primary		
Jeffrey (1972)	Expressive	Initial Acquisition [b]	Shaping/fading; Modeling	Primary		
Schroder & Baer (1972)	Expressive [a]	Initial Acquisition [b]	Shaping/fading; [c] Modeling	Primary		
Barton (1972)	Expressive	Appropriate Usage		Primary/token		
Griffiths & Craighead (1972)	Expressive	Initial Acquisition [b]	Modeling	Token		Multiple baseline
Garcia, Guess, & Byrnes (1972)	Expressive [a]	Grammar, Syntax	Modeling	Primary		Reversal of contingency
Guess & Baer (1973)	Receptive, Expressive	Grammar, Syntax		Token		
Twardosz & Baer (1973)	Expressive [a]	Appropriate Usage	Shaping/fading; Modeling [b]	Token		Multiple baseline
Striefel & Wetherby (1973)	Receptive [a]	Initial Acquisition [b]	Shaping/fading	Primary		
Baer & Guess (1973)	Expressive [a]	Grammar, Syntax	Modeling	Primary/token		Reversal of contingency

[a] Study included analysis of generative property of specific language behavior trained.
[b] Initial acquisition of specific words or phonemic elements.
[c] Optional: Used only if other interventions failed to elicit desired response.
[d] Systematically paired with social reinforcement.

5. REHABILITATION

alternating procedures: In one condition, each of the three words would be trained to criterion before the next was introduced; in the second condition, the three words would be trained concurrently until all three had reached criterion. The two procedures were equally effective in producing correct imitations of the words being trained. However, generalization to probe items was significantly greater following concurrent training.

In 7 studies, contingent reinforcement of responses was the only intervention employed. In these studies, no antecedent events preceded the presentation of the stimulus to which the subject(s) responded (Guess et al., 1968; Guess, 1969; Barton, 1970; Peine et al., 1970; Baer & Guess, 1971; Barton, 1972; Guess & Baer, 1973).

Experimental Control

Several research designs were employed in these 23 studies, the complexity of which probably reflects the complexity of the language behaviors being investigated. Behavior analysis researchers commonly use an A-B-A design (baseline—intervention—return to baseline) to demonstrate the effectiveness of their interventions. However, in most of the studies reported here, such a design was either not practical or not desirable.

The method of reversing contingencies was employed by several of these investigators and involves the switch of contingent reinforcement to a previously unreinforced, and usually incorrect, response after the correct response has been successfully trained. In the studies which used this design, reestablishment of the normal contingencies for correct responding consistently succeeded in reinstituting the previously established patterns of correct responding. In a multiple baseline design, experimental control is demonstrated through successive application of the intervention to two or more subjects, behaviors or settings. As the intervention is applied to each, a change in the pattern of responses is interpreted as indication of the effectiveness of the technique employed.

Implications

Suggestions for Classroom and Clinical Practice

In the past five years, a large amount of behavior analysis research has appeared dealing with the language development of severely retarded subjects. Perhaps the most striking implication to be drawn from all these studies is that it is definitely possible to improve the language skills of severely retarded children and adults through the application of systematic instructional techniques and reinforcement contingencies. However, for the teacher or clinician who is applying such behavior management techniques, some more specific inferences can be made.

In order for a response to be reinforced, it must first exist in the student's repertoire.

This is an obvious fact, but one we can easily forget in our enthusiasm for behavior modification. In several of the studies discussed here, the investigators found it necessary to develop a systematic shaping procedure in order to initially establish the desired behaviors. The use of modeling and physical prompting, which could be gradually faded out as the behavior came under reinforcement control, was reported as a successful approach in several of these studies.

Several implications for the scheduling of consequent events can be drawn from the research reviewed here. The selection of effective reinforcers is certainly one critical component in a program designed to strengthen or extend a desired behavior once it has been initially acquired. While we frequently assume that primary reinforcers are the most potent, the study by Barton (1972) demonstrated that tokens were significantly more effective than primary reinforcers in modifying the social speech of the four severely retarded women included in that study. In selecting a reinforcer for any one student, the teacher or clinician should experiment with a wide variety of reinforcers—both primary and secondary—to determine which is most reinforcing for that particular person. Similarly if a time out procedure is to be used effectively, it must take the form of time out from a truly reinforcing reinforcement, not just time out from the activity or attention.

The conflicting findings regarding generalization which were reported in these studies indicate clearly that we should not expect generalization to occur automatically. The practice of gradually fading from a one to one to a variable ratio schedule of reinforcement, employed in many of these investigations, may prove to be a useful practice for the clinician or teacher who wishes to promote generalization across settings, as well as maintenance over time. Although it may be possible to reinforce a desired response every time it occurs, in a clinical or classroom setting, this behavior will disappear if it is not reinforced when it occurs in other settings. If the behavior is placed on an intermittent schedule, it will be more resistant to the inevitable instances of nonreinforcement in uncontrolled situations.

One potential means for fostering generalization to new responses is indicated by the findings of Schroeder and Baer (1972). In their study, generalization was found to be greater after several words had been trained concurrently, as opposed to a sequential teaching procedure. Certainly, this would be an easy technique to apply in both clinical and classroom settings and one with which the teacher or clinician may wish to experiment.

Directions for Future Research

From the results of the studies discussed here, it would seem that the possibility of modifying the language behavior of severely retarded subjects through the use of operant

procedures has been clearly established. Far from exhausting the need for research in this area, however, these studies have revealed many unanswered questions which call for further investigation.

Certainly, there is a need to extend the range of ages and settings involved in future language training research. With the current trend towards early screening and intervention for handicapped children, more studies involving severely retarded subjects under the age of seven would be relevant. Similarly, as the move towards deinstitutionalization progresses, we look increasingly towards research conducted in public school, group home, foster home, and natural home environments.

It is somewhat surprising that every study discussed here involved the use of some tangible reinforcement. It would seem worthwhile to investigate the possible application of purely social reinforcement in the form of contingent praise or physical contact (e.g., hugging, patting). As has been noted earlier, this type of reinforcement has all too often been lacking in the environments of institutionalized subjects. It seems possible that this might provide a source of very potent reinforcement. Similarly, the effects of different antecedent events, without any elaborate reinforcement contingencies, would seem to merit investigation. Certainly, in studies of language *acquisition*, the efficiency of waiting for the subject to emit a desired response, which has not yet been mastered, and then reinforcing it, may be questioned. Although most studies have employed antecedent strategies as a "last resort," it is hoped that future investigators will focus more direct attention on these antecedent instructional interventions.

It should be noted that only a few of the studies described here have reported data on either maintenance over time or generalization of learned responses to new settings. Since the reason for training language skills is to have those skills applied in the subject's daily living, it is hoped that future investigators will analyze intervention strategies employed in training or modifying specific language behaviors in order to identify those variables which are most effective in promoting maintenance. Similarly, analyses of data obtained through the systematic manipulation of antecedent or consequent events are needed to determine the efficacy of different intervention strategies in terms of response generalization—both to untrained responses *and* to new settings.

The 23 studies which have been discussed here represent an exciting avenue of research which holds great promise for the severely retarded individual. As future investigators find answers to the many new and difficult questions raised by the present studies, we may hope to see this promise realized and the door of two-way communication finally opened to those who have been shut out for so long.

Subtitles for TV and Films

Because of technical advances and changing attitudes, hearing-impaired persons can now enjoy films and TV programs that their handicap had previously denied them

The first of the two sight and sound revolutions that occurred during the last half-century was launched in October of 1927 by Al Jolson in *The Jazz Singer,* a silent film with four talking and singing interludes. The second revolution was television, the post-World War II *enfant terrible* that became a "boob tube" to its detractors and a "window on the world" to its boosters. Whether for praise or for scorn, TV's impact on the world is undeniable. In the United States alone it reaches more than 70 million homes. The average family watches TV six hours and seven minutes daily.

Both developments, of course, were cause for rejoicing. But not for everyone. It was no fun for those who heard nothing when Jolson got down on one knee and sang "My li'l maa-haa-hammy" in the movies. And it was no less than frustrating to those who could not understand the story behind the news commentaries that gave early television its sense of awe and immediacy because they could not hear the comments. Sound films and TV brought no cheers from the deaf.

Today, this situation is changing. Hearing-impaired persons throughout the nation can now understand and enjoy many of the same high-quality commercial films which their handicap had previously denied them. Moreover, they have access to hundreds of educational films and other types of audiovisual materials prepared especially for them. On public television, there literally is "good news" for the deaf. "The Captioned ABC News," produced at WGBH in Boston under a contract with OE's Bureau of Education for the Handicapped, uses the sound and picture of the regular ABC evening news with Harry Reasoner and Barbara Walters. By special arrangement with the American Broadcasting Company, WGBH tapes the shows presented each evening at 6 o'clock (Eastern Standard Time) Monday through Friday, removes all of the commercial segments, and, to communicate the newscast's sound portion, adds electronically printed captions of one, two, or three lines. The commercial breaks are then filled with weather, sports, features, and news of special interest to the hearing-impaired, and the complete captioned package is fed to the Public Broadcasting Service (PBS) about five and one-half hours after the start of the original broadcast. Available to the deaf also throughout the PBS schedule is a weekly selection of such shows as the "Adams Chronicles" and the "Upstairs, Downstairs" series.

This is not to imply that video offerings for the hearing-impaired anywhere near approximate what's available for persons who don't have a hearing problem. Currently, the total fare for the deaf amounts to about eight hours a week. But, as Al Jolson was fond of saying, "Stick around, folks; you ain't seen nothin' yet!"

Permitting the quantum jump from famine to what appears will be a pretty good feast is the development of new techniques in captioning—the use of subtitles similar to those in foreign movies that help an audience understand what it's all about. But the similarity ends there. Captioning for the hearing-impaired, both on films and videotape (even though the processes are different), is far more sophisticated. Its techniques permit excellent readability, regardless of the background in the picture. The letters are optically reinforced to make them stand out; conventional subtitles used by most foreign-film distributors, for example, tend to wash out when they are superimposed over light or white backgrounds. Culturally and educationally, there are advantages because each presentation is adapted especially for the average hearing-impaired adult or child, depending on the program type. Adjustments in the language level and reading rate make the original sound portion more understandable and en-

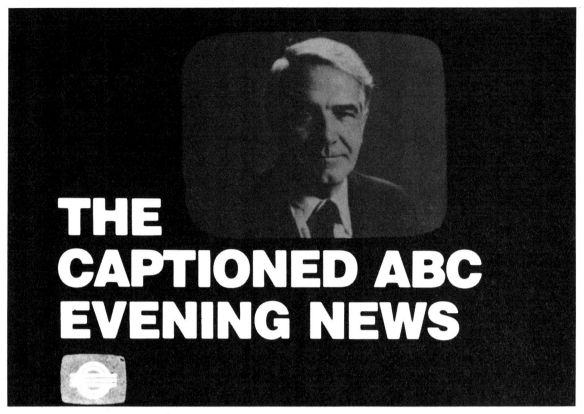

THE CAPTIONED ABC EVENING NEWS

joyable, thus any youngster with a learning disability is motivated to become a better reader.

There are two methods of captioning; in both, subtitles are superimposed on the picture. Far and away the most prevalent one, by virtue of its being until recently just about the only one, is "open" captioning. Anyone tuning in a program using open captions will see the subtitles whether he wants them or not. They're superimposed on the film and there's no way a viewer can blot them out. WGBH uses open captioning in its evening news, and since many people with normal hearing listen to the program, there is the ever-present possibility of complaints from them about the captions interfering with their enjoyment of the program. So far this has not been a major problem, but it could become one.

The second method sidesteps this problem. A recent decision by the Federal Communications Commission permits allocation on line 21 of a TV receiver screen (the first nonvisual line above the picture) for a process developed by PBS by which electronic translations of the audio portion can be transmitted and become visible on the home screen only when decoded by a special device incorporated into the TV set. Thus a hearing viewer would see nothing but the picture; a hearing-impaired viewer, by switching in a little black box (the decoder) would see the subtitles. By the turn of a switch the decoder can be disengaged and

the set returned to standard viewing; that is, no subtitles would be visible. The FCC decision in favor of the "closed" captioning system will most certainly help narrow the program-availability gap for the 13.4 million nonhearing Americans.

PBS has been refining and testing the closed system since 1972 under a contract with the Bureau of Education for the Handicapped. During the experimental phase in 1974, decoding equipment was installed at test sites in 12 major cities throughout the country, and PBS broadcast 13 of its most popular prime-time shows with closed captions.

As part of its evaluation of the project, Gallaudet College of Washington, D.C., surveyed 1,400 of the hearing-impaired viewers and found that 90 percent would not have been able to understand the programs without the special visual service. Moreover, 94 percent said they could purchase a home decoder if it were available.

The costs of closed captioning, PBS officials state, are relatively modest and the only major expense is the captioning equipment, which runs between $25,000 and $50,000—but this is a one-time cost to the TV producers. Officials also say that the home decoders, which were developed by the National Bureau of Standards and found workable in tests run during the 1974 experiments, can be marketed within a year at a cost of approximately $100 each.

In July of 1975, PBS began on a regular

Five nights a week it's good news for the hearing-impaired when "The Captioned ABC Evening News" comes into their sets via public television.

222

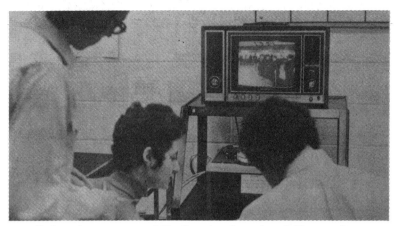

Today, there are over 800 educational captioned-films available in 60 centers which distribute them nationwide to schools and classes for the deaf.

weekly basis to feed some of its programs in both the open and closed formats to all of its 267 member stations. Such prime-time series as "Feeling Good," the Nova science series, "Masterpiece Theatre," the "Adams Chronicles," and "Once Upon a Classic" have been telecast a total of four hours each week in prime time. The closed caption telecasts are currently viewed on the campuses of large residential schools for the deaf, where the decoder units used during the experimental phase have been installed as part of the school's closed-circuit TV system. These programs have proved to be welcome supplements to the captioned newscasts.

News captioning is a complicated and time-consuming job, and producing the nightly news show at WGBH is especially complicated because of time-imposed constrictions. Each weekday evening in the shadows of the Harvard playing fields, a five-person captioning team goes into action at 6 o'clock. On the command of a microwave signal from the ABC-TV transmission relay at the downtown Boston Prudential Center, the ABC evening news begins coming in on a special line. During the next five hours the team will make audiotape and videotape recordings of the news; type scripts of what is said on the news; edit the scripts into caption form; type the copy into a computerized machine called a Vidifont, which produces the captions; check the typing; practice timing changes from one caption into the next; write sports, weather, updates, and other important news; type that information into a second computerized Vidifont system; proofread the captions; and then work with the technical staff to broadcast the captioned news, live, to PBS viewers.

The 16 staff members of WGBH's caption center fill the remainder of their time producing the features and other inserts that replace the nightly six minutes' worth of commercials cut from the ABC news. One staffer is also involved in evaluating the center's efforts by means of questionnaires and meetings with panels of deaf persons who were invited to the studios of many local public-service TV stations across the country.

A third area of expanded staff activity focuses on producing videotaped programs for holidays and special occasions. These are shown in place of the news. In 1974, for example, the staff captioned "Godspell Goes to Plimoth Plantation" for Thanksgiving and followed it with other specials for Christmas and New Year's Eve. In February of 1975 the caption center produced and broadcast a half-hour documentary on the VIII World Winter Games for the Deaf at Lake Placid.

The Office of Education, with the cooperation of various associations for the deaf, began experimenting with captioning techniques in the 1950s. The signing in September 1958 of Public Law 85-905, "an act to provide for a loan service of captioned films for the deaf," provided the needed federal resources. Motion pictures subsequently were leased from all of the major film companies, then captioned and distributed to groups of deaf and hearing-impaired persons all over the country. Today, there are approximately 450 theatrical films in the captioned-film lending library in Indianapolis and over 800 educational captioned-films available in the 60 centers which distribute them nationwide to schools and classes for the deaf.

Each year an average of 50 to 60 theatrical films and many more educational films are captioned for distribution. All of the major film companies send prints of their new films to the National Association for the Deaf, where screening groups made up of a cross-section of the deaf population view each

5. REHABILITATION

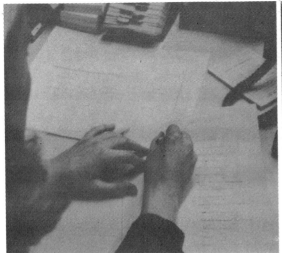
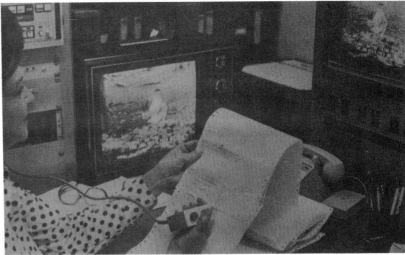

film, evaluate it, and recommend whether or not it should become a part of the captioned-film loan program. Teachers of the deaf—some of whom are themselves deaf—evaluate educational films that are captioned for classroom use. A group of deaf people wishing to obtain film services must register with the Educational Media Distribution Center in Washington, D.C.

Chief of OE's Captioned Films and Telecommunications Branch is Malcolm J. Norwood, who has been deaf since early childhood. Dr. Norwood has been the guiding spirit of the entire captioning program from its very start, and it was under his direction that the venture into television began in 1971 with a grant to the WGBH Educational Foundation—Boston's public television affiliate.

Under the grant, a two-year contract provided for the captioning of the station's gourmet cooking show, "The French Chef," and 26 other public television productions. In the succeeding months, eight captioned versions of the popular program featuring Julia Child were made available to public television stations across the country via PBS, and the entire series with captions was shown later in Boston and many other cities.

Following the successful completion of these captioned shows, WGBH received another demonstration contract under the Education of the Handicapped Act to begin telecasts of "The Captioned ABC News" on December 3, 1973. This authority, as amended, has subsequently been the basis for funding all of OE's TV captioning activities, currently pegged at about a half-million dollars a year for the work at WGBH and nearly $1.3 million to date for developing the closed system at PBS.

What little other programing that has existed on TV for the hearing-impaired has been mostly in the form of news programs that provide the anchorman with a "silent partner"—a person who interprets the news in sign language. But "signing" the news hasn't helped the millions of persons who don't use the language of signs, including some profoundly deaf who have never learned manual translation, or those who have experienced a loss of hearing with age and who really don't think of themselves as hearing-impaired. However, in an effort to serve the total hearing-impaired audience in the best possible way, the Presidential Debates last year were interpreted in sign language simultaneously on PBS and then were telecast with open captions on the following night over many PBS stations.

TV captioning for the deaf is not a simple matter of dubbing onto the video portion of a transcript some of the words spoken on the audio portion. It's much more complicated than that. Here are some points that the WGBH caption center takes into account:

□ The average low-verbal deaf person has a fourth- to sixth-grade reading ability, and the academic and language achievement of the average deaf student leaving school is at least a year behind his hearing counterpart. Yet there is a prevalent misconception that deaf persons must be good readers—a sort of "compensation" by nature for the loss of hearing.

□ Some deaf persons don't know many of the idioms and figures of speech that others routinely pick up through their ears. They must deal with language nuances without the benefit of such auditory cues as vocal inflections. Thus language that presents two distinct meanings is to be avoided. For example, it is advisable to write "unrehearsed" rather than "off the cuff" in describing an extemporaneous speech. And again, when an ABC newscaster said, "Today begins that annual December dance on Capitol Hill known as the adjournment frenzy," the captioned version read: Every December, Con-

At station WGBH in Boston, the captioning team takes notes on the evening news, adjusts the language level for easy comprehension, breaks sentences into sequences of phrases, and finally inserts the electronically printed captions into a tape of the newscast.

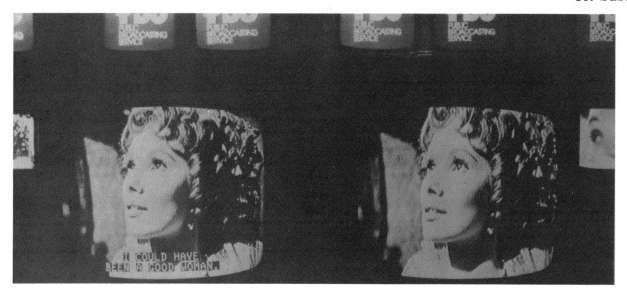

gress is very busy as it tries to finish before Christmas.

□ Experts say that the reading rate for the average deaf adult watching TV should not exceed 140 words per minute. The ABC evening news has a speaking rate that averages 165 words, with some stories approaching 185. The verbatim transcript of the show is edited for the captioned version to adjust not only the language but also the reading rate. The captioned show averages 120 words (about 15 captions) per minute, recognizing that there is more to be "seen" in the picture than just the caption.

□ Captions are flashed on the picture for several seconds at a time. How does a deaf person know who is saying what? Solution: In group shots, captions are positioned on the screen according to who is speaking. If the voice is off-camera, the words are shown at the top of the screen.

When "The Captioned ABC News" began in December of 1973, eight stations on the Eastern Educational Television Network carried the program. Today the show is viewed on approximately 120 stations, making it available to about half the hearing-impaired population of the United States.

Initially distributed on PBS in August of 1974, the captioned news is carried by about half of its stations, which constitute the world's largest television system. Phillip W. Collyer, director of the caption center at WGBH, points out that, although ABC provides its captioned news at no cost, the decision to present the program rests with each individual PBS station. Should a station decide it wants to use the program, it must apply for permission to the local ABC affiliate. "It is this excellent cooperative effort," says Mr. Collyer, "that has permitted the growth of the show over its first three years."

For years, a number of other countries have been looking into the operation of OE's programs of captioning for the deaf. None was successful in establishing anything similar until early 1975 when the National Film Board of Canada received authority to establish a program with an initial budget of $50,000 (OE's was $78,000 at the start). Included in the planning is a national news program on television modeled after WGBH's "Captioned ABC News."

The immediate job ahead is to launch the expansion of the closed system into the non-public TV programing areas and the homes of the hearing-impaired. First priority, of course, is the production of the needed electronic hardware, encoders and decoders. Negotiations with a number of manufacturers is now in progress. The next priority is to train captioners; OE currently is offering such training assistance to the commercial networks, TV producers and production agencies, and advertising agencies as a start in urging them to caption their programs as normal procedure.

Then, perhaps the next advance for the benefit of hearing-impaired persons who watch TV is "real time" or near-instant captioning. PBS engineers have developed a feasibility study that concludes such communication to be in the future, although no one yet is prepared to say how far into the future. Still, it's not farfetched to suppose that, when the next sight and sound revolution comes along, those with hearing handicaps will not be left sitting cheerless and frustrated. More likely they'll be right up front, cheering and rejoicing—and benefiting—along with everyone else.

Open captioning (in which captions are visible whether the viewer wants them or not) causes some viewer complaints. But another method, closed captioning, would show the captions only in homes equipped with a special decoder, a development that should increase the availability of programs for deaf Americans.

Time-Intensity Trade for Speech:

A Temporal Speech-Stenger Effect

MICHAEL J.M. RAFFIN,

DAVID J. LILLY,

AARON R. THORNTON

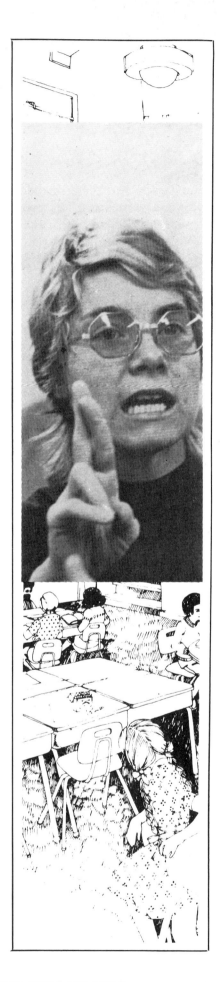

When the same acoustic signal is presented simultaneously to both ears, and when both signals are at equal sensation levels, the subjective percept is a sound image that appears to be inside the head, usually in the median plane. Several factors may affect the apparent position of the sound image within the head. Venturi (1796) probably was the first investigator to postulate that this percept is dependent upon differences in interaural intensity. Shaxby and Gage (1932) showed experimentally that interaural differences in the phase (or time of arrival) of the signal also may affect the apparent position of the sound image within the head. Subsequent studies have corroborated this interaction between interaural time and interaural intensity differences. In general, a time advantage in one ear can compensate for an intensity advantage in the other ear. Studies that deal with these reciprocal compensatory relations often are considered under the heading of "time intensity trade" experiments (Hafter and Carrier, 1972).

Three psychophysical procedures have been used to study the stimulus parameters involved in the lateralization produced by interaural time and interaural intensity differences for pure tones, noise, and click stimuli. The matching method requires the subject to use a "pointer" to indicate the apparent location of a test signal presented with certain interaural time and intensity differences (Moushegian and Jeffress, 1959; von Bekesy, 1930). The scaling method utilizes a visible scale set in front of the listener to represent his perceived auditory "space." The listener reports the number on the scale that corresponds most closely with the position of the perceived auditory image. As the image is displaced further from the median plane, the subject

"Time-intensity Trade for Speech: A Temporal Speech — Stenger Effect," Michael J.M. Raffin, David J. Lilly, Aaron R. Thornton, *Journal of Speech and Hearing Research*, Vol. 19 No. 4, December 1976. ©1976 Journal of Speech and Hearing Research.

must assign an increasingly larger number to its position (Sayers, 1964; Sayers and Lynn, 1968; Sayers and Toole, 1964; Toole and Sayers, 1965). The centering method utilizes the ability of a listener to offset an interaural intensity difference by an opposing interaural time difference to produce a sound image perceived in the center of the head (Blodgett, Wilbanks, and Jeffress, 1956; David, Guttman, and van Bergeijk, 1958, 1959; Deatherage and Hirsh, 1959; Harris, 1960; Shaxby and Gage, 1932). This method yields a traditional measure of binaural interaction—the binaural trading ratio. This ratio is determined by the interaural time difference necessary to cancel a given interaural intensity advantage. Computationally, the binaural trading ratio (in μsec/dB) provides a measure of interaural time divided by an equally effective amount of interaural intensity.

David et al. (1959) point out that experimental results obtained with click stimuli cannot be used to predict pure-tone data. The binaural trading ratio for pure tones ranges from 0.3 μsec/dB to 2.5 μsec/dB (Moushegian and Jeffress, 1959; Shaxby and Gage, 1932; Whitworth and Jeffress, 1961). For clicks presented at similar sesnsation levels, the binaural trading ratio falls between 100 and 800 μsec/dB (David et al., 1959).

Implicit in the use of the binaural trading ratio is the assumption that functionally identical values for interaural time difference and interaural intensity difference in some way involve an identical neural representation. Consequently, models of binaural interaction typically postulate a transformation of time and intensity into a single neural code (van Bergeijk, 1962). Support for this view comes from the fact that subjects in some experiments reported hearing a fused auditory image that could be centered with appropriate balance of interaural time differences and interaural intensity differences (David et al., 1959; Harris, 1960).

In exception to this generalization are the data of Banister (1926), Whitworth and Jeffress (1961), and Hafter and Jeffress (1968). When presented with binaural stimuli, their subjects reported hearing two separate images rather than a fused image. One image was amenable to changes in position through interaural intensity differences, whereas the other image was moved principally by changes in interaural time differences. Accordingly, some investigators argue that no combination of interaural time and interaural intensity differences can bring both images to the median plane of the head at the same time (Gilliom and Sorkin, 1972; Hafter and Carrier, 1972). Hafter and Jeffress (1968) propose that subjects (in experiments whose results indicate the perception of a single image) might actually hear two images but, owing to the nature of the instructions, center on only one of the images.

Clinically, only the lateralization produced by an interaural intensity difference has been incorporated into an audiometric test. When Stenger (1900, 1907) presented identical tones to the two ears of listeners with normal hearing, they reported the presence of a sound image in the median plane. When the intensity of the signal presented to one ear was increased, while the intensity of the signal presented to the other ear remained unchanged, the signal appeared to lateralize completely to the ear receiving the more intense signal. Under these conditions, most listeners were unable to discern whether the less intense signal was present or absent. This effect commonly is referred to as the Stenger effect.

The Stenger test is particularly valuable for patients who exhibit unilateral hearing loss with no evidence of organic disease (Politzer, 1909; Priest, 1945). Unfortunately, this procedure is not applicable for all patients with unilateral hearing impairment. Patients with diplacusis binauralis, for example, often are unable to demonstrate the Stenger effect for pure tones. Moreover, the pure-tone Stenger procedure can yield spurious test data with some clinical audiometers that use a separate oscillator for each channel. If these two oscillators are not phase locked, binaural beats may be perceived when the signals (nominally at the same frequency) are presented simultaneously to both ears (Hopkinson, 1972). To circumvent these potential problems, the pure-tone Stenger test has been modified so that speech may be used as the test stimulus (Johnson, Work, and McCoy, 1956; Taylor, 1949).

For most patients, the conventional (intensive) pure-tone or speech Stenger tests can provide evidence regarding the existence of unilateral nonorganic hearing loss (Menzel, 1962). In addition, these tests can be used to estimate the magnitude of the nonorganic component for some patients (Menzel, 1960, 1965). Ventry and Chaiklin (1965), however, have shown that the intensive Stenger procedures are most valuable for the patient who exhibits a large difference between auditory threshold in the better ear and alleged threshold in the poorer ear.

Our review of the literature failed to reveal any time-intensity trade experiment for speech. Published research for noise, for clicks and for pure tones, however, suggests that it should be possible to demonstrate a time-intensity trade for speech signals. If interaural time differences and interaural intensity differences both affect the apparent location of the speech signal within the head, and if the image is fused, then a clinical application of these phenomena may be realized. Specifically, systematic manipulation of interaural time differences for speech may be used to circumvent some of the problems inherent to the conventional intensive Stenger test.

Any investigation of the time-intensity trade for speech, however, must be designed to evaluate also the presence of a potential "ear effect." For example, if time-intensity trade data for speech signals vary according to which ear is stimulated first, then a straightforward clinical application of this time-intensity trade might be difficult. Kimura (1961a, b) found a right-ear superiority for recall of verbal material. Additional research documents the predominance of right-ear scores over left-ear scores in the recognition of dichotically presented speech for right-handed individuals (Bartz et al., 1967; Berlin et al., 1973; Broadbent and Gregory, 1964; Bryden, 1963; Cooper et al., 1967; Gerber and Goldman, 1971; Lowe-Bell et al., 1970; Satz et al., 1965; Studdert-Kennedy and Shankweiler, 1970). Other studies show a failure of left-handed listeners to demonstrate a preference for either ear, which may relate, in part, to the fact that left-handed individuals may show mixed cerebral dominance for speech (Benton, 1970; Branch, Milner, and Rasmussen, 1964; Cyr, Daniloff, and Berry, 1971; Hecaen and Ajuriguerra, 1964; Knox and Boone, 1970; Penfield and Roberts, 1959).

Because the present experiment is concerned with potential clinical application of the time-intensity trade for speech, lateralization produced by interaural time disparities will be referred to as a "temporal speech–Stenger effect" in the remainder of this report. The primary goals of this experiment were:

1. To determine if a time-intensity trade could be demonstrated for speech signals.
2. To determine whether subjects demonstrate an "ear effect" for the temporal speech–Stenger effect.
3. To determine the magnitude of the interaural time delay that produced maximum lateralization effect while still maintaining the percept of a single fused image.
4. To determine whether the magnitude of the temporal speech–Stenger effect exceeds the uncertainty usually associated with clinical audiometric measurements.
5. To determine whether intrasubject and intersubject variability for the temporal speech–Stenger effect is comparable to corresponding measures obtained for the intensive speech–Stenger effect.

METHOD

Subjects

Five young adults, between 24 and 30 years of age, were selected as subjects for this study. All subjects had equal air- and bone-conduction thresholds of 10 dB hearing level (HL) (ANSI, 1969) or less at octave frequencies from 250 through 4000 Hz. Air-conduction thresholds for these subjects also were 10 dB HL or less for 125, 1500, 3000, 6000, and 8000 Hz. In addition, the speech-reception threshold (SRT) for each subject did not exceed 5 dB HL. No subject had a history of ear disease. Two male subjects and one female subject were right handed. One male and one female were left handed.

Apparatus and Calibration

A speech audiometer (Grason-Stadler, Model 162) was used to determine the SRT for each subject and to control the signal levels in the main experiment. The output of a magnetic tape recorder (Magnecord, Model 1020) was fed to the auxiliary input of the audiometer. All of the data for this experiment were gathered with the subject seated in a double-walled sound-insulated test room (Industrial Acoustics, Model 1204-A). The magnetic tape recorder was calibrated to conform with specifications promulgated by the National Association of Broadcasters (NAB, 1965). One channel of the speech audiometer was fed directly to a dynamic earphone (Telephonics, TDH-39) mounted in a neoprene cushion (Telephonics, MX-41/AR). This channel was designated as the "lagging" channel in the main experiment. The second channel of the speech audiometer was fed to an impedance-matching transformer (United Transformer, Type LS-33), through the experimenter's attenuator, through the subject's attenuator, through a second impedance-matching transformer (United Transformer, LS-33), and then to a second (matched) earphone (Telephonics, TDH-39) mounted in a cushion (Telephonics, MX-41/AR). All of the attenuators used in this experiment were found to be linear ($\pm$ 0.2 dB) within the range of attenuation values required for the study. A remote monitoring circuit, that was part of a method-of-adjustment system, was used to determine the setting on the subject's attenuator.

Selection of Speech Materials

Since the speech–Stenger test often is performed with spondaically stressed CID W-1 words (Hirsh et al., 1952), these words also were used to construct the temporal speech–Stenger test tape. Because of published research indicating that these words were not recorded at equal levels (Lilly, Sung, and Franzen, 1966), and that they are not equally intelligible when presented auditorily (Bowling and Elpern, 1961; Curry and Cox, 1966; Beattie, Svihovec, and Edgerton, 1975), the words *hothouse, drawbridge, northwest, inkwell, farewell,* and *duckpond* were deleted from the master list. The remaining 30 words were used in the recording of our experimental speech–Stenger test tape.

Recording of Speech Materials

Initial Master Tape. A male talker with general American speech was seated in an anechoic chamber as he read the 30 selected W-1 words. A microphone (Bruel and Kjaer, Type 4131) was affixed on a stand 20 cm from the talker's mouth. The output of this microphone was amplified and fed to the input of a 1-dB step attenuator. This attenuator allowed the words to be recorded at a level near 0 VU while the talker maintained a comfortable level of speaking. From the attenuator, the signal was fed to the auxiliary input of the tape recorder. A second VU meter was placed in front of the speaker so that he could monitor himself.

5. REHABILITATION

Experimental Test Tape. Figure 1 is a block diagram of the instrumentation used for recording the temporal speech–Stenger test tape. A tape deck (Sony, Model TC-650) was used to play back the initial master tape. Although the reproduced equalization of this tape deck was calibrated optimally, it met the NAB (1965) frequency-response criteria only for the range from 100 through 7500 Hz.

The output of the tape deck was fed to an attenuator (Hewlett-Packard, Model 350-D), a power amplifier (Langevin, Model AM-50), and then to a

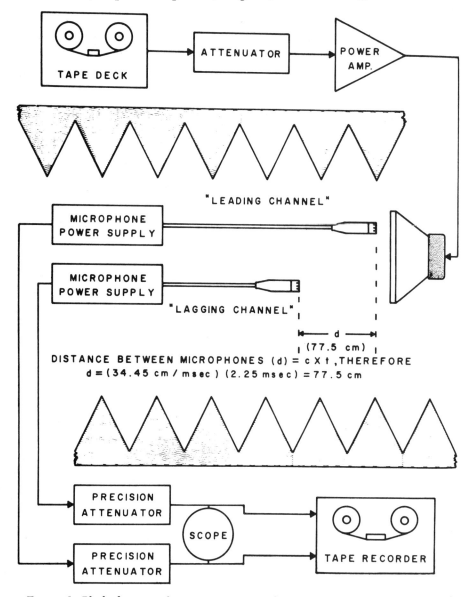

FIGURE 1. Block diagram of instrumentation used for recording the temporal speech–Stenger test tape. Computational example shows approximate distance (d) between the two microphones (77.5 cm) for an interchannel time delay (t) of 2.25 msec. Abbreviation (c) denotes speed of sound in air.

loudspeaker (KLH, Model 32) located within the anechoic chamber. Two microphones (Bruel and Kjaer, Type 4131) with their respective power supplies (Bruel and Kjaer, Type 2801) were used to transduce the acoustic signals from the loudspeaker. The output from each microphone power supply was led out of the chamber through a 0.1-dB step (precision) attenuator to one of the two channels of the tape recorder. These attenuators were used to set the VU meters for each channel to 0 VU for each carrier phrase and for each syllable of each word. The materials thus recorded showed fluctuations no greater than ±0.75 VU.

Deatherage (1966) found that multiple images are perceived when the interaural time delay exceeds 2 msec for nonspeech stimuli. In a pilot study, we found that multiple images were not perceived for speech stimuli until the interaural time delay was 3 msec. In addition, we found that interaural time delays of between 2 and 3 msec produced the maximum lateralization effect. Accordingly, six interaural time delays were chosen for the experiment (0.00, 1.00, 2.00, 2.25, 2.50, and 2.75 msec). For the 0-msec time-delay list, each of the two microphones was placed exactly the same distance from the loudspeaker. A 1000-Hz calibration tone was played through the loudspeaker, and the output of the two microphones was monitored on a dual-beam oscilloscope (Tektronix, Type 502A). This calibration tone also was recorded at 0 VU for each channel. For each subsequent list, as the interchannel time delay increased, one of the microphones was moved further away from the loudspeaker. This microphone (the lower one in Figure 1) and its associated channel on the tape recorder was defined as the "lagging channel." The position of the upper microphone in Figure 1 remained fixed. This microphone and its associated channel was defined as the "leading channel."

The distance between the two microphones was computed for each time delay. An example of this computation is provided in Figure 1 for the 2.25-msec interchannel time delay. When each experimental test list was recorded, the relative interchannel phase of the 1000-Hz calibration tone always was used to adjust precisely each interchannel time delay. Identification phrases for each time-delay list later were spliced to the beginning of each list. The calibration tone recorded at 0 VU was spliced to the beginning of the experimental test tape.

Procedure

A method of adjustment was used to gather data for the experiment. Each subject was instructed to adjust the image of a speech stimulus until it was perceived to be in the center of his head. These adjustments were made by controlling the level of the signal in the leading channel. In addition, each subject was instructed to report immediately any confusion in image localization or the perception of multiple images. After each trial, the subject reset his attenuator knob to some random position chosen by the experimenter. The settings of the experimenter's attenuators also were chosen at random within a range of values that would allow for median-plane localization (within the subject's attenuator range). Resetting the subject's attenuator after each trial also helped to minimize positional references that the subject might have established for the knob.

The channel in which the stimulus lagged was chosen as the reference channel. Each of the time delays (0.00, 1.00, 2.00, 2.25, 2.50, and 2.75 msec) was presented at 10, 25, 40, 55, and 70 dB HL. For each of the 30 resulting conditions, each subject was given five trials for the right ear leading and five trials for the left ear leading. For all trials, the same earphone was used with the leading channel. Each subject, therefore, completed the experiment after 300 judgments of median-plane localization. The choices of leading ear, time delay, and level of presentation in the reference channel were each selected at random for each subject.

RESULTS

Table 1 provides a summary of the group data. Means, standard deviations, and ranges are listed for all experimental conditions. To determine the interactions of time delay, level of presentation, and ear effect, two four-way (time delay × level of presentation × ear × subject) analyses of variance

5. REHABILITATION

TABLE 1. Summary of group data, obtained on five normal-hearing listeners.

Interaural Time Delay (msec)	Level of Presentation (dB HL)	Mean (dB)	Standard Deviation	Range
0.00	10	1.4	1.31	−0.1– 3.1
	25	1.0	0.69	0.1– 1.6
	40	1.2	0.53	0.5– 1.9
	55	1.2	0.84	0.2– 2.1
	70	1.2	1.85	−0.2– 4.3
1.00	10	7.0	2.02	4.2– 9.6
	25	14.0	2.42	12.2–18.2
	40	17.3	4.01	14.6–24.0
	55	20.2	3.70	15.7–25.7
	70	20.4	5.09	16.4–29.2
2.00	10	9.7	0.61	9.1–10.4
	25	18.96	2.83	14.7–22.4
	40	21.5	2.54	18.6–25.2
	55	23.7	1.45	22.3–26.0
	70	26.9	5.79	21.8–36.8
2.25	10	9.94	1.27	8.8–12.1
	25	21.5	1.89	18.4–23.4
	40	25.6	1.48	23.3–27.0
	55	27.3	0.77	26.8–28.5
	70	29.9	5.16	26.3–38.9
2.50	10	6.6	1.38	4.4– 8.2
	25	15.9	3.26	12.3–19.7
	40	18.4	3.30	15.4–22.5
	55	23.2	1.81	20.1–24.6
	70	28.7	6.02	23.0–36.7
2.75	10	5.58	1.74	3.7– 8.2
	25	11.6	2.21	10.0–15.5
	40	15.5	1.89	12.7–18.0
	55	18.2	1.30	16.3–19.9
	70	24.1	7.97	15.8–37.3

(ANOVAs) (Lindquist, 1956; Winer 1962) were computed using the Statistical Analysis System (Service, 1972). A 0.01 level of confidence for these analyses was chosen prior to the collection of data. Because the data from published research were inconclusive with regard to the left-ear dominance for left-handed individuals, it was decided that the first ANOVA would be computed with the ear variable defined as the right versus the left ear for all listeners ($df = 20{,}80$; $F = 0.709$; $p < 0.8062$). For the second ANOVA, the ear variable was defined as the dominant versus the nondominant ear based on the individual's handedness ($df = 20{,}80$; $F = 1.476$; $p < 0.1136$). The results of the ANOVA for simple effects also failed to demonstrate the presence of an ear effect ($df = 1{,}4$; $F = 0.618$; $p < 0.5208$) for the task of median-plane localization using speech signals.

The results of three-way analyses of variance (time delay × level of presentation × subject) revealed a time delay by level of presentation interaction. As a result of this significant interaction ($df = 20.80$; $F = 10.612$; $p < 0.0001$), additional ANOVAs were computed (Myers, 1973). These analyses revealed that the introduction of a time delay produces a significant effect ($p < 0.0002$) at each level of presentation, and that there was no effect of level of presentation with a time delay of 0.00 msec. For all other interaural time delays, a significant effect was noted ($p < 0.0004$).

The group data also are plotted in Figures 2 and 3. Figure 2 shows the interaural intensity difference (IID, in dB) required to obtain an image localized in the median plane as a function of level of presentation (in dB HL) for each interaural time delay (ITD, in msec). The effect is negligible at a time delay of 0.00 msec regardless of level of presentation. For all other time delays, the magnitude of the effect increases with level of presentation. At 10 dB HL, the magnitude of the ITD effect is between 5 and 10 dB. It was not expected that this magnitude would exceed 10 dB at 10 dB HL, since an effect greater than 10 dB would have required the signal in the leading channel to be attenuated to some infrathreshold level. Although the ITD effect tends to increase with level of presentation, the effect asymptotes at 55 dB HL with an interaural time delay of 1.00 msec.

Figure 3 shows the magnitude of the effect (the interaural intensity difference required to obtain an image localized in the median plane) as a function of interaural time delay (in msec) for each level of presentation (in dB HL). It should be noted that for all levels of presentation, a maximum effect occurs at 2.25-msec time delay. At this interaural time delay, a mean effect of about 30 dB was obtained at 70 dB HL in the reference ear. The magnitude of the effect increases slowly from 0.00 to 2.25 msec interaural time delay and then decreases rapidly with larger interaural time delays. This pattern was noted for all levels of presentation.

To determine whether the maximum effect (for an interaural time delay of 2.25 msec at each level of presentation) was significantly greater than the effect obtained with the other time delays, a Tukey Studentized range technique (Tukey, 1949) at the 0.05 level of confidence was computed. This technique is used to calculate a "critical difference" between means against which

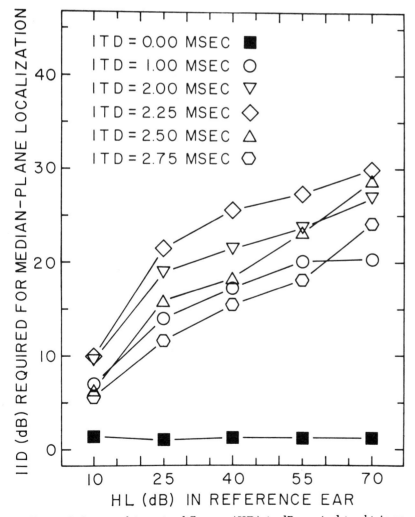

FIGURE 2. Interaural intensity difference (IID) in dB required to obtain an image localized in the median plane as a function of level of presentation in dB hearing level (HL) in the reference (lagging) ear for each interaural time delay (ITD).

5. REHABILITATION

the differences between means for each interaural time delay may be compared. The results of this analysis are found in the Appendix. The critical difference for each level of presentation is indicated in parentheses. It may be noted that at 10 dB HL, there is no significant difference in the effect at the 2.00-msec time delay and the effect at the 2.25-msec time delay. However, the magnitudes of the effect noted at these time delays both are greater than

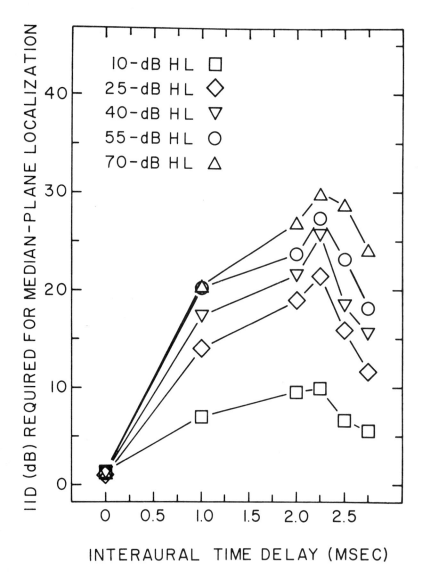

FIGURE 3. Interaural intensity difference (IID) in dB required to obtain an image localized in the median plane as a function of interaural time delay (in msec) for each level of presentation in dB hearing level (HL) in the reference (lagging) ear.

those obtained at the other time delays. Again, at 25 dB HL, the 2.25-msec time delay shows an effect which is not significantly greater than that obtained with the 2.00-msec time delay. At 40 dB HL, the magnitude of the effect obtained at the 2.25-msec time delay is greater than that obtained at any other interaural time delay. Similar results were observed at 55 dB HL. At 70 dB HL, however, the magnitude of the effect is not significantly greater at a time delay of 2.25-msec than it is at the 2.00, the 2.50, or the 2.75-msec time delay. The appendix also reveals that, regardless of the level of presentation, all interaural time delays produce a significant effect compared to the results obtained with the 0.00-msec time delay.

All subjects reported hearing multiple images at 2.75-msec interaural time delay. Specifically, subjects reported hearing the speech signal at the ears while simultaneously hearing it "inside the head." Two subjects reported hearing multiple images at an interaural time delay of 2.50 msec at 55 and 70 dB HL. No subject reported the perception of multiple images at any of the levels of presentation for an interaural time delay of 2.25 msec.

The present study also was designed to investigate selected aspects of the intensive speech–Stenger effect. Specifically, when the interaural time delay was 0.00 msec, any lateralization of the signal could be attributed only to differences in interaural intensity. Examination of the bottom curve in Figure 2 shows that, on the average, the subjects in the present study achieved a median-plane localized image with interaural intensity differences of less than 2 dB when the interaural time difference was 0.00 msec.

Data obtained at 0.00-msec interaural time delay also permitted us to compare intrasubject and intersubject variability for the intensive speech–Stenger effect with that obtained for the maximum temporal speech–Stenger effect (2.25-msec interaural time delay). A test described by Walker and Lev (1953, p. 205) for the comparison of two variances based on related scores was used. It was found that neither the intrasubject variance nor the intersubject variance differed significantly ($p < 0.05$) for the intensive speech–Stenger or for the temporal speech–Stenger.

DISCUSSION

The results of the present experiment indicate that an interaural time advantage to one ear may be offset by an interaural intensity advantage to the other ear for speech stimuli. These findings are in agreement with the results of published research using nonspeech stimuli (Deatherage and Hirsh, 1959; Pinheiro and Tobin, 1969).

A maximum temporal speech–Stenger effect was observed with an interaural time delay of 2.25 msec. This interaural time delay did not produce the perception of multiple images. Other investigators (Deatherage, 1966; Harris, 1960) suggested that, with nonspeech stimuli, multiple images are perceived with interaural time delays greater than 2 msec.

The results obtained in the present study, at 2.25-msec interaural time delay, yield binaural trading ratios of approximately 75 μsec/dB at 70 dB HL, 105 μsec/dB at 25 dB HL, and 226 μsec/dB at 10 dB HL. The binaural trading ratio computed in this experiment at 70 dB HL (75 μsec/dB) is greater than the 25 μsec/dB calculated for high-pass filtered noise bursts at a comparable level (David et al., 1959). The binaural trading ratio computed for the present experiment at 25 dB HL (105 μsec/dB) is only slightly larger than the binaural trading ratio reported by Harris (1960). At 20 dB SL, he computed a binaural trading ratio of 90 μsec/dB for high-pass filtered clicks. The results of the present study for low-level signals also may be compared with the results presented by David et al. (1959). For high-pass filtered noise bursts, presented at 10 dB SL, they computed a binaural trading ratio of 200 μsec/dB. For speech stimuli presented at 10 dB HL, a binaural trading ratio of 226 μsec/dB was computed from the data of the present investigation.

Changes in the binaural trading ratio for speech signals, as a function of level of presentation, agree with the patterns observed for noise bursts and pure tones. That is, as the level of presentation increases, the binaural trading ratio decreases (David et al., 1959; Deatherage and Hirsh, 1959). Differences in the absolute values of the binaural trading ratios of this experiment and those of experiments using nonspeech stimuli may be attributed to differences

5. REHABILITATION

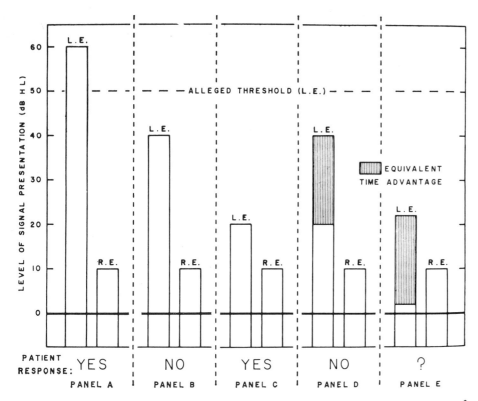

FIGURE 4. Hypothetical clinical situations that might arise during the administration of a speech–Stenger procedure to a patient. In this example the patient's hypothetical thresholds are assumed to be 0 dB hearing level (HL) bilaterally. The patient, however, gave speech reception thresholds of 0-dB HL for the right ear (R.E.), and 50-dB HL for the left ear (L.E.). Panels A, B, and C refer to the hypothetical results that might be obtained with the conventional (intensive) speech–Stenger procedure. Panels D and E refer to hypothetical results that might be obtained with the temporal speech–Stenger procedure. A time advantage of 20 dB is assumed (a time advantage of at least 22 dB was computed from the results of the present experiment).

in the nature of the stimuli used (speech versus nonspeech) or to differences in the calibration reference levels (SL versus HL for pure tones versus HL for speech).

For a time delay of 2.25 msec, none of the subjects showed a range of scores greater than 10 dB. If the uncertainty usually associated with clinical audiometric measurement is assumed to be ± 5 dB, then none of the subjects exhibited greater variability with the maximum temporal speech–Stenger effect (2.25 msec interaural time delay) than might be expected for other clinical audiometric procedures. Furthermore, since the magnitude of the maximum temporal speech–Stenger effect is at least 22 dB (at 25-dB HL), we suggest that the magnitude of the maximum temporal speech–Stenger effect exceeds the uncertainty usually associated with clinical audiometric measurements. An increase in intrasubject and intersubject variability, however, coincided with the reported perception of multiple images. It appears that the presence of perceived multiple images contributes some confusion to the task of median-plane localization. Neither intrasubject nor intersubject variability for the maximum temporal speech–Stenger effect was greater than comparable measures for the intensive speech–Stenger effect.

Because the magnitude of the maximum temporal speech–Stenger effect is greater than the uncertainty usually associated with clinical audiometric measurements, and since neither intrasubject nor intersubject variability is greater than that obtained with the intensive speech–Stenger effect, an investigation of the maximum temporal speech–Stenger effect for clinical applications appears warranted. In addition, it may be advisable to verify the magnitude of the temporal speech–Stenger effect with a large number of subjects (only five subjects were used in the present experiment) suitably matched to patient groups. It also may be necessary to investigate whether interaural time and interaural intensity differences are additive.

A Potential Clinical Application

The intensive speech–Stenger test often is used clinically to help determine whether a unilateral hearing impairment is nonorganic. If interaural time and interaural intensity effects are additive, it may be possible to combine both effects and thus produce a clinical speech–Stenger procedure that is more sensitive than the intensive speech–Stenger test. This potential clinical application is illustrated in Figure 4. The five panels in Figure 4 depict hypothetical clinical situations that might arise during the administration of a speech–Stenger procedure to a hypothetical patient. For the purposes of this example, it is assumed that the patient has given threshold responses of 50 dB HL in his left ear (LE) and 0-dB HL in his right ear (RE). With the intensive speech–Stenger test, a signal often is presented simultaneously to both ears at some level above the patient's alleged speech-reception thresholds. In Panel A of Figure 4, both signals are presented at 10 dB SL. If the threshold in his left ear actually is 0 dB HL, the patient perceives the signal primarily in the left ear. Since this signal is at a level greater than his claimed threshold, he probably will respond. When the level of the signal in the left ear is decreased to 40 dB HL, while the signal level in the right ear remains unchanged (as shown in Panel B of Figure 4), the patient still perceives the signal essentially in his left ear. However, the patient now may realize that the signal level is below his alleged threshold, and he probably will not respond (even though a signal still is present in his right ear at 10 dB SL). As the level of the signal in the left ear is decreased to a point where the interaural intensity difference is between 10 and 30 dB, the patient may perceive a signal in his right ear. When this happens, then he may again begin to respond. This hypothetical situation is represented in Panel C of Figure 4. It is at this point that the examiner must estimate the patient's actual threshold when only the intensive speech–Stenger effect is used. Now, if the interaural intensity difference favoring the left ear is 10 dB (for example), if an interaural time delay of 2.25 msec is introduced to the right ear, and if the two are additive, then the patient again will perceive the signal in the left ear (and may not be aware of the suprathreshold signal in the right ear). This condition is illustrated in Panel D of Figure 4. The shaded area represents the equivalent interaural time advantage in dB. Finally, Panel E of Figure 4 suggests that the signal level in the left ear may be reduced to near actual threshold before the patient detects the suprathreshold signal in the right ear and begins to respond. Thus with the application of the temporal speech–Stenger effect, it may be possible to reduce the amount by which the examiner must estimate the patient's actual threshold.

INDEX

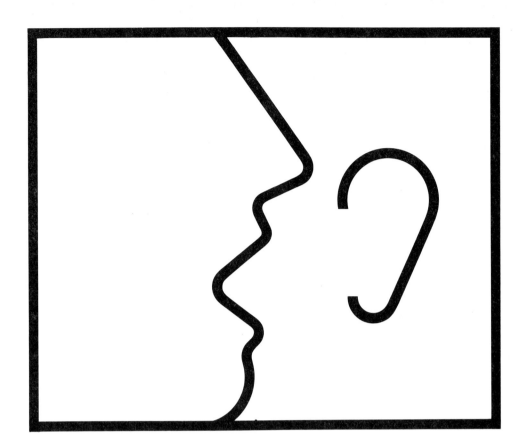

acculturation mode, 205
Acoupedic Program,The (Denver), 5
acquisition, of language and speech, 12
  of esohpageal speech subsequent to
  learning pharyngeal speech, 86-89
active treatment, 15
air injection, 87
alaryngeal speech, 86, 87
Alaska, 14
Alexander Graham Bell Association, 5
alveolar pressure, 69
American Indians hearing loss, 14
American Organization for the Education of
  the Hearing Impaired, 153
American Sign Language, 161-166
American Speech and Hearing Association,
  123
Ameslan, 162
  signs, 163
amplification, 5, 10, 13
  devices, 39
  early, 11, 12
  opposition to early, 14
  wide range, 11
ancillary paramedical personnel, 15
aphasia, 59 103-107, 110-117, 124-128
  definition, 103
  motor, 104
  sensory, 103
apraxia, 76
articulation, 112

Articulation Test, 122
Association Method, The, 40
attention span, 7
audiogram, 6, 17
audiological services, 15
audiologist 13, 15, 21, 121, 194
audiometric data, 33
audiometric techniques, 104
audiometry, 15
audition, 10
auditory approach, 4, 10-20, 16
auditory behavior, 23
auditory behavior response, 21-24
Auditory Discrimination test, 122
auditory dysfunction, 32-37
auditory figure ground, 110
auditory/oral program, 152-155
auditory perception, 110
auditory processing, 5
auditory recall, 111
auditory skills, 144
auditory stimuli, 38, 204
auditory system, 17
auditory techniques, 12
auditory training, 11, 12, 26, 27, 38-41, 39,
  149, 177
  early, 18, 41
  at home, 25-28, 26
aural behavior, 21
aural training, 8
autistic, 161-166

autistic children and their mothers, 133-138
background noise, 7
Bekesy, sweep-frequency audiometry, 32
  fixed-frequency audiometry, 33, 34
Berrien Springs, 16
binaural hearing aids, 13
binaural system, 9
binaural trading ratio, 227
Binet Intelligence Scale, 209
body language, 94
brain injury, 120
breathing exercises, 112
breathstream, 70
Brown, Constance, Hearing and Speech, 15
Bureau of Education for the Handicapped,
  222

Caesar, Julius, 214
captioned ABC News, 221
carrier wave transmission, 29
Central Institute for the Deaf, 103
central nervous system, 103
cerebral dominance, 76
cerebral palsy, 120, 211
Child, Julia, 224
Churchill, Winston, 108
cleft lip, 120
cleft palate, 120
cochlear dysfunction, 32
cochlear structures, 32
Columbia-Presbyterian Medical Center, 215

communication, 59
  ability, 146
  deficiencies, 204-210
Concorde, 214
consonant injection, 87
Cooke, Alistair, 108

deaf as a bilingual person, 41
deaf infant, 21
decibel, 104, 203, 214
developmental criteria, 21
diplacusis binauralis, 227
discoordination of phonation with articulation and respiration, 68-77
disfluencies, 79, 80
dysacusic children, 110-117
dysarthria, 59, 76
dyslexic children, 213

early detection, 10
early intervention, 5
  infant, 11
earmold fitting, 15
Education of the Handicapped Act, 224
educational planning, 106
electret microphone, 16
electro-acoustic modification, 30 184
electrodermal (EDR), 103
electroencephalic responses,(EER), 103
element association method, 179
encouraging normal speech, 119
environmental noises, 39
Eskimo, 16
esophageal sound, 87
esophageal speech classes, 87
esophagus, 87
expressive language, 218

Fay, Dr. Thomas H., 215
female language, 129-132
Folk-Linguistics, 129-132
Franklin, Benjamin, 109
fundamental frequency, 89
fused image, 228
future efforts, 41

Gallaudet College, 222
galvanic skin resistance, 103
Gentile study, The, 19
gesuural mode, 206
glossal press, 87
glottal airflow, 69

headphones, 30
HEAR Foundation, 11
HEAR Training Unit, 12
hearing aids, 5, 6, 9, 11, 14, 16, 26, 142, 184-191, 192-194
  battery type, 143
  literature, 31
  longitudinal study, 184-191
  receivers, 30
  repair, 15
  types of, 193
  use of, 105
hearing impaired child, 4-9, 167
  severely hearing impaired, 13
  infants, 142
hearing impairment, 167-174

hearing screening programs, 13
Hearing Test, 122
hearing therapists, 121
Heathrow Airport, 216
how to protect your hearing, 202-203

inductance loop amplification, 29
infant hearing screening clinic, 22
influence of environment, 199
information processing, 167-174
inheritance, 11
integrated preschool, 142
intellectual training, 8
intelligibility, 88
intensity, 110
interaural time delay, 228
intervention techniques, 218
intonation, 94, 150
intraoral pressure, 87
intrasubject variability, 228

jaw exercises, 112
Jespersen, Otto, 129

Kaiser-Permanente Foundation, 203
Kleffner, Dr. Frank, 103
Kostic, Dr. Djordje, 11

language, 177
  and communication, 41
  and reading, 180
  development, 117
  disability, 103
  expressive, 20
  learning, 30
Language Development Test, 122
language methodology, 134
language screening, 15
laryngeal reflex, 76
larynx, 120
lateral lisps, 59-62
lateralization, 227
learned speech, 110
learning disability, 12
learning to listen, 142-148
Lindsay, John, 108
linguistic components of language, 149
linguistic performance, 133
linguistic production in schizophrenic mothers, 135
linguistic stereotypes, 129-132
lip exercises, 112
lipped speech, 70
lipread, 69
  artificial lipreading, 178
loop auditory training systems, 29-31
low frequency amplification, 17

malocclusion, 120
manual symbols, 12
maternal rubella, 6, 11, 23
McGinnis, Mildred, 40
mean length of utterance (MLU), 135
memory span, 145
Meniere's disease, 203
methodology, 23, 116-117, 169, 196-197
  research, 218
Metropolitan Toronto School for the Deaf, 5
middle ear, 203

Midland School of New Jersey, 110
Minnesota, Picture Vocabulary Test (MPVT), 100
misarticulation, 60
"Mommy Talk," 129-132
monolingual children, 116
monosyllables, 39
Mother Tongue, 108-109
motor aphasia, 103
motor incoordination, 103
multisensory approach, 25
Myklebust, Dr. Helmer, 103

National Association for Hearing and Speech Action, 194
National Bureau of Standards, 222
National Film Board of Canada, 225
National Institute of Occupational Safety and Health, 215
New Jersey State Health Department, 108
neck-type electrolarynx, 87
neoglottis, 87, 88
nerve deafness, 203
noise, 214-216
noise-induced hearing loss, 32-37
normal development of speech, 118
normality, 5, 9
normal learning environment, 5
normal speech, 5

operant behavior, 115
operant conditioning, 117
optimal language learning, 13
oral articulatory movements, 69
oral methods, 10
organic problems, 120
otologists, 194
otosclerosis, 203

palatal paresis, 87
pantomimed speech, 68
parent-child relationships, 122
parent-infant programs, 13
parental interaction, 147
parental involvement, 16
pharyngeal fistula, 87
pharynx, 86
phonation, 69, 150
phonemes, 69, 150
phonetic articulation, 70
phonetic association, 126
phonetically balanced words, 104
Phonologic prosthesis, 205
phonology, 149
physical exercises, 112
physiologic and aerodynamic analysis of stuttering, 68
Picture Vocabulary Test (PPVT), 100
pitch, 26, 70, 71, 110, 203
play therapy, 105
Porch Index of Communication Ability, 127
postsurgical complications, 87
Premack's system, 207
preschool hearing impaired, 29-31
prevention, 15
profanity, 131
prosthetic methods, 205
prosthetic training, 205
psycholinguistic research, 133

Public Broadcasting Service (PBS), 222
pure-tone thresholds, 33

reading lips, 168
receptive language, 218
receptive learning, 177
recognition of verbal labels of pictured
    objects, 195-201
Regional Conference on the Auditory
    Approach, 10
regular classes, 18
    classroom teacher, 19
    school, 19
rehabilitation, 15
reinforcers, 115
research in deaf education, 14
residual hearing, 10, 13, 25, 26, 28, 31,
    40, 41
    maximizing, 40
responding behavior, 135
response recording, 22
retarded deaf children, 206
rock music concerts, 203

Schafer, R. Murray, 215
schizophrenia, 133
self-correction, 120
self-reinforcement, 54
semantic association, 126
sense of touch, 26
sensorineural loss, 11
sequence of words, 145
severely retarded, 217-220
similar phrases, 28
social behavior, 142
social development, 176
socioacusis, 214
songs, 96
sound stimuli, 115
special education, 211-213
speech, 8, 17, 41, 124, 177
    causation, 120
    deviation, 59

disability, 103
natural, 18
pathologists, 21, 59
pathology, 60
rhythm, 26
screening, 15
tests, 34
therapy, 79, 156-160
speech and hearing clinic, 143
speech discrimination tests, 35
    scores, 36
speech-language dichotomy, 149
speech materials, 229-230
speech motor skills, 112
speech reception threshold, 114-117
speech sounds, 119
speech therapists, 121, 122, 123
stimuli, 22
stuttering, 54, 59, 63-67, 68-77, 71, 78-85
subtitles for TV and films, 221-225
subglottic respiratory processes, 69
syntax, 150
synthetic mode, 206

tangible reinforcement, 114-117
Tangible Reinforcement Operant Condition-
    ing Auditometry (TROCA), 115
target behaviors, 217
teachers of deaf, 21
teaching aural language, 149-155
teaching language for the severely retarded,
    207
teaching methods, 105
teaching the nonverbal child, 176-181
tempo, 110
temporal patterning, 40
Temporal Speech-Stenger Effect, 226
thematic summaries, 100
therapy, 8, 86
Thorndike and Lorge, 63
throat, 120
time-intensity, 226-237

time sequence, 165
tongue, 86, 87
tongue exercises, 112
tongue thrust, 44-53
Tracy Clinic, 106
tympanometry, 15

unisensory approach, 5
University of Minnesota Speech and Hearing
    Clinic, 50
University of Southern California Center for
    the Study of Communicative Disorders, 72
University of Washington Regional Primate
    Center, 211

velum, 87
verbal behavior, 78, 128
verbal communication, 7
verbal elaboration, 100
verbal interaction, 146
verbal-tangible reward, 78-85
vicarious punishment, 54-58
videofluoros copy, 87
video measures, use of, 73
videotapes, use of, 55
Vidifont, 223
vision, 25
visually presented picture and word stimuli,
    167-174
vocabulary development, 119
vocabulary development of educable re-
    tarded children, 100-102
vocal tract, 70
    movements, 69
voice production exercises, 112

Waardenburg's syndrome, 23
Washington University of St. Louis, 216
Wechsler Intelligence Scale, 209
Wedenberg, Erik, 40
whispering, 68, 72
word-association task, 54
word-frequency level, 65, 66, 67
word retrieval, 124-128

STAFF

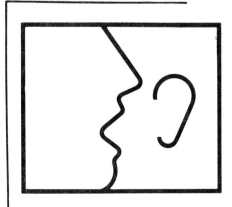

Publisher	John Quirk
Editor	Dona Chiappe
Editorial Ass't.	Carol Carr
Permissions Editor	Audrey Weber
Director of Production	Richard Pawlikowski
Director of Design	Donald Burns
Customer Service	Cindy Finocchio
Sales Service	Diane Hubbard
Administration	Linda Calano
Index	Mary Russell

Cover Design

Li Bailey of Enoch and Eisenman Inc. New York City.

Appendix: Agencies and Services for Exceptional Children

Alexander Graham Bell Association for the Deaf,
Inc.
Volta Bureau for the Deaf
3417 Volta Place, NW
Washington, D.C. 20007

American Academy of Pediatrics
1801 Hinman Avenue
Evanston, Illinois 60204

American Association for Gifted Children
15 Gramercy Park
New York, N.Y. 10003

American Association on Mental Deficiency
5201 Connecticut Avenue, NW
Washington, D.C. 20015

American Association of Psychiatric Clinics for
Children
250 West 57th Street
New York, N.Y.

American Bar Association
Commission on the Mentally Disabled
1800 M Street, NW
Washington, D.C. 20036

American Foundation for the Blind
15 W. 16th Street
New York, N.Y. 10011

American Medical Association
535 N. Dearborn Street
Chicago, Illinois 60610

American Speech and Hearing Association
9030 Old Georgetown Road
Washington, D.C. 20014

Association for the Aid of Crippled Children
345 E. 46th Street
New York, N.Y. 10017

Association for Children with Learning Disabilities
5200 Brownsville Road
Pittsburgh, Pennsylvania 15210

Association for Education of the Visually
Handicapped
1604 Spruce Street
Philadelphia, Pennsylvania 19103

Association for the Help of Retarded Children
200 Park Avenue, South
New York, N.Y.

Association for the Visually Handicapped
1839 Frankfort Avenue
Louisville, Kentucky 40206

Center on Human Policy
Division of Special Education and Rehabilitation
Syracuse University
Syracuse, New York 13210

Child Fund
15 Windsor Street
Hartford, Connecticut 06120

Children's Defense Fund
120 New Hampshire Avenue NW
Washington, D.C. 20036

Closer Look
National Information Center for the Handicapped
1201 Sixteenth Street NW
Washington, D.C. 20036

Clifford W. Beers Guidance Clinic
432 Temple Street
New Haven, Connecticut 06510

Child Study Center
Yale University
333 Cedar Street
New Haven, Connecticut 06520

Child Welfare League of America, Inc.
44 East 23rd Street
New York, N.Y. 10010

Children's Bureau
United States Department of Health, Education
and Welfare
Washington, D.C.

Council for Exceptional Children
1411 Jefferson Davis Highway
Arlington, Virginia 22202

Epilepsy Foundation of America
1828 "L" Street NW
Washington, D.C. 20036

Gifted Child Society, Inc.
59 Glen Gray Road
Oakland, New Jersey 07436

Institute for the Study of Mental Retardation
and Related Disabilities
130 South First
University of Michigan
Ann Arbor, Michigan 48108

International Association for the Scientific Study
of Mental Deficiency
Ellen Horn, AAMD
5201 Connecticut Avenue NW
Washington, D.C. 20015

International League of Societies for the Mentally
Handicapped
Rue Forestiere 12
Brussels, Belgium

Joseph P. Kennedy, Jr. Foundation
1701 K Street NW
Washington, D.C. 20006

League for Emotioally Disturbed Children
171 Madison Avenue
New York, N.Y.

Muscular Dystrophy Associations of America
1790 Broadway
New York, N.Y. 10019

National Aid to the Visually Handicapped
3201 Balboa Street
San Francisco, California 94121

National Association of Coordinators of State
Programs for the Mentally Retarded
2001 Jefferson Davis Highway
Arlington, Virginai 22202

National Association of Hearing and Speech
Agencies
919 18th Street NW
Washington, D.C. 20006

National Association for Creative Children and
Adults
8080 Springvalley Drive
Cincinnati, Ohio 45236
(Mrs. Ann F. Isaacs, Executive Director)

National Association for Retarded Children
420 Lexington Avenue
New York, N.Y.

National Association for Retarded Citizens
2709 Avenue E East
Arlington, Texas 76010

National Children's Rehabilitation Center
P.O. Box 1260
Leesburg, Virginia

National Association for the Visually Handicapped
3201 Balboa Street
San Francisco, California 94121

National Association of the Deaf
814 Thayer Avenue
Silver Spring, Maryland 20910

National Cystic Fibrosis Foundation
3379 Peachtree Road NE
Atlanta, Georgia 30326

National Easter Seal Society for Crippled Children
and Adults
2023 W. Ogden Avenue
Chicago, Illinois 60612

National Federation of the Blind
218 Randolph Hotel
Des Moines, Iowa 50309

National Paraplegia Foundation
333 N. Michigan Avenue
Chicago, Illinois 60601

National Society for Autistic Children
621 Central Avenue
Albany, N.Y. 12206

National Society for Prevention of Blindness, Inc.
79 Madison Avenue
New York, N.Y. 10016

Orton Society, Inc.
8415 Bellona Lane
Baltimore, Maryland 21204

President's Committee on Mental Retardation
Regional Office Building #3
7th and D Streets SW
Room 2614
Washington, D.C. 20201

United Cerebral Palsy Associations
66 E 34th Street
New York, N.Y. 10016

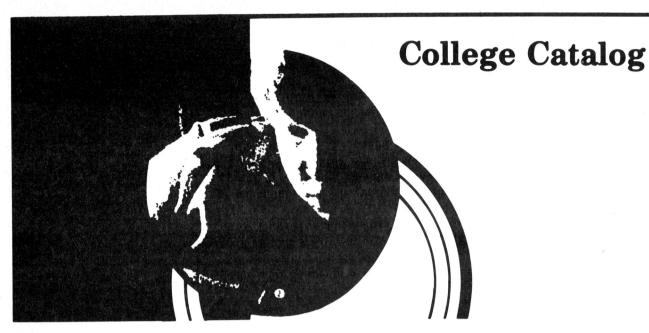

College Catalog

SPECIAL LEARNING CORPORATION

The Special Learning Corporation has developed a series of readers designed for the college student in preparation for teaching exceptional children. Each reader in this high quality series closely follows a college course of study in the special education field. Sending for our free college catalog will provide you with a complete listing of this series, along with a selection of instructional materials and media appropriate for use in special education.

For further information please contact:

College Catalog Division
Special Learning Corporation

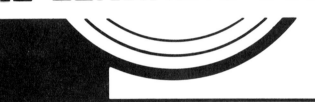

SPECIAL LEARNING CORPORATION
42 Boston Post Rd. Guilford, Conn. 06437

1978 Catalog
SPECIAL LEARNING CORPORATION

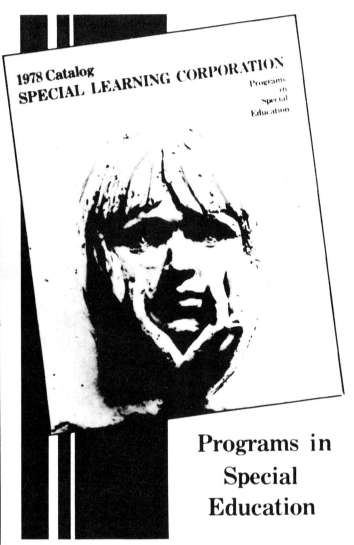

Programs in Special Education

Table of Contents

Basic Skills

I.   Language Arts

II.   Self-instructional Special Education Math

III.   Mathematics

IV.   Special Education Materials

V.   Early Childhood Education

VI.   Bi-lingual Programs-L.A. and Math

VII.   College and Professional Books

VIII.   Media-cassettes, films filmstrips

IX.   Social Learning

X.   Science

XI.   Testing Materials

XII.   Mainstreaming Library

- special education ● learning disabilities ● mental retardation
- autism ● behavior modification ● mainstreaming ● gifted and talented
- physically handicapped ● deaf education ● speech and hearing
- emotional and behavioral disorders ● visually handicapped
- diagnosis and placement ● psychology of exceptional children

Special Learning Corporation

42 Boston Post Rd. Guilford, Connecticut 06437 (203) 453-6212

COMMENTS PLEASE:

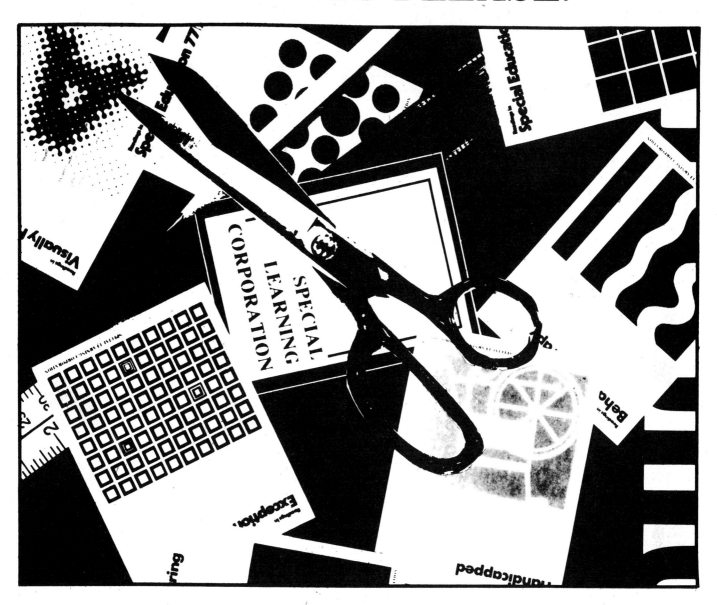

SPECIAL LEARNING CORPORATION

42 Boston Post Rd.

Guilford, Conn. 06437

SPECIAL LEARNING CORPORATION

COMMENTS PLEASE:

Does this book fit your course of study?

Why? (Why not?)

Is this book useable for other courses of study? Please list.

What other areas would you like us to publish in using this format?

What type of exceptional child are you interested in learning more about?

Would you use this as a basic text?

How many students are enrolled in these course areas?

_____ Special Education _____ Mental Retardation _____ Psychology _____ Emotional Disorders
_____ Exceptional Children _____ Learning Disabilities   Other _____

Do you want to be sent a copy of our elementary student materials catalog?

Do you want a copy of our college catalog?

Would you like a copy of our next edition? ☐ yes ☐ no

Are you a ☐ student or an ☐ instructor?

Your name _____ school _____

Term used _____ Date _____

address _____

city _____ state _____ zip _____

telephone number _____

S/H